Psychoactive Herbs in Veterinary Behavior Medicine

Psychoactive Herbs in Veterinary Behavior Medicine

Stefanie Schwartz

Blackwell Publishing

Stefanie Schwartz, DVM, MSc, DACVB, Diplomate, American College of Veterinary Behaviorists, is Director of Behavior Services, VCA South Shore Animal Hospital, South Weymouth, Massachusetts, Clinical Assistant Professor, Department of Clinical Sciences, Tufts University, North Grafton, Massachusetts, and national consultant to Antech Diagnostic Laboratories.

Blackwell Publishing Professional
2121 State Avenue, Ames, Iowa 50014, USA

Orders: 1-800-862-6657
Office: 1-515-292-0140
Fax: 1-515-292-3348
Web site: www.blackwellprofessional.com

Blackwell Publishing Ltd
9600 Garsington Road, Oxford OX4 2DQ, UK
Tel.: +44 (0)1865 776868

Blackwell Publishing Asia
550 Swanston Street, Carlton, Victoria 3053, Australia
Tel.: +61 (0)3 8359 1011

First edition, 2005

ISBN-13: 978-0-8138-2299-0

Library of Congress Cataloging-in-Publication Data

Schwartz, Stefanie.
Psychoactive herbs in veterinary behavior medicine / Stefanie Schwartz.— 1st ed.
p. cm.
Includes bibliographical references and index.

1. Psychotropic plants—Therapeutic use. 2. Veterinary diet therapy. 3. Veterinary psychopharmacology. 4. Alternative veterinary medicine. I. Title.

SF756.85.S36 2005
636.089′578—dc22

2004029267

MIX
Paper from responsible sources
FSC® C013604
FSC www.fsc.org

For my Julia

Butterfly dance on
Blossom, tasting sunshine joy
Kiss rain, laugh, dream, grow

Contents

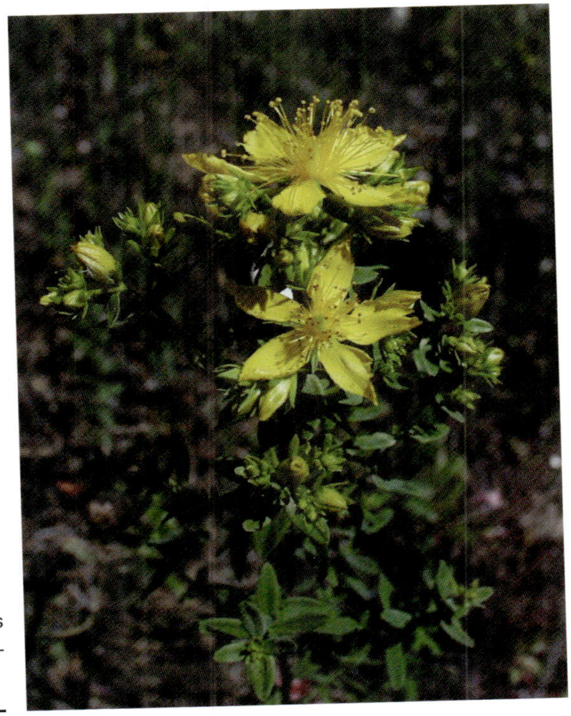

PLATE 1-1. Leaves and blooms of *Hypericum perforatum*. (Photo courtesy of Prof. George Ellmore)

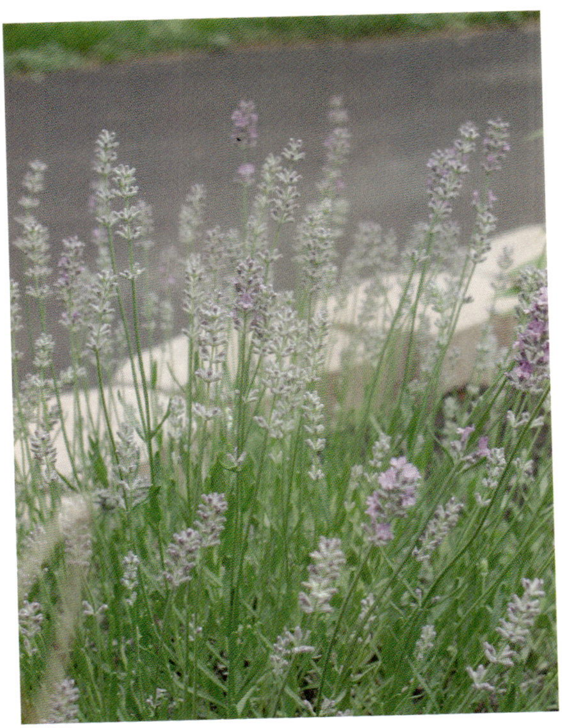

PLATE 1-2. *Lavandula angustifolia* (*L. officinalis*) showing characteristic gray-green lanceolate leaves and terminal blossoms. (Photo courtesy of Daniel Wallace)

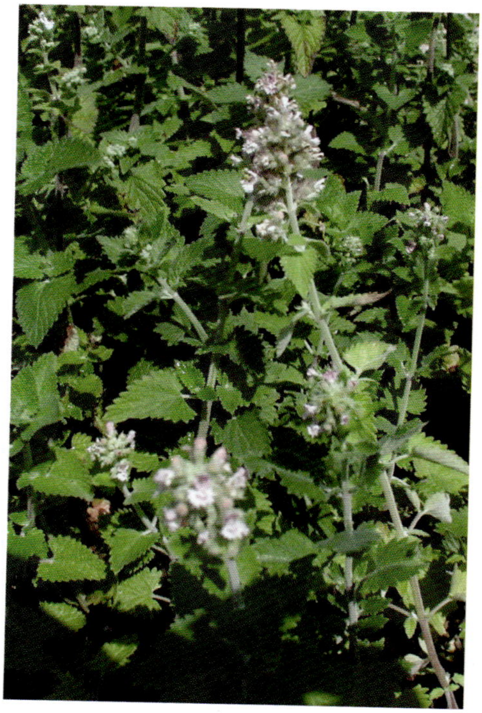

Plate 1-3. Leaves and blooms of *Nepeta cataria* (catnip). (Photo courtesy of Dr. Stefanie Schwartz)

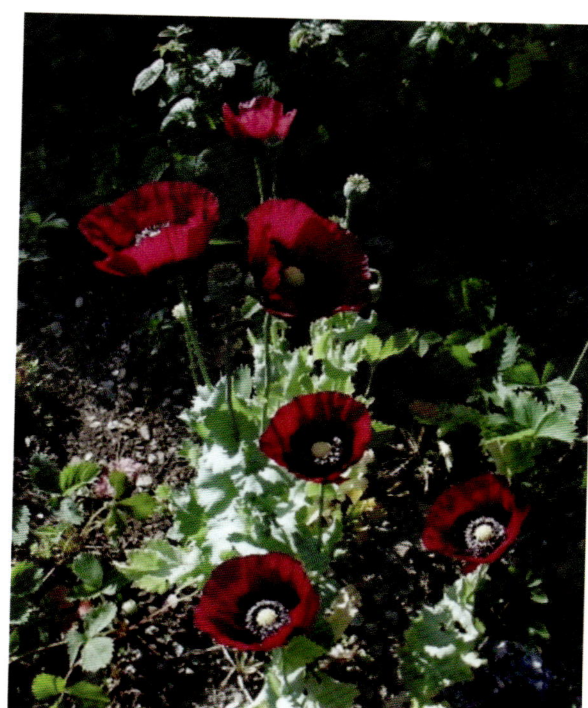

Plate 1-4. Aerial parts of *Papaver somniferum* showing poppy flower and seed capsules. (Photo courtesy of Prof. George Ellmore)

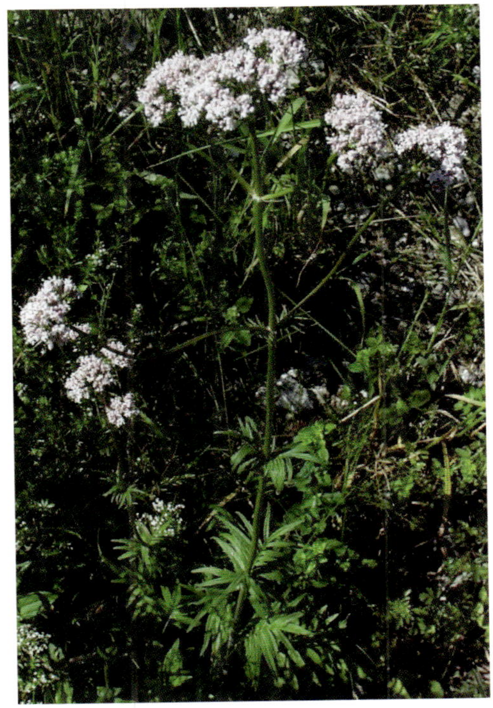

PLATE 1-5. *Valeriana officinalis* in bloom. (Photo courtesy of Prof. George Ellmore)

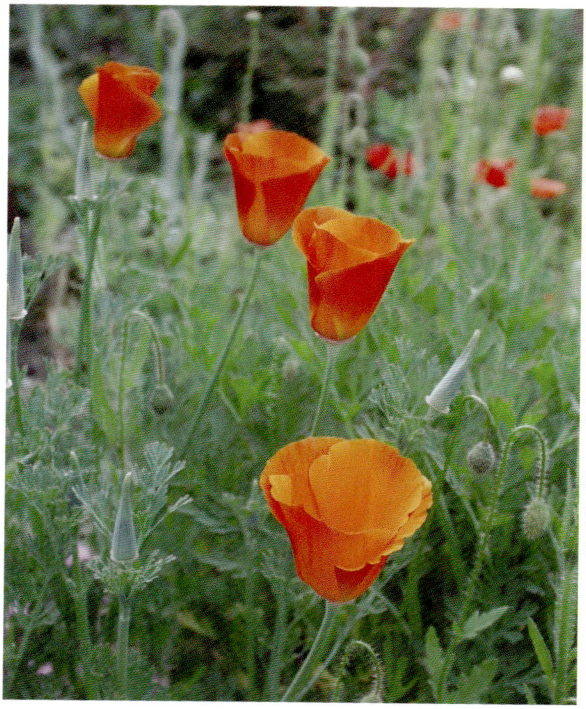

PLATE 2-1. Flowers of *Eschscholzia californica.* (Photo courtesy of Prof. George Ellmore)

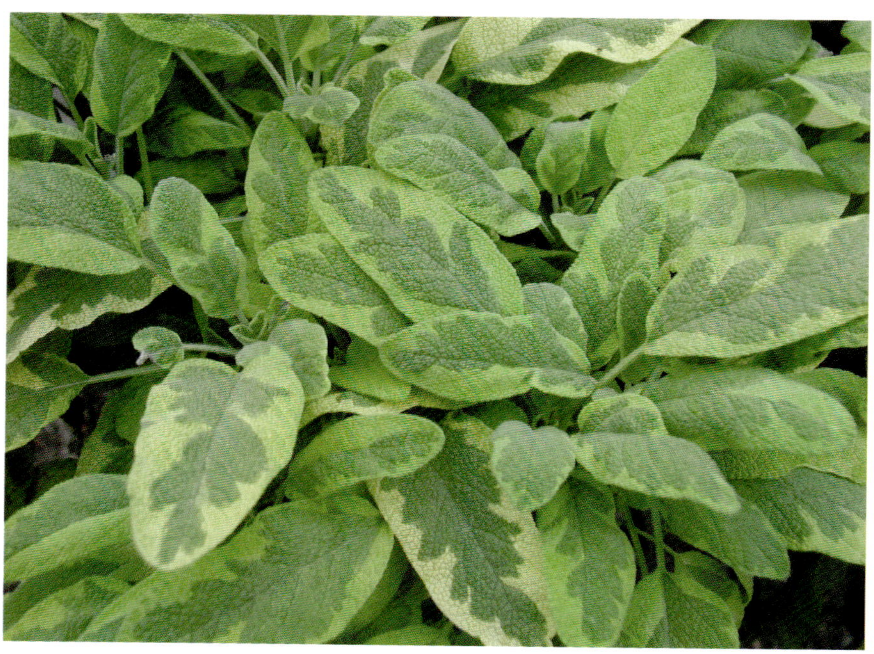

PLATE 2-2. Bicolor variety of *Salvia officinalis.* (Photo courtesy of Dr. Stefanie Schwartz)

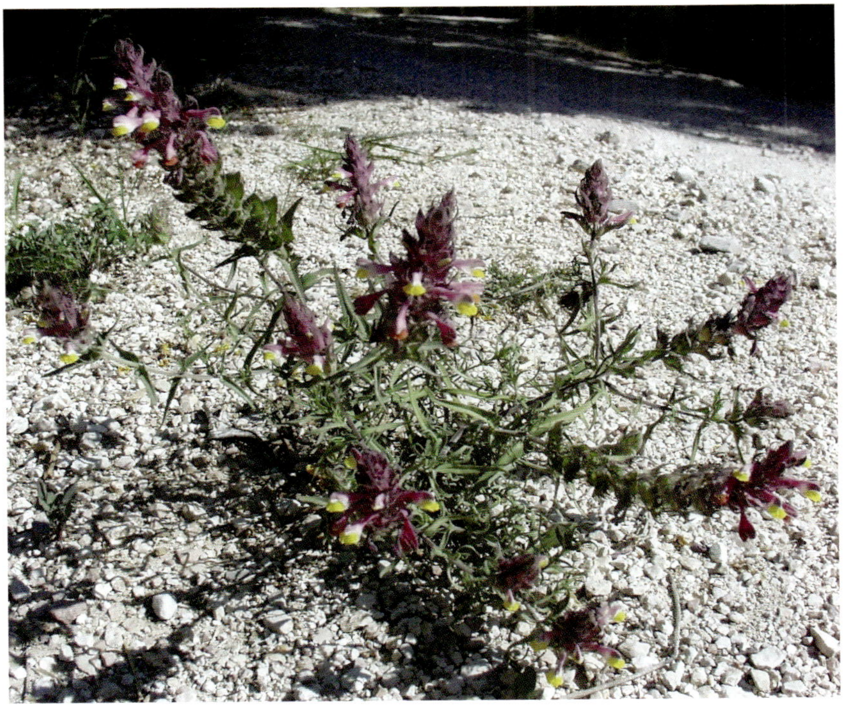

PLATE 2-3. Heavily branched *Scutellaria alpina, a* European *Scutellaria* species, in bloom. (Photo courtesy of Prof. George Ellmore)

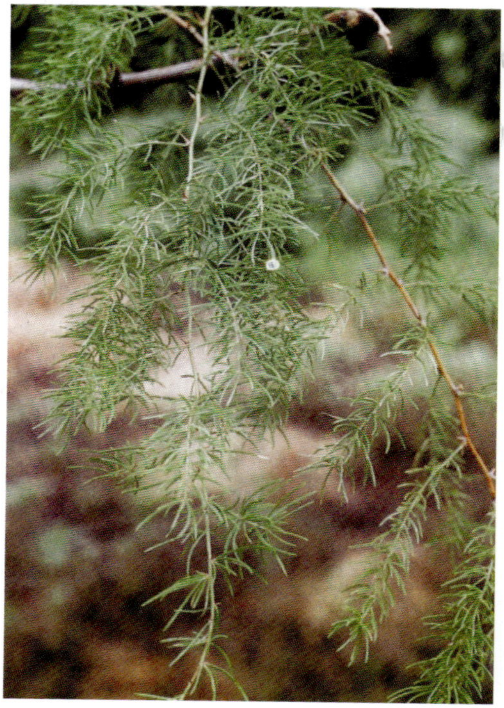

PLATE 3-1. *Asparagus racemosus* with flowering branch. (Photo courtesy of Dr. Jayvir Anjaria)

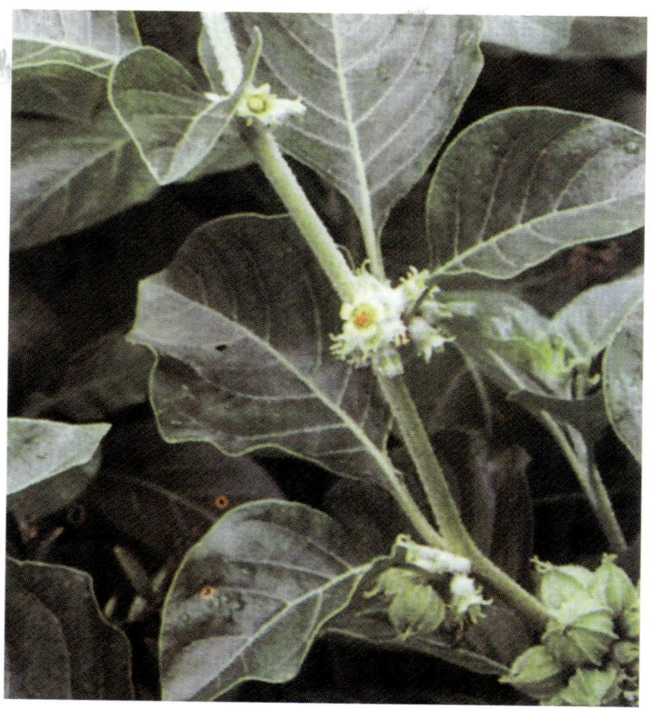

PLATE 3-2. *Withania somnifera* leaves. (Photo courtesy of Dr. Jayvir Anjaria)

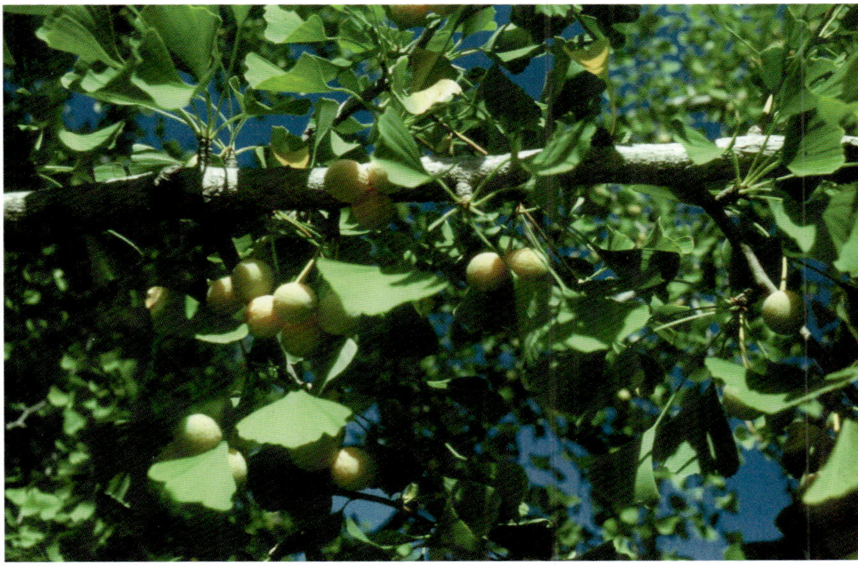

PLATE 4-1. Leaves and fruit of the female *Ginkgo biloba* tree. (Photo courtesy of Prof. George Ellmore)

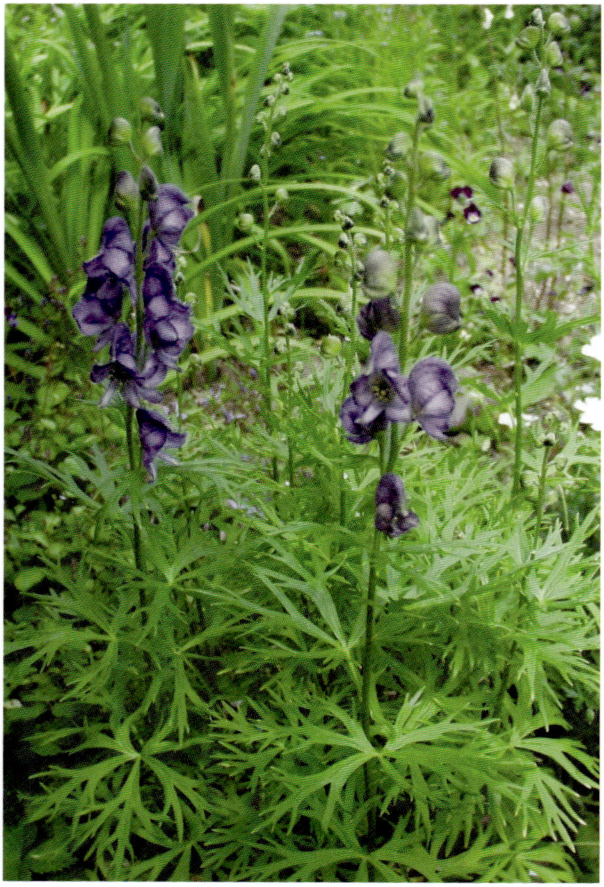

PLATE 4-2. *Aconitum napellus.* (Photo courtesy of Prof. George Ellmore)

Preface

"What nature delivers to us is never stale.
Because what nature creates has eternity in it."
—*Isaac Bashevis Singer* (1904-1991)

When I was invited to write this book, little did I know the odyssey upon which I was about to embark. This is the first book to investigate and synthesize scientific data about psychoactive herbs relevant to the specialty of veterinary behavior. Many of the herbs discussed have impressive proof to substantiate their use; others, less so; some have no proof at all, at least not yet. Let us not forget the many mainstream medicines that are plant derived (e.g., vincristine, yohimbine, penicillin, digoxin, codeine, morphine, ipecac, theophylline, atropine) and appreciate the potential of many other gifts from Nature that will surely take their places in our future psychotropic pharmacopoeias. Literally and figuratively, herbal medicine is all about going back to our roots. It is about remembering where we came from and incorporating the best of the past to produce a synthesized and brilliant future.

In order to understand medicinal herbs used in other systems of healing, it became necessary to explore the cultures, history, and even religions from which the systems emanate. This fundamental perspective is important to understanding the application of many of the herbs and is integrated in the text to enrich the reader's experience. My journey began as a scientific expedition. It evolved into a virtual (with the help of the Internet and e-mail) global voyage and a metaphysical passage. I am extremely grateful to have had this opportunity.

The staggering scope of this investigation brought me in touch with physicians, veterinarians, scientists, and healers around the world. I have spent many long hours, late into the night and early morning while the rest of the household slept, referencing and cross-referencing in fascination and in frustration, doing countless Internet searches, reading hundreds of journal articles and dozens of books, and waiting for e-mail replies from across the world or across the country and sometimes just across the state.

I undertook this project at the same time as another new one, the birth of my first child, Julia. I had written books before, but that was before I became a mother. I was often sleep deprived, either because of my baby, or the book, or both. But nature and inspiration give us strength, and I was nourished by the joy of watching both baby and book grow and flourish. In some ways, each may have distracted me from the other at times. But in so many more ways, I realize that they were meant to begin together; ultimately, Julia's arrival has put me in touch with instincts and insight that assisted me in my journey into the world of psychoactive herbs. This book is dedicated to my daughter with greatest eternal love.

Early on in my veterinary education, I recall being taught that our patients heal themselves. Treatment may be almost redundant, or quite possibly detrimental. The placebo effect and cases of spontaneous remission, with or without veterinary or medical intervention, imply that the therapy offered might have had little to do with the patient's recovery (or demise). What, then, is our role? What is it exactly that we do if we are not really needed? As clinicians, we are channeling the knowledge discovered by others who came before us. Most of us did not invent the medicines we prescribe or the techniques we perform, nor do we have diseases named in our honor; we are just passing information along. Yet, if this is all that medical or veterinary practice requires then surely a computer can replace us all. So, what is our purpose?

We forget that medicine is an art, not just a science. The healing power of touch, a soothing voice and a comforting hand, do not go unnoticed whether your patient is an elderly person or aging pet, a terrified child or a puppy who is alone, vulnerable, and afraid. More and more, we are coming to understand that we may be channeling far more than information; we may be channeling the life force of healing itself, whether it is called *prana*, *qi*, or divine spirit. Medicinal plants are part of Nature's bridge to all that surrounds us and goes beyond.

Regardless of what you accept as true, believe at least that we are vehicles whose purpose it is to promote healing. We must remain open and humbled by the simple truth of how little we really know about medicine and the miracle of life. With this, we can be more present and in tune with the needs of others who need us, professionally or personally. Skeptics will also be more open to what Western medicine currently calls "alternative" or "complementary" medicine, healing systems that have grown from Eastern, historical, or aboriginal traditions. Mysterious does not mean worthless; anecdotal does not necessarily mean ineffective. After all, a controlled study has never been done to test whether parachutes actually prevent death and trauma, yet we accept this as an obvious conclusion (Smith, Pell 2003). Ultimately, if a remedy is effective, does it matter where it came from? Will our patients, or their guardians, really care about which geographical region or culture is responsible for their rejuvenation? There is no doubt that scientific validation is essential; investigation of plants and the ethnobotanical cures of other medical practices are ongoing. Anecdotal remedies may prove useful, but they should be scientifically proven whenever possible.

The history of Western medicine is relatively brief compared to the ancient Eastern traditions, many of them thousands of years old. Western medicine, however great its teachings may be, arose rapidly like the rising sun. From the Western perspective at least, it may have temporarily eclipsed the lunar, older wisdom of Eastern medicine, but just as the sun's shadow continues to travel across the sky, so have the ancient Eastern healing traditions patiently waited for us to revive their teachings. This applies not only to the perceived polarity of East and West but also includes the suppression of indigenous knowledge by colonial forces. The British discouraged traditional Ayurvedic medicine when they invaded India, for example, and in some ways the United States and Canada continue to suppress Native American healing practices (and culture) to this day.

Traditional herbal remedies by native peoples around the world were used to tonify, purify, and sanctify. Many of these applications surround us on a daily basis, although we may not be aware of it. For instance, the use of stimulants such as *Nicotinia tabaca* (tobacco), *Erythroxylum coca* (cocaine), *Coffea arabica* (coffee), and *Cola acuminata* (cola), among others, in traditional medicine and ritual has become widespread and common practice in modern times. However, their modern application is very different from indigenous uses; we stimulate ourselves to avoid rest or self-examination. Another example is *Ephedra sinica* (*Ma huang*), a mainstay in traditional Chinese herbal formulas that has recently been banned in the United States much to the chagrin of Chinese herbalists. Consider, however, the possibility of accidental (or intentional) ingestion of these and other herbal supplements by family pets in which toxicity and fatal reactions have been reported (Ooms, Khan, Means 2001). The ban of over-the-counter ephedra was a regrettably appropriate action following reports of adverse effects and fatalities associated with its commercial use as a weight-control supplement in people. Such prostitution of ancient herbal remedies exceeds the applications outlined by traditional wisdom and experience; we must pay attention to the source.

As the popularity of herbal remedies continues to rise, commercial marketing will drive it higher. An important lesson learned early in my research is the increasing sensitivity and resentment of indigenous people to unlicensed exploitation of their knowledge, efforts, plant life, and generosity. Around the world, herbal wisdom is increasingly realized as lucrative intellectual property that deserves to be respected and should benefit the keepers of these ancient secrets.

For so long, Western or "modern" medicine has pushed aside the importance of the patient's responsibility in his or her own illness and in self-healing. Many conventional physicians (and some veterinarians) assumed a godlike omnipotence that is precariously based on the potency of a drug rather than their own role as healers. Bedside manner and simply spending time talking to and *caring* for the patient have been replaced, for example, with pharmaceutical media campaigns for antidepressant drugs that flash images of smiling patients, now recovered or in remission from their disease, frolicking in fields of daisies. The message is that we need not discern what caused the patient's depression when a simple pill will easily disguise the symptoms and, incidentally, avert the opportunity to truly heal the patient.

The use of medicine in veterinary behavior practice, whether the medicine is derived from conventional or alternative practices, is not meant to mask the symptoms. Misbehavior frequently originates in lifestyle deficiency and maladjustment. There is no remedy, herbal or synthetic, that can fix underlying problems such as a lack of exercise, attention, security, structure, and guidance. In the vast majority of cases, misbehavior is a sign that a pet's needs are not being met. The domestication of companion species demands that they be "civilized," inhibiting their species-specific instincts to accommodate human standards. However, it is also our responsibility to afford them some opportunity to express certain of their natural instincts within the boundaries we have imposed upon them for our own purposes. A permanent resolution of behavior problems will require a well-formed plan of behavior modification and lifestyle changes. For this reason, I have included outlines of the basic approaches to the most common behavior problems of small animal practice; referral to veterinary behaviorists is always best. A list of the most common synthetic psychoactive drugs used in veterinary behavior is included in an addendum for the reader's information.

As a board-certified veterinary behaviorist, I strive to restore psychological and physical balance to my patients' lives. Another realization made as I wrote this book is that I have always practiced holistic medicine but did not know it.* Holistic medicine is not apart from Western medicine; it is a natural evolution of a healing tradition that is still in its infancy, particularly when it is compared to the more ancient Eastern philosophies. There is truth to be found in both Eastern and Western medicine, and a synergy to be developed and nurtured.

Scientific data will continue to confirm or refute the efficacy of herbal remedies for their traditional or novel applications, and will surely impact future editions of this book. For example, there is an increasing interest in the use of herbal medicines by nonhuman animals and the intriguing evidence that some species may self-medicate (Huffman 2003). This book does not provide exhaustive information on traditional Eastern or Western healing methods or their philosophies, although it may motivate readers to continue with their own exploration. It is my hope that this book will serve in some small way as a catalyst toward synthesizing the medical philosophies and practices of the East and West, contemporary or modern with classical or traditional. I hope that it will also promote interest in the controlled study of psychoactive herbs for use in veterinary behavior medicine. The future of our planet will depend upon all peoples working together to pool our resources and to share knowledge; perhaps we have already begun to enact this destiny. Ultimately, we are all just beginning to uncover the profound secrets of Nature. In many ways, we are all children, trying to return to the Garden of Eden.

I acknowledge the influence of Dr. Katherine Houpt, a founding member of the American College of Veterinary Behaviorists based at Cornell University in Ithaca, New York. Dr. Houpt unknowingly fanned my growing interest in psychoactive herbs to treat veterinary patients by inviting me to contribute a paper on the subject many years ago to the Web site of the International Veterinary Information Services (www.ivis.org). I am grateful for her support throughout my many years in practice as a veterinary behaviorist, even before the ACVB became a reality.

I am very grateful to Dr. Susan Wynn of Woodstock, Georgia, who is Executive Director of the Veterinary Botanical Medicine Association. It is an honor to be part of a group of open-minded and open-hearted veterinarians with enormous skill, passion, and compassion. Dr. Wynn has been completely supportive and enthusiastic about this book from its inception. She offered extremely helpful comments on the manuscript and contributed several photos. She was also instrumental in introducing me to a rich and generous network of veterinary herbalists around the world. Through Dr. Wynn and the VBMA, I was put in touch with Dr. Phil Rogers of Dublin, Ireland, who "dabbles" in acupuncture, TCM, as well as holistic and alternative medicine. This brilliant, modest man has been my mentor and my friend, welcoming my queries and providing clarification and details that I lacked in order to produce the chapter on Oriental medicine. That chapter is dedicated to him, and to the memory of his beloved son Killian John.

I networked with experts around the world and eventually "met" Prof. Jayvir Anjaria of Ahmedabad, India, who is an enormously respected leader in medicinal plant research and veterinary medicine, and consultant in pharmaceutical and medicinal plant formulations. Author of "Ethnovet Heritage: Indian Ethnoveterinary Medicine, an Overview" (Anjaria, Parabia, Dwivedi 2002), Prof. Anjaria also graciously provided many of the photos in this book. During the course of our communication, Prof. Anjaria guided and nurtured my efforts and "adopted" me as his daughter. Prof. Anjaria put me in contact with two other distinguished experts for additional input: Prof. Arun Baxi, Dean of the Institute of Ayurvedic Pharmaceutical Science, Gujarat Ayurved University, India; and my dear Dr. Minoo Parabia, an expert in Taxonomy, EthnoBotany, and Ayurveda, and Professor of Biosciences and Director of the Shri Bapalal Vaidya Botanical Research Centre, South Gujarat University, India. The section on Ayurvedic medicine is dedicated with reverence and love to "Daddy" Jayvir, who is as close to *jivanmukti* as I have known.

It is difficult to describe the profound experience it has been to be graced with the attention and efforts of these and other busy, distinguished professionals, who responded to the e-mails of a stranger thousands of miles away. The power of the Internet became a glorious tool with which I was encouraged, instructed, and inspired. I hope some day to thank each of them, face to face, and that they will be proud of what they helped me create. Another lesson learned by writing this book is how intimately we really (not just "virtually") are all connected, if we are only open to the possibilities.

I am also very thankful for the support and enthusiasm of the library staff at Tufts University School of Veterinary Medicine, and specifically, Mrs. Jane

Cormier. Janie became my personal champion in this project; she was consistently helpful and kind as she located countless journal articles, often based on oblique and partial references, with true devotion to my compulsive pursuit of so many unanswered questions. Janie also put me in touch with botanist Prof. George Ellmore of the Biology Department at Tufts University in Medford, Massachusetts. He gallantly provided me with additional botanical images and even e-mailed digital photographs to me during his summer trip to France, making his an international effort.

Life depends so much on to whom we are born. I am the fortunate product of my beautiful father, a physician who has always inspired me with his own holistic tendencies, and my magnificent mother, who still channels more life energy than she knows.

Most of all, I thank my husband, Danny Wallace, for his patience, indulgence, support, patience, humor, friendship, understanding, and love. He brought me tea (mostly Earl Grey tea, containing oil of bergamot *Citrusauranthium bergamia*, but sometimes mint tea, *Mentha viridis*) when I didn't know I needed it; amused little Julia when I could not; walked our two dogs; entertained our five cats when they wanted to sit on my computer keyboard or books; and reminded me to get some sleep when I could no longer focus my eyes. He makes so many things possible, and so many impossible things either unimportant, or dreams come true.

> "Man & creatures merely come and go in circles, spirals, and in time, and medicine dreamed by mortal minds can never foil the long-term dream of God."
>
> *—Phil Rogers, Dublin, Ireland*

*"Holistic veterinarians are those who offer or refer for all therapies (both conventional and alternative) which are potentially safe and effective, assess and treat the whole patient's lifestyle, genetics, environment, and history, provide long-term relief where possible, and who spend sufficient time educating clients so that animal owners are satisfied that they understand their animal's condition, prognosis, and treatment plan." (Dr. Susan Wynn, personal communication 2004)

References

Anjaria J, Parabia M, Dwivedi S. Ethnovet Heritage: Indian Ethnoveterinary Medicine, An Overview. Pathik Enterprise Publishers; Ahmedabad, India. 2002.

Huffman MA. Animal self-medication and ethno-medicine: exploration and exploitation of the medicinal properties of plants. Proc Nutr Soc. 2003;62:371–381.

Ooms TG, Khan SA, Means C. Suspected caffeine and ephedrine toxicosis resulting from ingestion of an herbal supplement containing guarana and ma huang in dogs: 47 cases (1997–1999). JAVMA. 2001;218:225–229.

Smith GSC, Pell JP. Parachute use to prevent death and major trauma related to gravitational challenge: systematic review of randomized controlled trials. BMJ. 2003;327:1459–1461.

Disclaimer and Overview of Risks

This book is intended for licensed doctors of veterinary medicine, students enrolled in schools of veterinary medicine, and other scientists with an interest in herbal medicine. Nonprofessionals, pet owners, and amateur enthusiasts are advised not to practice medicine on nonhuman animals or people unless permitted by law. Herbal medicine is an evolving science. Medicinal herbs are not approved for the treatment of specific disease, although data are accumulating to support the application of particular herbs in medicine and veterinary medicine. Every effort has been made to present accurate facts; however, new knowledge continues to emerge and may change some of the information presented in this book. The author and publisher are not responsible for omissions or errors.

One of the major consequences of the release of information regarding medicinally beneficial plants is the overzealous harvest of wild plants. Around the world, many plants have been excessively collected and border on extinction, or have already been eradicated. The reader is reminded of the fragility of this planet's ecosystems and the finite supply of wild botanical specimens; please behave responsibly. Commercial sources are provided for your convenience among the list of Internet resources in the addendum.

The author has strived to synthesize information from a wide range of disciplines. Scientific data is presented either to support or refute the clinical use of specific plants or botanical remedies. In many cases, clinical data and controlled studies are scarce and cannot fully substantiate the clinical benefit of herbal preparations. Side effects are recognized and new ones will likely continue to emerge.

The use of herbal remedies and the doses of herbal preparations remain largely uninvestigated for use in companion animals. Suggested doses are based on extrapolation of human data or animal studies and from rare veterinary texts. Fresh herbs may require two to three times the amount of dried herb, and depending on the ingredients and method of preparation, herbal extract often requires less than 50% of the dose of dried herb (Dr. Phil Rogers, personal communication 2004). The author's conservative rule of thumb is to advise an initial canine or feline dose of one half the recommended human dose on the product label. The use of herbal remedies ideally deserves the direction of experienced veterinary herbalists. It is preferable to use a product that contains the lowest available concentration of the prescribed herb and to use single herb preparations in order to better dose and isolate the effects of specific herbs. This method facilitates the recognition of benefits and the distinction of any adverse effects specific to each herb. Experienced veterinary herbalists should be consulted to discuss choices of traditional herbal "cocktails" (polyherbal formulas). Please contact the Veterinary Botanical Medical Association at http://www.vbma.org for a list of practitioners in your area.

Gradual withdrawal from concomitant herbal or synthetic psychoactive remedies is usually necessary before the addition of another herbal or synthetic medicine. A washout period of at least one week is suggested between therapies. Potential interaction with any other medication must also be considered.

This book is not meant to replace a referral to a board-certified veterinary behaviorist. The number of veterinary specialists in this field is growing in North America, Europe, and beyond. Reliance on psychopharmacology alone, whether the substances are considered conventional or alternative, is not a sound approach. Misbehaving pets suffer from any combination of lifestyle deficiencies, latent health problems, genetic predispositions, and maladaptive, learned patterns. These not only impact the quality of their and their guardians' lives but also can alter a pet's longevity. Any complaint or concern regarding a pet's misbehavior or emotional well-being, regardless of how unimpressive it may seem to anyone other than the pet's guardian, deserves immediate attention. A delay in referral may well result in the destruction, abandonment, or relinquishment of even the most beloved companion animal. Please take advantage of the training of qualified veterinary behavior specialists in your area. For a list of veterinary behaviorists who are board-certified by the American College of Veterinary Behaviorists, please visit http://veterinarybehaviorists.org/.

Foreword

Almost the moment a veterinarian gains a reputation for having knowledge in herbal medicine, he or she will be consulting with people who want alternatives to psychoactive drugs or behavior modification techniques. The patients are often dogs with chronic, serious anxiety or aggression syndromes, or cats with long-standing, habitual, inappropriate elimination problems. Until now, we have done our best to cull the myriad traditional sources of information and do our own personal scientific literature reviews to identify potentially useful herbs for these conditions.

Psychoactive herbal medicines are not, in fact, substitutes or alternatives to conventional psychoactive drugs. Herbal medicine is a completely different way of thinking, because the plants are complex compounds that offer multiple targeted, synergistic mechanisms of action. Just as cocktail therapy is gaining recognition in the treatment of other serious problems such as cancer and HIV, herbal medicine may well be the way of the future for many of today's medical problems.

In this book, Dr. Stefanie Schwartz has accomplished a first. Never before has a veterinary specialist comprehensively reviewed the considerable scientific literature on herbal medicine and applied it to the specialty. Dr. Schwartz introduces the reader to the major traditional systems of medicine and reviews those herbs that have been used for emotional or behavioral problems within those cultural systems.

I have postgraduate scientific training but have spent the last few years studying traditional texts in herbal medicine. Before reading this book, I was concerned that the science supporting herbal medicine, which is relatively meager considering the traditional knowledge base, would drown out our hard-won traditional study and experience. Dr. Schwartz has been sensitive to both. As more veterinarians realize the potential offered by use of herbs in their practices, the dialogue between science and tradition will be facilitated and broadened. Dr. Schwartz has taken the first step here in this book.

She states, "As clinicians, we are channeling the knowledge discovered by others who came before us." It is clear that she came to understand the common, and still useful, aspects of these traditional systems—personal involvement, community support, practitioner sensitivity and experience, *and* herbal medicines. And she has the scientific and specialized expertise to lend a new perspective on our traditions. This text should be a well-thumbed and dependable volume for anyone who manages small animal behavior problems; I'm certain it will be for me.

Susan G. Wynn, DVM
Registered Herbalist, American Herbalist Guild
Executive Director, Veterinary Botanical Medicine Association
Acworth, Georgia
USA

* * *

Dr. Stefanie Schwartz, author of *Psychoactive Herbs in Veterinary Behavior Medicine,* is one of a growing number of physicians and veterinarians worldwide who see the strengths and shortcomings of western allopathic medicine. She writes, "Early on in my veterinary education, I recall being taught that our patients heal themselves." All great systems of complementary or holistic medicine use this principle.

Surgery, drugs, herbs, acupuncture, and other treatments heal little, if anything. At best, they help the body to heal itself. At worst, they remove a damaged organ (and thereby remove any functional use of that organ), or they hide or suppress symptoms (thereby forcing the damaged organism to cry for help by expressing *dis*-ease in different symptoms). For example, stress may be expressed as distress with the development of a stomach ulcer. Symptomatic or surgical treatment of the ulcer does not address the cause of the ulcer (*stress*). The distressed organism may seek a new way to express distress, for example, by developing hypertension or a heart attack.

Similarly, if a dog develops behavioral dysfunction, we should not suppress the symptoms or punish the dog for expressing them. Instead, we should try to address the basic causes for the symptoms and alleviate them. At the same time, we may need to help the dog cope with any unresolved causes or persistent patterns of misbehavior by strengthening basic constitution or vital energy. Properly used, herbal medicine is an effective way to do that. Herbal medicine has a very ancient tradition in all great cultures. It is often relatively inexpensive and, used properly by trained herbalists, safe.

Dr. Schwartz is a knowledgeable, deep-thinking, compassionate, and caring colleague. In addition to having more than twenty years in private behavior practice, she is academically affiliated with Tufts University School of Veterinary Medicine and is national consultant for Antech Laboratories. She possesses practical expertise in veterinary matters and animal behavior and a deep knowledge of herbal medicine.

This great work deserves to be read widely, especially by those who are so unthinking as to believe in the "quick fix" or a "pill for every ill." As a student of herbal medicine for many years, I can say that this book has shown me that I have much to learn. I recommend it highly to colleagues who want to improve their success rates in clinical practice and to understand *how* herbal medicine can help them to do this.

In the Author's Preface, Dr. Schwartz writes: "We forget that medicine is an art, not just a science. The healing power of touch, a soothing voice and a comforting hand do not go unnoticed. . . . More and more, we are coming to understand that we may be channeling . . . the life force of healing itself, whether it is called *prana*, *qi*, or divine spirit. . . . We must remain open and humbled by the simple truth of how little we really know about medicine and the miracle of life." I concur; medicine is a divine vocation. The most gifted healer is still a fallible and imperfect human who merely attempts to manifest God's healing love. This book is a great work of dedication, critical assessment, scholarship, and love. It stems from the author's love of life, and love of animals and human beings.

Phil Rogers MVB, MRCVS
Dublin, Ireland

Psychoactive Herbs in Veterinary Behavior Medicine

CHAPTER

1

Western Psychoactive Herbs

"For some patients, though conscious that their condition is perilous, recover their health simply through their contentment with the goodness of the physician." —*Hippocrates* (c. 460–40 BC)

Agaricus Species and Other Medicinal Mushrooms

Medicinal fungi have long been part of traditional use in Asian cultures for cooking and for healing purposes. Today, medicinal properties of mushrooms have been the focus of intensive research, particularly in Japan, China, Korea, and Russia. For example, *Ganoderma lucidum* (Reishi), a sacred mushroom in ancient China, has at least 80 different biologically active components that are valued for their antivirus, anticancer, hypotensive, hypoglycemic, and immunotropic properties. Dietary fiber in mushrooms may help to absorb organic waste in the digestive tract. Their high content in amino acids is also recognized (Wasser 2002; Mizuno 2002). *Agaricus muscarius* extract is used in homeopathic preparations for the treatment of a variety of complaints including behavioral symptoms such as rage, fury, raving, delirium, idiotic faces, nervousness, headaches associated with sex or pain, emotions, mania, and insanity. There is no proof of its psychoactive benefit. Homeopathy is an alternative system of healing developed by the eighteenth-century German physician Samuel Hahnemann. In homeopathy, the patient is treated with substances that are capable of producing clinical signs in healthy individuals that are similar to those of the patient to be treated (AVMA 2000). Although some homeopathic preparations contain plant material, homeopathy is distinct from herbal medicine. Principles of homeopathy are applied to animals by veterinary homeopaths. This book does not investigate homeopathic preparations.

The majority of mushroom preparations are marketed as dietary supplements or "nutraceuticals" primarily for improving resistance to disease. Worldwide sales of Reishi-derived products in 1995 exceeded US$1.628 billion and overall medicinal mushroom products sell in excess of US$6 billion each year (Wasser 2002).

In the United States, Agaricus (meaning "gilled mushroom") accounts for approximately 90 percent of mushroom production (half of these are grown in the state of Pennsylvania alone), primarily for the food industry. *Agaricus bisporus* has two brown strains: Portabello and Crimini. Crimini is actually the same fungus that is harvested before it opens its gills (Fig. 1-1).

Clinical Effects

A number of polysaccharide antitumor drugs have been developed from mushrooms including the *Shiitake* (*Lentinus edodes*) and *Reishi* (*Ganoderma lucidum*) (Fig. 1-2). The water-soluble antitumor polysaccharide first isolated from the Shiitake was named "lentinan" and has been shown to arrest chemical and viral tumor growth. Another compound derived from the turkey tail mushroom (*Trametes versicolor*) marketed under the name of Krestin® now accounts for 25 percent of the anticancer drug market in Japan and, by 1993, its U.S. sales topped $350 million (Wasser 2002).

Agaricus blazei from Brazil has drawn interest since epidemiologists discovered that the local consumption of the fungus was associated with an extremely low rate of disease. The mushroom was first discovered in Florida in 1944 and has become a medicinal phenomenon (Mizuno 2002). In comparative studies, this mushroom had the most potent anticancer effect compared to shiitake, reishi, and

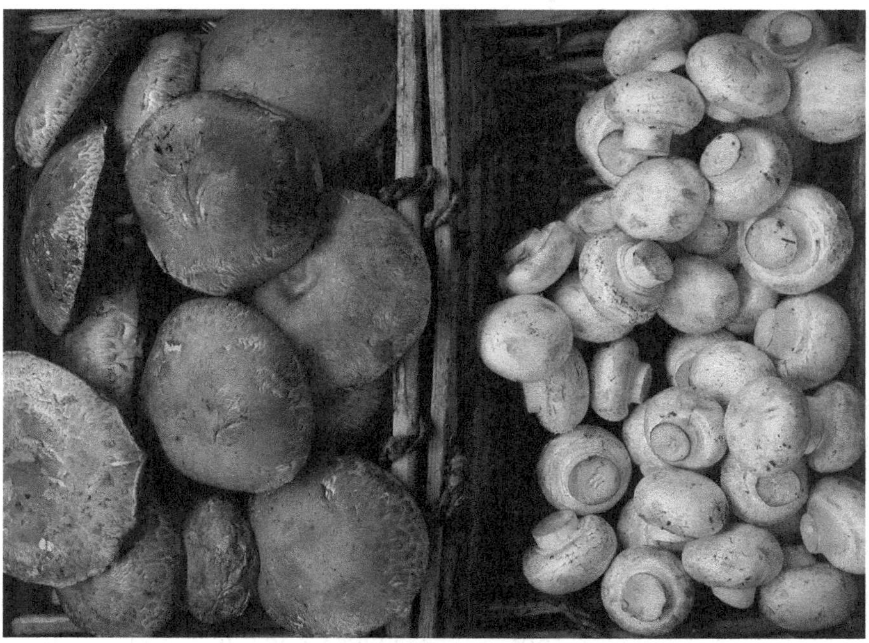

FIGURE 1-1. Portabello (left) and Crimini mushrooms (right) are both stages of *Agaricus bisporus*. (Photo courtesy of Dr. Stefanie Schwartz)

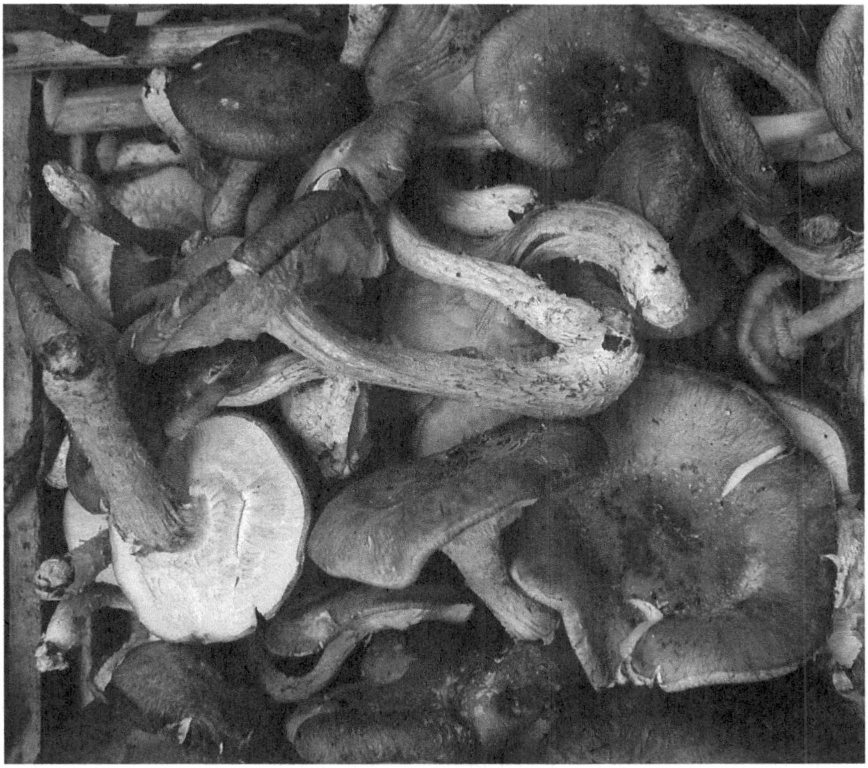

FIGURE 1-2. *Lentinus edodes* (Shiitake mushrooms). (Photo courtesy of Dr. Stefanie Schwartz)

other medicinal fungi. Antiviral (including HIV and western equine encephalitis virus) and immune-boosting properties have also been identified. This mushroom has proven effects against colon, breast, ovarian, lung, and liver cancer, among others (Mizuno 2002; Wasser 2002; Oshiman, Fujimiya, Ebina et al. 2002; Takaku, Kimura, Okuda 2001; Sorimachi, Ikehara, Maezato et al. 2001). It may also help to improve senile dementia (Mizuno 2002).

Adverse Effects

In one study, *Agaricus muscarius* caused a cataleptic response in rats (Sukul, Bal, Bhattacharyya 1986). Interestingly, the more dilute preparation had a prolonged cataleptogenic effect compared to a more concentrated preparation. In another report, Agaricus-induced catalepsy was potentiated by the selective dopaminergic antagonist bromocriptine and by the mixed agonist apomorphine (Sukul, Klemm 1986).

Side effects associated with therapeutic doses of medicinal mushrooms are rare; however, individual sensitivities are always possible. For example, "shiitake dermatitis" is a photosensitized skin reaction characterized by flagellate skin lesions and associated with the consumption of shiitake mushrooms (Hanada, Hashimoto 1998).

Clinical Application in Veterinary Behavior Medicine

A. blazei may become of therapeutic benefit in the treatment of senile cognitive changes in aging pets, or for the treatment of canine and feline cognitive dysfunction syndromes. Nonetheless, in the absence of confirmed data regarding the usefulness of Agaricus species for emotional, psychiatric, or psychological conditions, it appears that, for now, the use of medicinal mushrooms in veterinary behavior practice is deferred pending proof of more specific and convincing psychotropic properties.

References

American Veterinary Medical Association. Guidelines for alternative and complementary veterinary medicine. In: 2000 AVMA Directory and Resource Manual, 48th ed. Schaumburg, Illinois: American Veterinary Medical Association: 66–67.

Hanada K, Hashimoto I. Flagellate mushroom (Shiitake) dermatitis and photosensitivity. Dermatology. 1998;197:255–257.

Mizuno T. Medicinal properties and clinical effects of culinary-medicinal mushroom *Agaricus blazei*. Internat J Med Mushrooms 2002;4:299-312

Oshiman K, Fujimiya Y, Ebina T et al. Orally administered beta-1,6-D-polyglucose extracted from *Agaricus blazei* results in tumor regression tumor-bearing mice. Planta Med. 2002;68:610–614.

Sorimachi K, Ikehara Y, Maezato G et al. Inhibition by *Agaricus blazei* Murill fractions of cytopathic effect induced by western equine encephalitis (WEE) virus on VERO cells in vitro. Biosci Biotechnol Biochem. 2001;65:1645–1647.

Sukul NC, Lemm WR. Influence of dopamine agonists and an opiate antagonist agarius-induced catalepsy, as tested by a new method. Arch Int Pharmacodyn Ther. 1988;295:40–51.

Sukul NC, Bala SK, Bhattacharyya B. Prolonged cataleptogenic effects of potentized homoepathic drugs. Psychopharmacology (Berl). 1986;89:338–339.

Takaku T, Kimura Y, Okuda H. Isolation of an antitumor compound from *Agaricus blazei* Murill and its mechanism of action. J Nutr. 2001;131:1409–1413.

Volk T, Ivors K. *Agaricus bisporus*: fungus of the month. http://botit.botany.wisc.edu/toms_fungi/apr2001.html

Wasser SP. Review of medicinal mushrooms advances: good news from old allies. HerbalGram. 2002;56:28–33.

Avena sativa

Avena sativa (Oat) is an annual grass and one of the earliest grains to become domesticated. Oats probably originated in Eurasia and North Africa, but spread quickly throughout Europe and are now grown around the world (Russo 2001; PDR 2000). The aerial portions of the plant including stem, leaf, and fruit are harvested and prepared fresh or dried. Oat bran, oat straw, and oatmeal are all derived from oats (Russo 2001; PDR 2000). Alternative names include wild oats, Milky Oat Seed, green oats, gruner hafer, farine d'avoine, herbe d'avoine (Russo 2001; PDR 2000). Milky oat seed is a special preparation of a milky secretion from oat seed with a brief shelf life of approximately one week. The milk must be immediately conserved as a tincture and is reputed to possess calming properties; it was also used to treat morphine and opium addiction in the 1800s (Tillotson, Tillotson, Abel 2001) although this eventually was found to be ineffective (Felter, Lloyd 1898).

Historical Perspective

Oats have been used in traditional folk medicine for a long list of troubles. Physical ailments for which oats have been used therapeutically, although without documented efficacy, include gout, neurasthenia, rheumatism, dermatopathy (seborrhea, dry skin), bladder disease, gastrointestinal disorder, diabetes, constipation, diarrhea, and frostbite (Russo 2001; PDR 2000). It was also used by nineteenth-century physicians to relieve nervous exhaustion associated with a variety of illnesses, cardiac weakness, and as an antispasmodic (for example, spasm of the neck of the bladder) (Felter, Lloyd 1898).

Ingredients

Compounds identified in *A. sativa* include polysaccharides (saccharose, beta-glucans), starch, peptides, B vitamins, amines, steroid saponins, and flavonoids (including apigenin, vitexin).

Clinical Effects

Recent research supports a cholesterol-lowering property of beta-glucan polysaccharides. Therapeutic benefits of *A. sativa* have also been linked to their fiber content and antioxidant properties. It has been shown to improve glucose tolerance, as well as GI and cardiovascular health (Hu 2003; Kris-Etherton, Hecker, Bonanome et al 2002; PDR 2000; Hallfrisch, Scholfield, Behall 1995; Braaten, Wood, Scott et al. 1994; Davidson, Dugan, Burns et al. 1991).

Adverse Effects

No recognized adverse effects or medical risks are associated with therapeutic dosages of *A. sativa* preparations (PDR 2000), although individuals may develop an allergic sensitivity (Jarvinen, Turpeinen, Suomalainen 2003).

Availability

A. sativa has also been applied to help patients suffering from anxiety, insomnia, stress, and opium and tobacco withdrawal (PDR 2000; Tillotson, Tillotson, Abel 2001). Traditionally, oat tea is prepared as a sedative for anxiety and sleeplessness, although there is no scientific validation of this purported effect (Russo 2001).

Clinical Application in Veterinary Behavior Medicine

There is sparse evidence to substantiate the psychoactive benefit of *Avena sativa* and, although administering oats in small quantity may not be harmful to pets, it is not considered a reliable psychoactive plant for veterinary behavior practice at this time.

References

Braaten JT, Wood PJ, Scott FW et al. Oat beta-glucan reduces blood cholesterol concentration in hypercholesterolemic subjects. Eur J Clin Nutr. 1994;48:465–474.

Davidson MH, Dugan LD, Burns JH et al. The hypocholesterolemic effects of beta-glucan in oatmeal and oat bran. A dose-controlled study. JAMA. 1991;265:1833–1839.

Felter HW, Lloyd JU. King's American Dispensatory. Ohio Valley Company, Cincinatti, OH. 1898. Available online at http://www.ibiblio.org/herbmed/eclectic/kings/

Hallfrisch J, Scholfield DJ, Behall KM. Diets containing soluble oat extracts improve glucose and insulin responses of moderately hypercholesterolemic men and women. Am J Clin Nutr. 1995;61:379–384.

Hu FB. Plant-based foods and prevention of cardiovascular disease: an overview. Am J Clin Nutr. 2003; 78(3 Suppl):544S–551S.

Jarvinen KM, Turpeinen M, Suomalainen H. Concurrent cereal allergy in children with cow's milk allergy manifested with atopic dermatitis. Clin Exp Allergy. 2003;33:1060–1066.

Kris-Etherton PM, Hecker KD, Bonanome A et al. Bioactive compounds in foods: their role in the prevention of cardiovascular disease and cancer. Am J Med. 2002;113 (Suppl 9B):71S–88S.

PDR for Herbal Medicines (2nd ed) Medical Economics Company Inc., Montvale, NJ 2000;551–553.

Russo E. Handbook of Psychotropic Herbs: A Scientific Analysis of Herbal Remedies for Psychiatric Conditions. The Haworth Press, Binghamton, NY 2001;134–136.

Tillotson AK, Tillotson HSH, Abel R. The One Earth Herbal Sourcebook. Kensington Publishing, New York, NY 2001;167–169.

Catha edulis

Catha edulis (khat, qat) is a bush native to East Africa and the Arabian Peninsula. Inhabitants chew its leaves as a sociocultural tradition across these regions. Similar to the traditional use of coca leaves in the Andes, the khat plant has psychostimulant effects and is used to relieve fatigue (Hassan, Guanid, El-Khally et al 2002; Kalix 1992). The use of khat may be growing as a recreational drug; for example, *C. edulis* has been detected in the urine of young people at "raves" in Europe (Brown, Jarvie, Simpson 1995).

Ingredients

The primary bioactive compound is thought to be cathinone (S-alpha-aminopropiophenone), an alkaloid that has similar effects to amphetamine on the CNS as well as sympathomimetic properties. As does amphetamine, cathinone triggers presynaptic catecholamines release. Human subjects report similar objective and subjective effects between amphetamine and cathinone (Widler, Mathys, Brenneisen et al 1994; Kalix 1992, 1991). Cathine, also known as norpseudoephedrine, has also been identified in *C. edulis* as well as in the ephedra plant (Kalix 1991).

Cathinone is more lipophilic and moves more readily into the CNS compared with cathine.

CNS Effects

C. edulis consumption has been associated with euphoria, alertness, and increased cognitive function; however, it has also been shown to provoke dysphoria and mild sedation. Increased blood pressure and heart rate were consistent findings in all subjects (Nencini, Ahmed, Elmi 1986). Recently, khat chewing has been linked with functional mood disorders attributed to its sympathomimetic action. It has been shown to cause symptoms of clinical depression and may exacerbated pre-existing psychiatric disturbance (Hassan, Guanid, El-Khally et al 2002; Awas, Kebede, Alem 1999).

Despite the perception of its positive role in North African and Middle Eastern communities, *C. edulis* use can become an addiction (Griffiths, Gossop, Wickenden et al. 1997). A potent reinforcing effect exceeding that of cocaine has been demonstrated in both monkeys and rats; a role of D_1-type dopamine receptors has been suggested (Gosnell, Yracheta, Bell et al. 1996). In fact, both cathinone and amphetamine increased dopamine levels in the anterior caudate-putamen and the nucleus accumbens, although the effect of amphetamine was greater than cathinone at higher doses (Pehek, Schechter, Yamamoto 1990).

Miscellaneous Effects

C. edulis increased sexual arousal in male rats; however, it did not promote erection or ejaculation and was not considered an aphrodisiac (Taha, Ageel, Islam et al. 1995). In a rodent study, khatamines including cathinone were shown to increase T3 and T4 levels, suggesting that thyroid stimulation may contribute to suppressed appetite, hyperthermia, and metabolic changes observed in khat chewers (Islam, Tariq, el-Feraly et al. 1990).

Adverse Effects

C. edulis toxicity has been reported (Al-Qirim, Shawwan, Zaidi et al. 2002). *C. edulis* consumption has been linked with oral cancer and has a pronounced genotoxic effect in the buccal mucosa (Kassie, Darroudi, Kundi et al. 2001). Short-term (3 months) and long-term (6 months) administration of *C. edulis* leaves have been associated with elevated alkaline phosphatase (ALP), alanine aminotransferase (ALT), aspartate aminotransferase (AST), as well as inflammatory lesions of the liver and kidneys (Al-Habori, Al-Aghbari, Al-Mamary et al. 2002a,b).

Cathinone has been linked with low sperm count and motility, as well as a rise in abnormal sperm in human males and in laboratory animals (Islam, Tariq, Ageel et al. 1990), but not in male rabbits (Al-Habori, Al-Aghbari, Al-Mamary et al. 2002a). Female reproductive toxicity in human and guinea pig subjects has also been demonstrated and associated with infant mortality (Jansson, Kristiansson, Qirbi 1988a,b).

Clinical Application in Veterinary Behavior Medicine

C.edulis is of interest to veterinarians for its potential therapeutic and abusive administration in pets. Pet guardians may intentionally or accidentally expose animals to *C.edulis*. Despite the risk of serious side effects, *C.edulis* deserves further study for its clinical potential as an alternative to amphetamine treatment in the rare cases of true canine hyperkinesis.

References

Al-Habori M, Al-Aghbari A, Al-Mamary M et al. Toxicological evaluation of *Catha edulis* leaves: a long term feeding experiment in animals. J Ethnopharmacol. 2002a;83:209–217.

—. Investigation into the toxicological effects of *Catha edulis* leaves: a short term study in animals. Phytother Res. 2002b;16:127–332.

Al-Qirim TM, Shawwan M, Zaidi KR et al. Effect of khat, its constituents and restraint stress on free radical metabolism of rats. J Ethnopharmacol. 2002;83:245–250.

Awas M, Kebede D, Alem A. Major mental disorders in Butajira, southern Ethiopia. Acta Psychiatr Scand Suppl. 1999;397:56–64.

Brown ER, Jarvie DR, Simpson D. Use of drugs at 'raves'. Scott Med J. 1995;40:128–171.

Gosnell BA, Yracheta JM, Bell SM et al. Intravenous self-administration of cathinone by rats. Behav Pharmacol. 1996;7:526–531.

Griffiths P, Gossop M, Wickenden S et al. A transcultural pattern of drug use: qat (khat) in the UK. Br J Psychiatry. 1997;170:281–284.

Hassan NA, Gunaid AA, El-Khally FM et al. The effect of chewing Khat leaves on human mood. Saudi Med J. 2002;23:850–853.

Islam MW, Tariq M, Ageel AM et al. An evaluation of the male reproductive toxicity of cathinone. Toxicology. 1990;60:223–234.

Islam MW, Tariq M, el-Feraly FS et al. Effect of khatamines and their enantiomers on plasma triiodothyronine and thyroxine levels in normal Wistar rats. Am J Chin Med. 1990;18:71–76.

Jansson T, Kristiansson B, Qirbi A. Effect of khat on maternal food intake, maternal weight gain and fetal growth in the late-pregnant guinea pig. J Ethnopharmacol. 1988a;23:11–17.

—. Effect of khat on uteroplacental blood flow in awake, chronically catherterized, late-pregnant guinea pigs. J Ethnopharmacol. 1988b;23:19–26.

Kalix P. Cathinone, a natural amphetamine. Pharmacol Toxicol. 1992;70:77–86.

Kalix P. The pharmacology of psychoactive alkaloids from ephedra and catha. J Ethnopharmacol. 1991; 32:201–208.

Kassie F, Darroudi F, Kundi M et al. Khat (*Catha edulis*) consumption causes genotoxic effects in humans. Int J Cancer. 2001;92:329–332.

Nencini P, Ahmed AM, Elmi AS. Subjective effects of khat chewing in humans. Drug Alcohol Depend. 1986;18:97–105.

Pehek EA, Schechter MD, Yamamoto BK. Effects of cathinone and amphetamine on the neurochemistry of dopamine in vivo. Neuropharmacology. 1990;29:1171–1176.

Widler P, Mathys K, Brenneisen R et al. Pharmacodynamics and pharmacokinetics of khat: a controlled study. Clin Pharmacol Ther. 1994;55:556–562.

Humulus lupulus

Humulus lupulus (Hops, hopfenzapfen) is a climbing perennial vine native to Europe but cultivated around the world. *H. lupulus* is used to add flavor and aroma to beer and ale. It grows 6 to 12 m (20–35 ft) tall. The female flower, the source of the bittering agent lupulin, blossoms conspicuously; a yellowish fruit cone grows from its center. The inconspicuous male flower is only 5 mm in diameter. Serrated leaves have three to five lobes and are opposite on the stem, which is covered in six rows of barbs (Anonymous 2003; Russo 2001). *H. lupulus* is a member of the *Cannabinaceae* family, which also includes hemp and *Cannabis spp* (Anonymous 2003; Siegel 1976).

Historical Perspective

H. lupulus has been used medicinally for hundreds of years. A twelfth-century abbess and herbalist named Hildegard von Bingen first described the use of the plant. It was popular in the 1600s as a purifying agent for a variety of ills. Long ago, the young shoots were eaten as vegetables. The dried flowers were used for the treatment of mania, toothache, earache, and neuralgia because of their mild narcotic, hypnotic, and sedative effects. It has been used to induce sleep and to calm nervousness. Unproven uses include appetite stimulation and intestinal inflammation (Anonymous 2003; Russo 2001).

Physicians continued to apply its traditional use as a soporiphic, sedative, and hypnotic through the 1800s but recognized that it had little effect. They did, however, advocate its use in various forms to treat a variety of respiratory, digestive, and dermatologic diseases. Consumption of beer, ale, and port were considered to be medicinal at least in part because of their hops content (Felter, Lloyd 1898).

Although it is related to *Cannabis sativa* (hemp, marijauana) *H. lupulus* has been suggested as a marijuana substitute; however, no hallucinogenic effect is reported (Anonymous 2003; Siegel 1976).

Native Americans were familiar with *Humulus lupulus*. The Mohegan prepared an infusion of the blossoms as a tonic for nerves and “nervous tension” (Tantaquidgeon 1928; Moerman 2002). Similarly, the Delaware used the blossoms to treat nervousness (Moerman 2002; Tantaquidgeon 1972). The Meskwaki used the root of *Humulus lupulus* to induce sleep (Moerman 2002; Smith 1928).

Contemporary herbalists use *H. lupulus* as a sedative and mild hypnotic. ESCOP endorses its use for the treatment of insomnia, tension, and restlessness, whereas the German Commission E approves of its use for anxiety, restlessness, and sleep disturbances (Russo 2001). There is also an accumulating evidence and interest in its endocrine, antitumor, and free radical scavenging properties (Anonymous 2003).

Ingredients

Compounds isolated from the plant include acylphloroglucinols (10%), alpha-bitter acids (e.g., humulone); beta-bitter acids (e.g., lupulone); volatile oil (< 1%, e.g., humulene); resins; tannins (proanthocyanidines); phenolic acids (e.g., caffeic acid, chlorogenic acid); flavonoids (e.g., xanthohumole) (PDR 2000). In addition to lupulin, novel odor-active compounds in hops extracts have been identified (Steinhaus, Schieberle 2000).

Until recently, it was thought that the medicinal parts of the plant were primarily in the whole dried female flower and fresh cones collected prior to seed ripening. These are dried at 30°C to 60°C (PDR 2000). However, recent research has confirmed that bioactive components were present in the leaves of adult plants, the female cones, as well as the male inflorescences, although in lower concentrations. A gradual increase in bioactive compounds (e.g., alpha-acids, beta-acids, desmethylxanthohumol, and xanthohumol) was observed as the female inflorescences developed into cones (De Keukeleire, Ooms, Heyerick 2003).

Cones from distinct populations that were accessible in both 1989 and 2001 were found to possess unique chemical attributes. This is thought to indicate a succession of genotypes, and suggests temporal cycling of plants. One variety contained a higher proportion of cohumulone in alpha acids, and cultivars of both American and European commercial *H. lupulus* generally contained higher concentrations alpha acids (Hampton, Nickerson, Whitney et al. 2002).

CNS Effects

A recent study of *Valeriana officinalis* extract and *H. lupulus* extract, used alone and in combination, revealed a partial agonistic activity at adenosine receptors that may explain their hypnotic effect (Muller, Schumacher, Brattstrom et al. 2002). *H. lupulus* extract has also shown high affinity for $GABA_{A,B}$, glycine, $CCK_{A,B}$, and Cl^- ion channel receptors among others (Cott 1995).

In a unique murine study, an airborne metabolite (2-methyl-3-butene-2-ol) induced a period of excitation followed by a prolonged eight-hour narcotic sleep (Hansel, Wohlfart, Coper 1980).

Anticancer Effects

Nitric oxide (NO) plays an important role in many inflammatory responses and is also involved in carcinogenesis. In a recent study, the inhibitory effect of extracts from *H. lupulus* extract on the production and inhibition of NO in mouse macrophage cells was investigated. The chalcones, including xanthohumol, significantly inhibited the production of NO by suppressing the expression of inducible NO synthase (Zhao, Nozawa, Daikonnya 2003). Xanthohumol was determined to exert an exceptionally broad spectrum of inhibitory mechanisms at the initiation, promotion, and progression stage of carcinogenesis. (Gerhauser, Alt, Heiss et al. 2002). Another component of *H. lupulus*, humulon, exhibited anticarcinogenic and anti-inflammatory effects (Yasukawa, Takeuchi, Takido 1995).

A selection of 159 native *H. lupulus* genotypes were analyzed and found to contain several bioactive components (e.g., xanthohumol, xanthogalenol, prenylflavonoids) associated with mammalian anticancer activity (Hampton, Nickerson, Whitney et al. 2002). It appears that the anticarcinogenic effect of the *H. lupulus* flavonoids is due to their potent, selective inhibition of human cytochrome P450 enzymes, which activate carcinogens. Their chemical structures resemble other plant-derived compounds, many present in the human diet, with cancer chemopreventive properties associated with cytochrome P450 inhibition (Henderson, Miranda, Stevens et al. 2000). Xanthohumol and isoxanthohumol, for instance, have shown promising *in vitro* chemopreventive activity against breast and ovarian cancer in humans (Miranda, Stevens, Helmrich et al. 1999).

Miscellaneous Effects

Recently, a phytoestrogen (8-prenylnaringenin) has been isolated from *H. lupulus* that is more potent than other established plant estrogens (Schaefer, Humpel, Fritzemeier 2003; Milligan, Kalita, Pocock et al. 2002; Milligan, Kalita, Pocock et al. 2000; Milligan, Kalita, Heyerick et al. 1999). This compound is found in dietary supplements marketed as breast enhancers (Coldham, Sauer 2001) and in products recommended for menopausal symptoms (Liu, Burdette, Xu et al. 2001). It is found in beer in concentration too low to be considered bioactive (Milligan, Kalita, Heyerick et al. 1999). This phytoestrogen has been shown to stimulate mammary cancer cells *in vitro* (Rong, Boterberg, Maubach et al. 2001). The unrestricted use of products containing *H. lupulus* extract by individuals predisposed to breast cancer and other estrogen-sensitive disease should be of concern.

Some native hop subspecies have exhibited natural repellence of insect and mite pests (Hampton, Nickerson, Whitney et al. 2002).

Proanthocyanidins from *H. lupulus* were found to be potent inhibitors of neuronal nitric oxide synthase activity. Among those identified and tested, procyanidin B3 showed the highest antioxidant activity, whereas a catechin trimer exhibited antioxidant activity considerably greater than that of alpha-tocopherol (Vitamin E) or ascorbic acid (Vitamin C) (Stevens, Miranda, Wolthers et al. 2002).

H. lupulus oil and extract exhibited antimicrobial activity against the Gram-positive bacteria (*Bacillus subtilis* and *Staphylococcus aureus*) and the fungus (*Trichophyton mentagrophytes var. interdigitale*); however, it was virtually inactive against the Gram-negative *Escherichia coli* and the yeast *Candida albicans* (Langezaal, Chandra, Scheffer 1992). Interestingly, a bacteria commonly found in beer that contributes to its spoilage (*Lactobacillus breva*) is resistant to the antibacterial effects of hop (Sakamoto, Van Veen, Saito 2002; Simpson, Smith 1992).

Agricultural by-products of *H. lupulus* may have potential for use in the removal of heavy lead (Pb-II) ions from contaminated aqueous solutions, and may be applied in removing heavy lead from contaminated waters (Gardea-Torresdey, Hejazi, Tiemann et al. 2002).

Adverse Effects

A case of systemic urticaria associated with exposure to *H. lupulus* has been reported (Pradalier, Campinos, Trinh 2002), but it appears to be an isolated incident. Reported side effects include "hop dermatitis" (more commonly seen in hop workers). In one interesting report, a woman who had worked in a hop plantation for more than thirty years developed contact dermatitis to the hop plant. Her symptoms recurred after leaving her job and it was subsequently determined that she used beauty creams containing hop extract. In addition, her husband continued to work at the plantation and may have been an ongoing source of exposure to his hop-sensitive wife (Spiewak, Dutkiewicz 2002). Rhinitis, conjunctivitis, asthma; contact urticaria (Estrada, Gozalo, Cecchini et al. 2002) have also been reported. *H. lupulus* pollen is one of the major causes of allergy in Asia (Park, Ko, Kim 1999; Sugaya, Tsuda, Ohguchi 1997) and is reported elsewhere (Hernandez Prieto, Lorente Toledano, Romo Cortina et al. 1998; Lewis, Dixit, Wedner 1991).

Reports of menstrual disturbance in female hop workers may be attributed to the presence of phytoestrogen 8-prenylnaringenin in the plant (Milligan, Kalita, Heyerick et al. 1999).

Five cases of malignant hyperthermia-like reactions to hops ingestion have been reported in dogs; four of the dogs were Greyhounds, suggesting that this breed may be particularly susceptible (Duncan, Hare, Buck 1997). The fifth dog was a Labrador Retriever. Only one of the five dogs survived despite routine cooling measures and other emergency treatments. Panting, pacing, hyperthermia, and seizure were among the associated clinical signs that developed within hours of hops consumption. The dogs had apparently consumed significant volumes of hops, used by home brewers of beer. One dog, for example, had ingested 600 ml of hops.

Availability and Dosage

H. lupulus is marketed alone or in combination with other herbal compounds. It may be found as a tincture in 60% ethanol, or in a liquid extract with 45% ethanol. The ground hop cones are steeped in boiling water for 10 to 15 minutes to yield approximately 0.4 gm per teaspoon of active ingredient. One cup of tea at bedtime for up to several days is advised to promote sleep. For anxiety and restlessness, one tablet or five drops of liquid or tincture can be taken up to three times a day (PDR 2000). No drug interactions are reported (Russo 2001).

Clinical Application in Veterinary Behavior Medicine

H. lupulus could be of clinical benefit to spayed or aging bitches with estrogen-deficient urinary incontinence. Although it has been used traditionally and by contemporary herbalists as a sedative and hypnotic, evidence to support its reliable clinical benefit is sparse at this time. Therapeutic doses of *H. lupulus* in dogs may not be associated with the severe hyperthermic reactions cited above; nonetheless, the use of *H. lupulus* deserves further study to determine whether its beneficial effects outweigh any risks.

References

Anonymous. *Humulus lupus*; Monograph. Altern Med Rev. 2003;8:190–192.

Coldham NG, Sauer MJ. Identification, quantitation and biological activity of phytoestrogens in a dietary supplement for breast enhancement. Food Chem Toxicol. 2001;39:1211–1224.

Cott J. Medicinal plants and dietary supplements: sources for innovative treatment or adjuncts? Psychopharmacol Bull 1995;31:131–137.

De Keukeleire J, Ooms G, Heyerick A et al. Formation and accumulation of alpha-acids, beta-acids, desmethylxanthohumol, and xanthohumol during flowering of hops (*Humulus lupulus L.*). J Agric Food Chem. 2003;51:4436–4441.

Duncan KL, Hare WR, Buck WB. Malignant hyperthermia-like reaction secondary to ingestion of hops in five dogs. JAVMA. 1997;21:51–54.

Estrada JL, Gozalo F, Cecchini C et al. Contact urticaria from hops (*Humulus lupulus*) in a patient with previous urticaria-angioedema from peanut, chestnut and banana. Contact Dermatitis. 2002;46:127.

Felter HW, Lloyd JU. King's American Dispensatory. Ohio Valley Company, Cincinatti, OH. 1898. Available online at http://www.ibiblio.org/herbmed/eclectic/kings/

Gardea-Torresdey J, Hejazi M, Tiemann K et al. Use of hop (*Humulus lupulus*) agricultural by-products for the reduction of aqueous lead(II) environmental health hazards. J Hazard Mater. 2002;91:95–112.

Gerhauser C, Alt A, Heiss E et al. Cancer chemopreventive activity of Xanthohumol, a natural product derived from hop. Mol Cancer Ther. 2002;1:959–969.

Hampton R, Nickerson G, Whitney P et al. Comparative chemical attributes of native North American hop, *Humulus lupulus var. lupuloides E. Small.* Phytochemistry. 2002;61:855–862.

Hansel R, Wohlfart R, Coper H. Sedative-hypnotic compounds in the exhalation of hops, II. Zeitschrift fuer Naturforschung 1980;35:1096–1097.

Henderson MC, Miranda CL, Stevens JF et al. In vitro inhibition of human P450 enzymes by prenylated flavonoids from hops, *Humulus lupulus*. Xenobiotica. 2000;30:235–251.

Hernandez Prieto M, Lorente Toledano F, Romo Cortina A et al. Pollen calendar of the city of Salamanca (Spain). Aeropalynological analysis for 1981-1982 and 1991-1992. Allergol Immunopathol (Madr). 1998;26:209–222.

Langezaal CR, Chandra A, Scheffer JJ. Antimicrobial screening of essential oils and extracts of some *Humulus lupulus L.* cultivars. Pharm Weekbl Sci. 1992;14:353–356.

Lewis WH, Dixit AB, Wedner HJ. Aeropollen of weeds of the western United States Gulf Coast. Ann Allergy. 1991;67:47–52.

Liu J, Burdette JE, Xu H et al. Evaluation of estrogenic activity of plant extracts for the potential treatment of menopausal symptoms. J Agric Food Chem. 2001;49:2472–2479.

Milligan S, Kalita J, Pocock V et al. Oestrogenic activity of the hop phyto-oestrogen, 8-prenylnaringenin. Reproduction. 2002;123:235–242.

Milligan SR, Kalita JC, Pocock V et al. The endocrine activities of 8-prenylnaringenin and related hop (*Humulus lupulus L.*) flavonoids. J Clin Endocrinol Metab. 2000;85:4912–4915.

Milligan SR, Kalita JC, Heyerick A et al. Identification of a potent phytoestrogen in hops (*Humulus lupulus L.*) and beer. J Clin Endocrinol Metab. 1999;84:2249–2252.

Miranda CL, Stevens JF, Helmrich A et al. Antiproliferative and cytotoxic effects of prenylated flavonoids from hops (*Humulus lupulus*) in human cancer cell lines. Food Chem Toxicol. 1999;37: 271–285.

Muller CE, Schumacher B, Brattstrom A et al. Interactions of valerian extracts and a fixed valerian-hop extract combination with adenosine receptors. Life Sci. 2002;71:1939–1949.

Park JW, Ko SH, Kim CW et al. Identification and characterization of the major allergen of the *Humulus japonicus* pollen. Clin Exp Allergy. 1999;29:1080–1086.

PDR for Herbal Medicines (2nd ed) Medical Economics Company Inc., Montvale, NJ. 2000;400–401.

Pradalier A, Campinos C, Trinh C. Systemic urticaria induced by hops. Allerg Immunol (Paris). 2002;34:330–332.

Rong H, Boterberg T, Maubach J et al. 8-Prenylnaringenin, the phytoestrogen in hops and beer, upregulates the function of the E-cadherin/catenin complex in human mammary carcinoma cells. Eur J Cell Biol. 2001;80:580–585.

Russo E. Handbook of Psychotropic Herbs: A Scientific Analysis of Herbal Remedies for Psychiatric Conditions. The Haworth Press, Binghamton, NY. 2001;123–125.

Sakamoto K, Van Veen HW, Saito H et al. Membrane-bound ATPase contributes to hop resistance of Lactobacillus brevis. Appl Environ Microbiol. 2002;68:5374–5378.

Schaefer O, Humpel M, Fritzemeier KH et al. 8-Prenyl naringenin is a potent ERalpha selective phytoestrogen present in hops and beer. J Steroid Biochem Mol Biol. 2003;84:359–360.

Siegel RK. Herbal intoxication: psychoactive effects from herbal cigarettes, tea, and capsules. JAMA. 1976;236:473–476.

Simpson WJ, Smith AR. Factors affecting antibacterial activity of hop compounds and their derivatives. J Appl Bacteriol. 1992;72:327–334.

Smith HH. Ethnobotany of the Meskwaki Indians. Bulletin of the Public Museum of the City of Milwaukee 1928;4:175–326.

Spiewak R, Dutkiewicz J. Occupational airborne and hand dermatitis to hop (*Humulus lupulus*) with non-occupational relapses. Ann Agric Environ Med. 2002;9:249–252.

Steinhaus M, Schieberle P. Comparison of the most odor-active compounds in fresh and dried hop cones (*Humulus lupulus L.* variety spalter select) based on GC-olfactometry and odor dilution techniques. J Agric Food Chem. 2000;48:1776–1783.

Stevens JF, Miranda CL, Wolthers KR et al. Identification and in vitro biological activities of hop proanthocyanidins: inhibition of nNOS activity and scavenging of reactive nitrogen species. J Agric Food Chem. 2002;50:3435–3443.

Sugaya A, Tsuda T, Ohguchi H. Marked increase of atmospheric pollen dispersion of ragweed (*Ambrosia spp.*): annual changes in atmospheric pollen counts of major allergen plants in autumn in Saitama Prefecture. Arerugi. 1997;46:585–593.

Tantaquidgeon G. Mohegan Medicinal Practices, Weather-Lore and Superstitions. SI-BAE Annual Report 1928;43: 264–270.

Tantaquidgeon G. Folk Medicine of the Delaware and Related Algonkian Indians. Pennsylvania Historical Commission Anthropological Papers, Harrisburg, PA. 1972.

Yasukawa K, Takeuchi M, Takido M. Humulon, a bitter in the hop, inhibits tumor promotion by 12-O-tetradecanoylphorbol-13-acetate in two-stage carcinogenesis in mouse skin. Oncology. 1995;52: 156–158.

Zhao F, Nozawa H, Daikonnya A et al. Inhibitors of nitric oxide production from hops (*Humulus lupulus L.*). Biol Pharm Bull. 2003;26:61–65.

Hypericum perforatum

Hypericum perforatum (St. John's Wort, also known as Amber, Goatweed, Klamath Wed, Tipton Weed, Hardhay, Saint John's Word, St. Johnswort, Johanniskraut) is a perennial member of the *Clusiaceae* (also called *Guttiferae*) family. It is native to Europe, western Asia, and northern Africa, although it has been introduced to Australia, New Zealand, and eastern Asia. It is also cultivated in Poland and

Siberia. A single plant can produce as many as 30,000 seeds, which are easily disseminated by wind to colonize new areas. In fact, it has naturalized to most other continents so successfully that it has become a weed (Russo 2001; Sumner 2000). There are almost 400 related species (Mills, Bone 2000; PDR 2000). The plant must be distinguished from other Hypericum species such as *H. hirsutum*, *H. barbatum*, among many others.

H. perforatum grows to 30 to 60 cm high, although it can grow as high as 1 m. A reddish stem is characterized by two raised edges. Branches are paired and oppose each other along the stem. The oval-shaped leaves, attached at the plant's base, are punctuated by translucent glandular dots (see color plate 1–1). Sparse, golden yellow flowers have five petals and appear in terminal cymes (Fig. 1-3). Bloom time occurs between June and September in the Northern Hemisphere. When the flowers are squeezed, an odorless, slightly bitter-tasting red juice is released (PDR 2000).

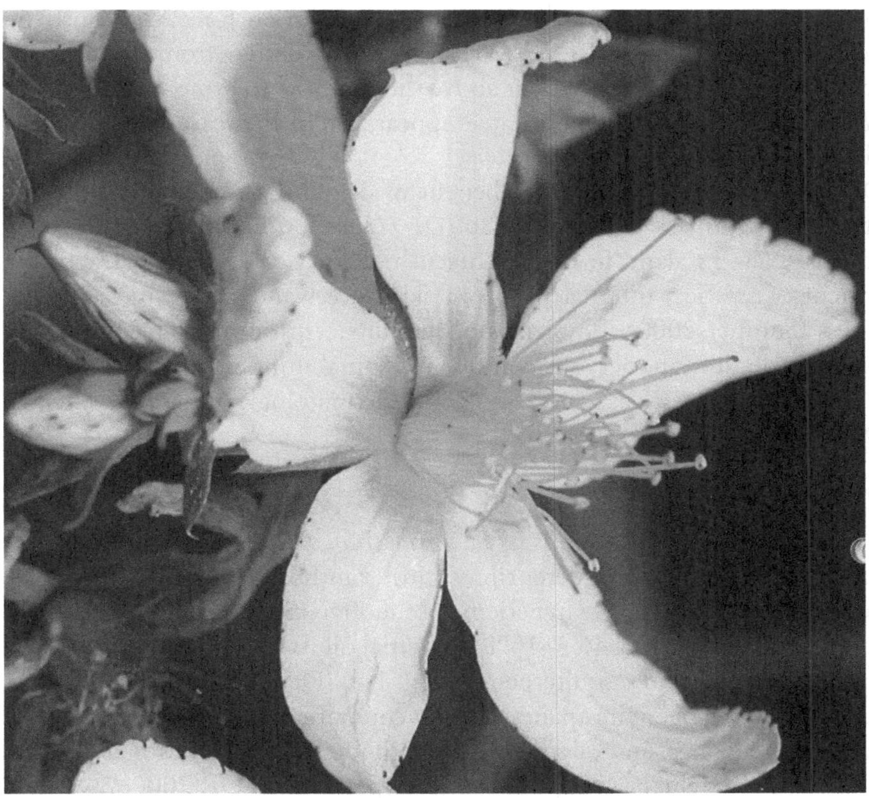

FIGURE 1-3. Close-up of *Hypericum perforatum* flower. (Photo courtesy of Prof. Jayvir Anjaria)

The medicinal parts of *H. perforatum* are the top aerial parts. The flowering plant, including fresh buds and flowers, is collected at the start of blooming. Quick drying and protection from light are required to preserve its active ingredients (Russo 2001; Mills, Bone 2000; PDR 2000).

Traditional uses include internal parasites, bronchitis and asthma, cholelithiasis, diarrhea, nocturnal enuresis, gout, rheumatism, stomach disorders, and myalgia. In Traditional Chinese Medicine (TCM), a solution of *H. perforatum* is used as a gargle to treat tonsillitis; dermatopathy is treated with topical application of *H. perforatum* (PDR 2000). Oral medication with *H. perforatum* is indicated for the treatment of depression, anxiety, and inflammatory lesions of the skin; wounds and burns respond to oily topical Hypericum preparations (PDR 2000).

Historical Perspective

Originally associated with Balder, the Norse god of light, the plant was named when Balder's day became St. John's day as Christianity spread through Europe (Sumner 2000). The plant's English name is linked with St. John because its bloom time commences close to the feast of St. John on June 24. "Wort" means "plant" in Middle English (Russo 2001). *Hypericum* derives from the Latin "above an icon" and refers to its placement above the doorway to protect against evil spirits. *Perforatum* refers to the perforated appearance of the leaves when held up to the light (Mills, Bone 2000).

Descriptions of the therapeutic benefit of drinking the herbal tea and herbal tincture are centuries old (Russo 2001). *H. perforatum* was introduced from Europe to New England in the seventeenth century as a medicinal herb for the treatment of sciatica, internal parasites, skin ulcers and burns, melancholy, and madness (Sumner 2000). Physicians of the nineteenth century recommended its use to treat depression, nervous complaints, spinal injuries, trauma, hemorrhage, and a variety of digestive, gynecologic, and dermatologic ailments (Felter, Lloyd 1898).

Ingredients

The principle active compounds of *H. perforatum* are the flavonoids (2-4%; e.g., hyperoside, quercitrin, isoquercitrin, rutin); xanthones (0.14–0.72%) and anthracenes (0.1–0.15%; e.g., hypericin, pseudohypericin) (naphthodianthrones); procyanidines and tannins (6.5–15%); essential oil (0.1–0.35%; e.g., aliphatic hydrocarbons, mono- and sesquiterpenes) (Fig. 1-4). Dry plant extract contains high concentrations of phenylpropanes (e.g., *p*-coumaric acid, caffeic acid), flavonol glycosides, biflavones, and oligomeric proanthocyanidins. Additional compounds include the phloroglucinols (2–4.5%; e.g., hyperforin) (PDR 2000; Awang 1991; Nahrstedt, Butterweck 1997). New compounds continue to emerge in *H. perforatum* extracts (Jurgenliemk , Nahrstedt 2002; Winkelmann, Heilmann, Zerbe et al. 2000).

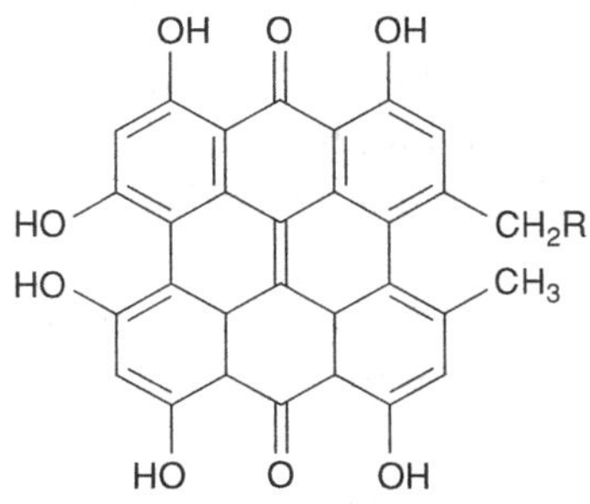

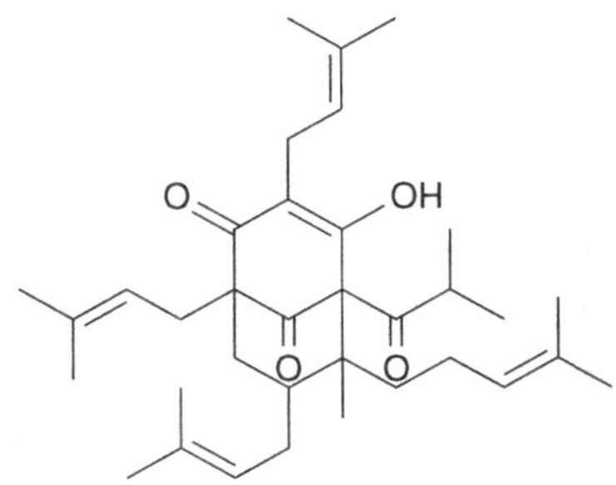

FIGURE 1-4. Active compounds of *Hypericum perforatum* (Mills, Bone 2002)

Hyperforin, found only in the flowers and fruit, is a lipophilic molecule that easily penetrates the CNS (Nahrstedt, Butterweck 1997). More than 40% of the naphthodianthrones (hypericin, pseudohypericin together are often referred to as "total hypericin") are extracted from the crude herb prepared by infusion (herbal tea) (Mills, Bone 2000).

A marked seasonal variation in the content of hypericin and pseudohypericin was demonstrated. During the summer months, the bioactive ingredients were between 300 and 500 times higher compared to winter months (Southwell, Campbell 2001). In the future, genetic manipulation and technological advances in agriculture may produce concentrations that are more consistent in the desired compounds of *H. perforatum* (Buter, Orlacchio, Soldati et al. 1998).

Neurological and CNS Effects

In electroencephalographic studies of 54 healthy volunteers, delta (cholinergic), theta (noradrenergic), and alpha (serotonergic) frequency values were emphasized, suggesting that hypericum preparations with a high hyperforin content have a shielding effect on the CNS. A peak pharmacodynamic effect was observed four and eight hours after administration (Schellenberg, Sauer, Dimpfel 1998).

Preliminary study of mouse neuromuscular junction and *H. perforatum* extract suggests a possible reduction of the degradation rate of ACh by acetylcholinesterase (AChE) (Re, Corneli, Sturani et al. 2003).

Hypericin (0.3%) and hypericin with (50%) flavonoids both caused increases of noradrenaline and dopamine in the rat diencephalons and a significant increase in the 5-HT content of the cortex. Hypericin with flavonoids induced an increase in noradrenaline content. Results indicated that flavonoids extend the effects of hypericin extract into brain regions (e.g., diencephalon and brainstem) that are involved in depression (Calapai, Crupi, Firenzuoli et al. 1999). The flavonol glycosides (e.g., hyperoside, rutin, quercetin) bind to benzodiazepine receptors, and some exhibit MAO_A inhibition. Their levels are so low, however, that they are felt to be clinically irrelevant to the extract's antidepressant effect (Nahrstedt, Butterweck 1997).

Experiments on the impact of herbal treatment for the consequences of learned helplessness in rats demonstrated that hyperforin exerted significant reuptake inhibition of serotonin (5-HT), dopamine (DA), GABA, and l-glutamate, but not for MAO receptors (Chatterjee, Bhattacharya, Wonnemann 1998). Elsewhere, serotonin and GABA systems were unaffected by hyperforin, but extracellular levels of dopamine, noradrenaline, serotonin and glutamate were enhanced, suggesting an underlying mechanism of reuptake inhibition by *H. perforatum* (Kaehler, Sinner, Chatterjee et al. 1999). In another report, the diglycoside flavonoid rutin was shown to be essential to the antidepressant effect of *H. perforatum* extract in rats (Noldner, Schotz 2002).

Although studies have failed to confirm significant MAO inhibition by hypericin (Baldt, Wagner 1994; Thiede, Walper 1994), a weak MAO inhibitor effect has been sustained by other studies (Muller, Schaefer 1996; Suzuki 1984). Until evidence that is more conclusive is available, prevailing opinion remains that the concomitant use of *H. perforatum* preparations with other MAOI drugs is contraindicated (PDR 2000). It has been demonstrated that hyperforin interferes with the storage of monoamines in synaptic vesicles rather than by selective inhibition of synaptic membrane or vesicular monoamine transporters (Roz, Mazur, Hirshfeld et al. 2002).

Chlorogenic acid, a derivative of the phenylpropane caffeic acid, may exert a stimulatory effect on the CNS (Nahrstedt, Butterweck 1997). Crude extracts contain a minute fraction of the endogenous inhibitory neurotransmitter GABA, but its concentration is not high enough to be biochemically, and therefore, clinically active. Biflavones have no proven biochemical activity despite their ability to bind to benzodiazepine receptors and to depress CNS function. This may be explained by their rapid metabolism or a failure to cross the blood brain barrier (Nahrstedt, Butterweck 1997).

In an important study in mice, *H. perforatum* extract LI 160 showed significant inhibition in the reuptake of serotonin, dopamine, and norepinephrine. It is the only compound known to exert a similar affinity for three neurotransmitter systems. An increase in serotonin 5-hydroxytryptamine type 2 (5-HT-2) binding sites and a decrease of beta-adrenoreceptor density in the frontal cortex (Muller et al. 1997) was also demonstrated. In another study, the extract had significant effects on adenosine, benzodiazepine, and $MAO_{A,B}$ and $GABA_{A,B}$ receptors. However, with the exception of GABA activity, it was concluded that *in vitro* concentrations would not be attainable by oral administration (Cott 1997).

One study of rat brain compared several species of Hypericum against flumazenil at the benzodiazepine receptor (BDZ-R) of the $GABA_A$ complex, which serves as a model for research into anxiolytic drugs. Their data found no competitive binding for hypericin, but a high inhibitory activity was demonstrated for amentoflavone, another extract component. Amentoflavone is present in the flowers but not in the leaves of *H. perforatum*; it is present in highest concentrations in the flower extracts of *H. olympicum* (Baureithel, Buter, Engesser et al. 1997). Amentoflavone is also present in *Ginkgo biloba*. Recently, amentoflavone's negative modulation of GABA receptors appeared to be independent of flumazenil-sensitive benzodiazepine sites (Hanrahan, Chebib, Davucheron et al. 2003). Overall, these findings suggest that GABA neurotransmission may be involved with beta-adrenergic down-regulation and dopamine modulation, contributing to our understanding of the mechanism of *H. perforatum*'s antidepressant effect.

Behavioral and Psychological Effects

H. perforatum is unique in that its mechanism of action resembles the pharmacology of other conventional antidepressants as well as novel mechanisms not typically associated with standard antidepressants. It has a well-documented inhibitory effect of the reuptake of monoamines serotonin, dopamine, noradrenaline, GABA, and glutamate (Butterweck 2003; Nathan 2001), although at least one other study did not support an effect on noradrenergic systems by *H. perforatum* extract (Franklin, Cowen 2001). Partial explanation for the antidepressant activity of *H. perforatum* includes inhibition of enkephalin activation by *H. perforatum* flavonoids (Denke, Schneider, Elstner 1999), and an increase in CNS dopamine levels via inhibition of dopamine beta-hydroxylase (Kleber et al. 1999).

Its monoamine reuptake inhibition, however, is distinct from other antidepressants in that it is exerted noncompetitively by enhancing intracellular Na+ ion concentrations. At the receptor level, chronic treatment with *H. perforatum* inhibits beta1-adrenoceptor but stimulates post-synaptic 5-HT1A receptors and 5-HT2 receptors. The active component constituent most responsible for the antidepressant effect is hyperforin, although other constituents such as hypericin, pseudohypericin, flavonoids and procyanidines also possess significant therapeutic properties of their own or exert a synergistic effect (Butterweck 2003; Nathan 2001; Muller 1998). A complementary or synergistic effect between components of *H. perforatum* extract is proposed (Butterweck, Christoffel, Nahrstedt et al. 2003; Williamson 2001).

The electric discharge of serotonergic neurons in the dorsal raphe nucleus of conscious cats was measured following systemic administration of two clinical preparations of *H. perforatum*; neither was found to exert any effect. This suggests that the mode of action of *H. perforatum* differs from that of conventional antidepressant drugs, which elevate brain serotonin (Fornal, Metzler, Mirescu et al. 2001).

Biochemical studies have shown that *H. perforatum* possesses only weak inhibition of MAO_A and MAO_B receptors but approximately equal affinity for inhibiting the reuptake of serotonin, dopamine, and noradrenaline (norepinephrine) (Butterweck 2003; Calapai, Crupi, Firenzuoli 2001). Other *in vitro* binding assays demonstrated significant affinity for adenosine, $GABA_A$, $GABA_B$, and glutamate receptors. *In vivo*, *H. perforatum* extract was associated with inhibition of beta-adrenergic receptors and stimulation of serotonin (5-HT) receptors in the rat frontal cortex. It also brought about changes in neurotransmitter concentrations in brain areas that are implicated in depression (Butterweck 2003).

Hypericin and pseudohypericin are photosensitizing plant pigments found in Hypericum species. It has been hypothesized that hypericin absorbs long wave light, thereby altering serotonin metabolism and improving depression. Hypericin's hypnotic effect could be the result of an ability to increase melatonin (Gruenwald 1997). In one report, nocturnal plasma melatonin was increased after three weeks of *H. perforatum* extract in 13 healthy volunteers. Unfortunately, this was not a controlled study, so results must be interpreted cautiously (Demisch, Sielaff, Nispel et al. 1991).

H. perforatum extract possess mild antidepressant, sedative, and anxiolytic properties. In a randomized, double-blind, comparative trial of 149 human patients with mild or moderate depression over a six-week period, a daily dose of *H. perforatum* extract (800 mg of a dry extract of *H. perforatum* in a 60% ethanol base) had an equivalent effect to 20 mg of the selective serotonin reuptake inhibitor fluoxetine (Harrer 1999). In another study, a commercial preparation of *H. perforatum* extract was compared to fluoxetine. Both compounds were effective in ameliorating complaints of depression. Patients and evaluating physicians found no therapeutic difference between the two groups although on standardized tests the herb was 78% to 83% as effective as the conventional antidepressant (Behnke, Jensen, Graubaum 2002).

Compared to the tricyclic antidepressant imipramine (25 mg TID, PO) *H. perforatum* extract (300 mg TID, PO) achieved comparable results between treatment groups of 135 clinically depressed patients. Moreover, the Hypericum group had fewer and milder side effects (Vorbach 1994). In a comparison study of LI 160 (300 mg TID) and amitriptyline (25 mg TID), *H. perforatum* was better tolerated and was not associated with sedation or impaired cognition, although both compounds were essentially equally beneficial to depressed patients (Wheatley 1997). In a recent double-blind study of healthy male volunteers, *H. perforatum* extract, amitriptyline, and placebo were compared. The antidepressant effects of amitriptyline and *H. perforatum* extract were comparable. Neither test impacted cognitive performance; however, amitriptyline did cause a decrease in heart rate variability and subjective sedation (Siepmann, Krause, Joraschky et al. 2002).

Recent data has shown that both *H. perforatum* and the prototypical antidepressant imipramine affected six common gene transcripts relevant to cellular ribosomes, microtubules, and mitochondria, in addition to the same glycolytic pathways and synaptic function, among other cellular processes (Wong, O'Kirwan, Hannestad et al. 2004). These data provide evidence that both synthetic and botanical medicines impact changes in the genetic expression of discrete brain regions.

In a recent report, *H. perforatum* was effective in relieving seasonal affective disorder and was as effective as therapy with bright light (Kasper 1997). Recently, it has shown promise for the treatment of premenstrual syndrome (Stevinson, Ernst 2000). It may prove of particular use for the treatment of depression in the elderly because of relatively few adverse effects compared to prescribed antidepressants (Vorbach, Arnoldt, Wolpert 2000). However, because geriatric patients often take a variety of prescription drugs, the potential for drug interaction with *H. perforatum* extract must be carefully considered (Gold, Laxer, Dergal et al. 2001).

H. perforatum was superior to placebo and possessed few side effects compared to placebo in a meta-analysis of 23 randomized trials of 1,757 patients with symptoms of mild to moderately severe depression (Linde 1996). However, interpretation of the data falls short of being irrefutable given the lack of standardization for trial duration, dosage regimen, diagnostic criteria, and compliance control of the clinical trials upon which this study was based. Nonetheless, *H. perforatum* extract LI 160 has been shown to exert a consistent and clinically significant therapeutic effect in a number of studies on depressed patients (Hubner, Lande, Podzuweit 1994; Sommer, Harrer 1994; Hansgen, Vesper, Ploch, 1994).

Despite positive results, at least one study suggested that *H. perforatum* preparations are not appropriate for cases of more serious depressive states (e.g., including delusions, suicidal tendencies, and resistance to therapy) (Volz 1997). However, results of another study support its effectiveness in patients suffering from severe depression (Vorbach 1997). In this study, photosensitivity reactions were not reported despite high doses (equivalent to 5.4 mg per day) of extract. In a recent study, young people aged 6 to 16 years with moderately severe major depressive disorder were treated with *H. perforatum* at an initial dose of 150 mg TID. Of the 34 subjects enrolled, 22 required an upward adjustment after four weeks to 300 mg TID. After eight weeks, 25 of the subjects had responded well to treatment of depression (Findling, McNamara, O'Riordan et al. 2003). In another study on 101 children under the age of twelve with depression, results were very promising with 100% resolution of signs within six weeks of beginning treatment with *H. perforatum* extract (300–1800 mg per day) (Hubner, Kirste 2001).

H. perforatum extract may exert an anxiolytic and antipanic effect, a finding that is consistent with other antidepressant drugs that are also effective on generalized anxiety disorder and panic disorders (Beijamini, Andreatini 2003).

Hypericin (450 mg BID of 0.3% extended release formulation) has been effective in the treatment of obsessive-compulsive disorder. In twelve subjects with a primary DSM-IV diagnosis of OCD, clinical improvement began within one week of the trial and progressed throughout the trial. Although 42% of subjects rated positive clinical effect, 50% of subjects were only minimally improved and 8% were unaffected (Taylor, Kobak 2000). *H. perforatum* merits further placebo-controlled and comparative study as a treatment for OCD.

Anti-inflammatory Effects

The high flavonoid content of oily *H. perforatum* preparations is responsible for its anti-inflammatory effects (Gulick 1999), which may be explained by inhibition of myeloperoxidase (Pabuccuoglu, Konyalioglu, Bas 2003). Recently, it has been suggested that *H. perforatum*'s anti-inflammatory effect is by virtue of cytokine modulation; depression may be alleviated by the release of corticotropin-releasing hormones. This is based on preliminary findings of *H. perforatum* suppression of interleukin-6 in depressed patients (Thiele, Brink, Ploch 1994). Suppression of interleukin-6 may inhibit corticotrophin-releasing factor and other adrenal hormones, thus deactivating the hypothalamic-pituitary-adrenal axis and providing a partial explanation for the herb's antidepressant effect as well (Nemeroff 1998). *H. perforatum* extract and hypericin exerted delayed effects on HPA axis control centers; however, hyperforin and hyperforin derivatives are not involved in the regulation of genes that control HPA axis function (Butterweck, Winterhoff, Herkenham 2003).

Hormonal Effects

H. perforatum was compared to *Cimicifuga racemosa* (Black Cohosh) in the treatment of menopausal symptoms in 812 patients. Psychological complaints were noted in 90% of subjects, including reduction in "hot flashes" and an increase in concentration after three weeks (PDR 2000). Another study found that 79% of menopausal women improved with *H. perforatum*; it also reported improved sexual well-being (Grube, Walper, Wheatley 1999).

Antimicrobial Effects

H. perforatum may have antifungal and antiviral properties (Nahrstedt, Butterweck 1997) and hyperforin has shown antibacterial properties that indicate its potential for topical treatment of infected wounds and other skin lesions (Schempp 1999). Hyperforin was effective against gram-positive bacteria including *Streptococcus pyogenes* and *Streptococcus agalactiae*, as well as against penicillin-resistant and methicillin-resistant *Staphylococcus aureus*. *H. perforatum* also showed antibacterial properties with *Escherichia coli*, *Pseudomonas aeruginosa*, and *Proteus vulgaris* (Mills, Bone 2000). Tannins are present in significant concentration and may account for some of the antimicrobial effects of *H. perforatum* (Nahrstedt, Butterweck 1997). The finding that tannic acids may inhibit the absorption of iron (Miller 1998) may also elucidate their mechanism of action.

Antimicrobial studies on three Hypericum species native to the Canary Islands and used in folk treatment to treat skin infections were shown to inhibit *Staph. aureus* and *epidermidis, Micrococcus luteus, Bacillus cereus*, and *Bordetella bronchiseptica* (Rabanal, Arias, Prado et al. 2002). The Hypericum genus includes at least 33 species with inhibitory properties of *Staph. aureus* (Gibbons, Ohlendorf, Johnsen 2002). In Africa, Hypericum species are among plants selected as toothbrush sticks. Given its antimicrobial properties, *H. perforatum* is useful for oral hygiene for those who cannot afford modern dental care (Kassu, Dagne, Abate et al. 1999).

The naphthodianthrones hypericin and pseudohypericin have antiviral properties, for example, against herpes simplex virus types 1 and 2, vesicular stomatitis virus, parainfluenza virus, vaccinia virus (Andersen, Weber, Wood et al. 1991), duck hepatitis B virus (Moraleda, Wu, Jilbert et al. 1993) and murine cytomegalovirus (Lopez-Bazzocchi, Hudson, Towers 1991). The mechanism of its antiviral activity may depend on the presence of a viral lipid envelope, given that the herb is ineffective against nonenveloped viruses such as poliovirus, adenovirus, and human rhinovirus. These substances also have a potent *in vitro* and *in vivo* effect against several retroviruses, including HIV (Lavie, Valentine, Levin et al. 1989; Meruelo, Lavie, Lavie et al. 1988; Kraus, Pratt, Tossberg et al. 1990).

The mechanism against retroviruses is unclear but a number of hypotheses have been suggested (Lavie, Valentine, Levin et al. 1989; Degar, Prince, Pascual et al. 1992; De Witte, Agostinis, Van Lint et al. 1993). It is currently thought that *H. perforatum*'s ability to modify viral capsid proteins is due to its photodynamic and lipophilic properties (Lavie, Mazur, Lavie et al. 1995; Wen, Chowdhury, Wills et al. 2002). Light-induced virucidal activity of hypericin was demonstrated against equine infectious anemia virus, which is related to the HIV virus (Carpenter, Fehr, Kraus et al. 1994). Hypericin's selective affinity for N-methyl-D-aspartate (NMDA) receptors supports its antiviral activity (Cott 1997). Elsewhere, however, its antiviral properties (specifically retroviruses) were not demonstrated in HIV-infected patients treated with hypericin and phototoxicity was reported as an adverse effect (Gulick 1999). Hypericin has demonstrated the ability to inhibit cytotoxic reactions of T cell-mediated illness (Lavie, Meruelo, Aroyo et al. 2000).

Antiaddictive Effects

Treatment with *H. perforatum* eases signs of nicotine withdrawal in mice, suggesting its potential for use and further study of *H. perforatum* in helping people to quit smoking (Catania, Firenzuoli, Crupi et al. 2003). Its ability to inhibit alcohol intake may also make it useful in prevention of relapse during withdrawal from alcohol dependence (Perfumi, Panocka, Ciccocioppo 2001; Rezvani, Overstreet, Yang 1999).

H. perforatum may reduce methadone blood levels and induce withdrawal symptoms, predisposing recovering addicts to failure (Eich-Hochli, Oppliger, Golay et al. 2003).

Anticancer Effects

H. perforatum or hypericin show antitumor activities *in vitro* against human colon and stomach cancer cells, as well as against murine leukemia cells (Brockmoller, Reum, Bauer et al. 1997). Tumor cell toxicity differed in hypericin and hypericin analogs (Wills, Park, Wen 2001). In a recent study, hypericin showed a selective destruction of urothelial tumors in rat bladder mucosa without damage to adjacent tissues (Kamuhabwa, Cosserat-Gerardin, Didelon et al. 2002; Orellane 2001). Elsewhere, the cytocidal effects of hyperforin and its cooperation with hypericin on leukemia cell growth inhibition in a synergistic manner have been reported (Hostanska, Reichling, Bommer 2003)

Photodynamic therapy (PDT) has become the focus of research for the treatment of cancer. PDT combines a photosensitizing agent (photosensitizer) which tumor cells uptake selectively, and visible light of the same wavelength as the absorption spectrum of the drug. Although each of these factors is innocuous used alone, the combined effect exerts a cytotoxic effect to tumor cells. Hypericin is a naturally occurring photosensitizer, and data supporting its effectiveness for the treatment of cancer is accumulating (Agontinis, Vanteighem, Merlevede et al. 2002; Wen, Chowdhury, Wills et al. 2002; Carpenter, Fehr, Kraus et al. 1994)

Adverse Effects and Drug Interactions

Between 1984, when the German Commission E approved its use, and 1994, German doctors prescribed more than 66 million daily doses of *H. perforatum* (De Smet, Nolen 1996). In 1980, however, the U.S. FDA declared *H. perforatum* unsafe because of reports of phototoxicity in grazing animals ("hypericism"). It was officially included in the United States Pharmacopeia National Formulary by 1998. In contrast, the UK's Committee on Safety of Medicines had no reports of adverse effects in a twenty-year period associated with *H. perforatum*. Furthermore, data obtained from the WHO Collaborating Centre for International Drug Monitoring collected over 20 years from Sweden, Ireland, Germany and Bulgaria reported only 57 adverse reactions (Ernst, Rand, Stevinson 1998).

Adverse effects associated with *H. perforatum* include gastrointestinal (diarrhea, anorexia, nausea, abdominal discomfort, dry mouth, constipation)(Vorbach 1997; Woelk 1994; Wheatley 1998); neurological effects (restlessness, fatigue, headache) (Wheatley 1998; Woelk 1994; Vorbach 1997) are difficult to interpret given that the herb was administered to depressed patients with these complaints. The tannic acid content of *H. perforatum* may inhibit the absorption of iron (Miller 1998). *H. perforatum* extract may prolong the effect of narcotic sleep aids (Okpanyi 1987) and shorten the effect of barbiturate sleep inducers (PDR 2000).

One of the best-known adverse effects associated with *H. perforatum* use is phototoxicity. *Hypericism* is the phototoxic reaction seen in grazing animals (horses, cattle, sheep, goats) that ingest the flowering herb. Unpigmented areas of the skin are affected; temperament changes are also reported (Southwell, Campbell 1991; Bourke 2000). The photosensitizing effect of *H. perforatum* is attributed to the naphthodianthrones (hypericin, pseudohypericin) that also are responsible for the red color of the herb's essential oil (Russo 2001). At high doses (3 g/kg, or the equivalent of 150 g for a 50 kg person) in animal studies (Duran, Song 1986; Brockmoller et al. 1997; Giese 1980; Southwell, Campbell 1991) and in people with HIV (Gulick 1999), *H. perforatum* causes a well-recognized photosensitivity characterized by sunburn-like lesions (rash, blisters) and inflammation of mucous membranes. At therapeutic doses in healthy patients, this reaction would not be expected to appear. Concomitant use of *H. perforatum* with other substances with a recognized photosensitization effect (e.g., quinolones, tetracycline, thiazides, sulfonamides) is not advised (Miller 1998). Pruritis has also been reported in patients taking *H. perforatum* extract (Woelk 1994; Wheatley 1998).

H. perforatum has significant antidepressant properties and so may have many common drug interaction profiles and side effects with conventional antidepressants. *H. perforatum* may trigger manic (Guzelcan, Scholte, Assies et al. 2001; Moses, Mallinger 2000; Nierenberg, Burt, Mathews et al. 1999) and hypomanic states (Schneck 1998). Antidepressants may cause psychosis in schizophrenic patients and can also trigger mania and hypomania. Two cases of possible schizophrenic relapses caused by concomitant use of *H. perforatum* have been described anecdotally (Lal, Iskandar 2000). Although by no means conclusive, the potential interference by *H. perforatum* extract and antipsychotic medication warrants serious attention.

The effects of *H. perforatum* preparations on reproductive health have not been investigated in depth; however, damage to oocytes and mutagenic effect on spermatocytes has been observed in hamster cells (Ondrizek et al. 1999a,b). *H. perforatum* may interfere with oral contraceptives and increase the possibility of unwanted pregnancy (Schwarz, Buschel, Kirch 2003). Use with oral contraceptives has been associated with breakthrough bleeding (PDR 2000). This may be attributed to the herb's induction of cytochrome 450 and enhanced metabolism of oral contraceptives (Ioannides 2002).

In laboratory studies, animals given 2 g/kg per day of dried *H. perforatum* for as long as one year showed no adverse reactions (Okpanyi, Lidzba, Scholl et al. 1990). Researchers in Iraq evaluated blood samples of sheep given different dosages of H. perforatum. Laboratory analyses showed decreased hemoglobin, red blood cell count, packed cell volumes, total protein, glucose, cholesterol, triglycerides, and serum alkaline phosphatase. Blood urea nitrogen, sodium, potassium, bilirubin (total and direct), aspartate aminotransferase, alanine aminotransferase, lactate dehydrogenase, and gamma glutamyltransferase were increased (Kako, al-Sultan, Saleem 1993).

Drug interactions have been reported, or are predicted to occur based on preliminary studies of its interactions with other compounds. *H. perforatum* extract may reduce theophylline levels (Nebel 1999) and digoxin (Cheng 2000; Andreas 1999). The impact on cardiac conduction by high doses of *H. perforatum* (1800 mg extract, 5.4 mg total hypericum) was compared to imipramine. A case of hypertensive crisis associated with *H. perforatum* has been recorded (Patel, Robinson, Burk 2002).

Data suggest that *H. perforatum* extract is safer for use in cardiac or elderly patients compared to some tricyclic antidepressants (Czekalla, Gastpar, Hubner et al. 1997). Reports also suggest that *H. perforatum* may potentiate the effect and toxicity of serotonin reuptake inhibitors (SSRIs). Therefore, its concomitant use with fluoxetine, paroxetine, sertraline, citalopram, clomipramine, and other SSRIs should be avoided (Means 2002; Gordon 1998; Lantz 1999). Similarly, it is contraindicated with MAOIs (Muller, Schaefer 1996; Suzuki 1984) and beta-sympathomimetic amines such as pseudoephedrine and *Ephedra sinica* (*Ma huang*) (Miller 1998). *H. perforatum* may potentiate the effects of selegiline (Anipryl®) and other MAO inhibitors(Means 2002). Concomitant medication with *H. perforatum* and amitriptyline decreases the plasma concentration of amitriptyline, possibly by induction of cytochrome P450 enzymes, and should be avoided (Johne, Schmider, Brockmoller et al. 2002). Herb-drug interactions may be related to modulation of cytochrome P450. A recent report suggests that *H. perforatum* produced significant increases on cytochrome P450 phenotypic ratios on female subjects, suggesting an apparent sexually dimorphic mechanism (Gurley, Gardner, Hubbard et al. 2002).

H. perforatum is a popular herbal product used by approximately 7% of patients with epilepsy. Short-term treatment with *H. perforatum* by epileptic patients did not affect therapeutic levels of the anti-epileptic carbamazepine (Burstein, Horton, Dunn 2000), however more long-term, controlled studies are needed (Spinella 2001).

The use of *H. perforatum* in transplant patients should be avoided. Heart transplant rejection due to interaction between *H. perforatum* and cyclosporine has been reported (Ruschitzka et al. 2000). Concomitant treatment of kidney transplant recipients with immunosuppressives and *H. perforatum* may increase the risk of transplant rejection (Mai, Stormer, Bauer et al. 2003; Bauer, Stormer, Johne et al. 2003).

Isolated case reports of patients taking nonstandard *H. perforatum* preparations are inconclusive, and further research is needed. Germany's Commission E approves of the use of *H. perforatum* oil for depression, anxiety, and other affective disturbances and cites no contraindications or drug interactions. The European Scientific Cooperative on Phytotherapy (ESCOP) recommends standardized preparations of *H. perforatum* for the treatment of mild to moderate depression, but also advises that treatment be discontinued after four to six weeks if no clinical response is achieved (Russo 2001).

There are no data to support recommendations for the restriction of tyramine-based foods by patients using *H. perforatum* (Ernst, Rand, Stevinson 1998). Because the herb has not been studied in pregnant or nursing mothers, it should be used with caution if at all in these states (Russo 2001). Laboratory studies did not find any mutagenic effects, however, suggesting that *H. perforatum* is safe for use during pregnancy (Okpanyi, Lidzba, Scholl et al. 1990). Prenatal exposure to a therapeutic dose of *H. perforatum* extract had no significant impact on certain cognitive tasks in mice offspring (Rayburn, Gonzalez, Christensen et al. 2001). Another report describing *H. perforatum* use by a nursing mother with postpartum depression did not reveal any adverse effects for either infant or mother (Klier, Schafer, Schmid-Siegel et al. 2002); however, long-term clinical studies are necessary.

Reports of side effects such as depression, vomiting, and diarrhea in dogs are on the rise, although the majority have not been serious. Several reports describe neurological signs such as seizure and suggest possible serotonin reactions associated with excessive doses (Means 2002).

Availability

H. perforatum is available in solid, semi-solid, liquid, powder, and oily preparations for internal and external use. Because each preparation may vary in total hypericin concentration, care must be taken in calculating the dose (Vorbach 1994; Woelk 1994). Hypericin and pseudohypericin are well absorbed by oral administration. Steady-state levels were reached after seven and four days respectively (Bone, Mills 2000). One study determined that steady state plasma levels of 100 to 150 ng/ml were reached 3.5 hours after oral administration of 300 mg *H. perforatum* extract WS 5572 containing 5% hyperforin to healthy human volunteers; the half-life was nine hours. Doses greater than 600 mg of the extract were not advantageous. Following administration of 300 mg/kg of the same extract to rats, maximum plasma levels of approximately 370 ng/ml were reached after three hours; half-life was six hours (Biber A, Fischer H, Romer Aet al. 1998). In a study of 348 patients with mild to moderate depression, three doses (0.17 mg, 0.33 mg, 1 mg; TID) of fresh *H. perforatum* extract were evaluated and found to be equally effective in controlling depressive complaints (Lenoir, Degenring, Saller 1999).

In cases of depression, treatment should be limited to no more than four to six weeks. Daily dosage recommendations vary between 200 and 1000 micrograms; in tablet or capsule form, the recommended dose of standard extract is 300 mg TID (PDR 2000). *H. perforatum* preparations standardized to 0.3 % hypericin (equivalent to LI 160 extract) at a dose of 300 mg TID have been recommended for the treatment of mild to moderate depression in human patients (Russo 2001). The dried herb may be taken in doses of 2 to 4 grams TID (Vorbach 1994; Woelk 1994). Traditionally, *H. perforatum* is taken as an infusion. To prepare the tea, 2 teaspoons (2–3 grams) of dried herb in 150 ml of boiling water are steeped for 10 minutes (PDR 2000).

Although hyperforin may be more stable in *H. perforatum* extract because of endogenous plant antioxidants (Orth, Rentel, Schmidt 1999), *H. perforatum* preparations have a limited shelf life (Bilia, Bergonzi, Morgenni et al. 2001). *H. perforatum* extracts are made with methanol solution and prepared in darkness. The extract LI 160 has been the preparation used in most clinical studies, however an extract (WS 5572) containing 5% hyperforin has recently been the focus of study (Lecrubier, Clerc, Didi et al. 2002; Russo 2001).

Data collected from six commercial samples of *H. perforatum* oil demonstrated that all hyperforin was gone by the end of five weeks (Maisenbacher, Kovar 1992). Another study showed that the active ingredient (hyperforin) had disappeared within 14 days (PDR 2000). Recently, several commercially available *H. perforatum* extracts were analyzed (Kopleman, NguyenPho, Zito et al. 2001). It was determined that their phytochemical properties differed greatly but they were all extremely sensitive to changes in storage conditions, particularly under conditions of elevated humidity.

Clinical Application in Veterinary Behavior Medicine

Studies indicate that the psychoactive effects of *H. perforatum* may be comparable to those of fluoxetine and other conventional antidepressant drugs. In addition, it has been effective in treating OCD, panic attack, and anxiety. *H. perforatum* is one of the most promising psychotropic herbs, although much more clinical research is needed to fully understand its mechanism and appreciate its clinical applications. It is likely to be of use in the control of behavioral disorders in veterinary behavior practice that are known to respond to tricyclic antidepressants, including house soiling, separation-related misbehavior, and aggression. It is also of interest in treating compulsive behaviors, fears and phobias, and anxiety-related disorders.

References

Agostinis P, Vantieghem A, Merlevede W et al. Hypericin in cancer treatment: more light on the way. Int J Biochem Cell Biol. 2002;34:221–241.

Andersen DO, Weber ND, Wood SG et al. In vitro virucidal activity of selected anthraquinones and anthraquinone derivatives. Antiviral Res. 1991;16:185–196.

Awang DVC. Herbal medicine: St. John's wort. Can Pharmaceut J. 1991;124:33–35.

Baldt S, Wagner H. Inhibition of MAO by fractions and constituents of Hypericum extract. J Geriatr Psychiatry Neurol. 1994;7(Suppl 1):57–59.

Bauer S, Stormer E, Johne A et al. Alterations in cyclosporin A pharmacokinetics and metabolism during treatment with St John's wort in renal transplant patients. Br J Clin Pharmacol. 2003;55: 203–211.

Baureithel KH, Buter KB, Engesser A et al. Inhibition of benzodiazepine binding in vitro by amentoflavone, a constituent of various species of Hypericum. Pharmaceutica Acta Helvetiae. 1997;72: 153–157.

Behnke K, Jensen GS, Graubaum HJ et al. *Hypericum perforatum* versus fluoxetine in the treatment of mild to moderate depression. Adv Ther. 2002;19:43–52.

Beijamini V, Andreatini R. Effects of *Hypericum perforatum* and paroxetine on rat performance in the elevated T-maze. Pharmacol Res. 2003;48:199–207.

Biber A, Fischer H, Romer A et al. Oral bioavailability of hyperforin from hypericum extracts in rats and human volunteers. Pharmacopsychiatry. 1998;31(Suppl 1):36–43.

Bilia AR, Bergonzi MC, Morgenni F et al. Evaluation of chemical stability of St. John's wort commercial extract and some preparations. Int J Pharm. 2001;213:199–208.

Bourke CA. Sunlight associated hyperthermia as a consistent and rapidly developing clinical sign in sheep intoxicated by St John's wort (*Hypericum perforatum*). Aust Vet J. 2000;78:483–488.

Brockmoller J, Reum T, Bauer S et al. Hypericin and pseudohypericin: pharmacokinetics and effects on photosensitivity in humans. Pharmacopsychiatry. 1997;30(Suppl 2):94–101.

Burstein AH, Horton RL, Dunn T et al. Lack of effect of St John's Wort on carbamazepine pharmacokinetics in healthy volunteers. Clin Pharmacol Ther. 2000;68:605–12.

Buter B, Orlacchio C, Soldati A et al. Significance of genetic and environmental aspects in the field cultivation of *Hypericum perforatum*. Planta Med. 1998;64:431–437.

Butterweck V. Mechanism of action of St. John's wort in depression: what is known? CNS Drugs. 2003;17:539–562.

Butterweck V, Winterhoff H, Herkenham M. Hyperforin-containing extracts of St. John's Wort fail to alter gene transcription in brain areas involved in HPA axis control in a long-term treatment regimen in rats. Neuropsychopharmacology. 2003;28:2160–2168.

Butterweck V, Christoffel V, Nahrstedt A et al. Step by step removal of hyperforin and hypericin: activity profile of different Hypericum preparations in behavioral models. Life Sci. 2003;73:627–639.

Calapai G, Crupi A, Firenzuoli F et al. Serotonin, norepinephrine and dopamine involvement in the antidepressant action of *Hypericum perforatum*. Pharmacopsychiatry. 2001;34:45–9.

Calapai G, Crupi A, Firenzuoli F et al. Effects of Hypericum perforatum on levels of 5-hydroxytryptamine, noradrenaline and dopamine in the cortex, diencephalon and brainstem of the rat. J Pharm Pharmacol. 1999;51:723–728.

Carpenter S, Fehr J, Kraus GA et al. Chemiluminescent activation of the antiviral activity of hypericin: a molecular flashlight. Proc Natl Acad Sci USA. 1994;91:12273–12277.

Catania MA, Firenzuoli F, Crupi A et al. *Hypericum perforatum* attenuates nicotine withdrawal signs in mice. Psychopharmacology (Berl). 2003;169:186-189.

Chatterjee SS, Bhattacharya SK, Wonnemann M et al. Hyperforin as a possible antidepressant component of hypericum extracts. Life Sciences 1998;63:499–510.

Cheng TO. St. John's wort interaction with digoxin. Arch Intern Med. 2000;160:2548.

Cott JM. In vitro receptor binding and enzyme inhibition by *Hypericum perforatum* extract. Pharmacopsychiatry. 1997;30(Suppl 2):108–112.

Czekalla J, Gastpar M, Hubner WD et al. The effect of hypericum extract on cardiac conduction as seen in the electrocardiogram compared to that of imipramine. Pharmacopsychiatry. 1997;30(Suppl 2):86–88.

Degar S, Prince AM, Pascual D et al. Inactivation of the human immunodeficiency virus by hypericin: evidence for photochemical alterations of p24 and a block in uncoating. AIDS Res Hum Retroviruses. 1992;8:1929–36.

Demisch L, Sielaff T, Nispel J et al. AGNP-Symposium, 1991. Cited in scientific Committee of ESCOP. ESCOP monographs: Hyperici Herba. European Scientific Cooperative on Phytotherapy, Exeter, 1996.

Denke A, Schneider W, Elstner EF. Biochemical activities of extracts from *Hypericum perforatum*. 2nd communication: Inhibition of metenkephaline- and tyrosine-dimerization. Arzneimittelforschung. 1999;49:109–114.

De Smet PA, Nolen WA. St. John's wort as an antidepressant. British Med J. 1996;313:241–242.

De Witte P, Agostinis P, Van Lint J et al. Inhibition of epidermal growth factor receptor tyrosine kinase activity by hypericin. Biochem Pharmacol. 1993;46:1929–1936.

Duran N, Song PS. Hypericin and its photodynamic action. Photochem Photobiol. 1986;43:677–680.

Eich-Hochli D, Oppliger R, Golay KP et al. Methadone maintenance treatment and St. John's Wort—a case report. Pharmacopsychiatry. 2003;36:35–37.

Ernst E, Rand JI, Stevinson C. Complementary therapies for depression: An overview. Arch Gen Psychiatry. 1998;55:1026–1032.

Felter HW, Lloyd JU. King's American Dispensatory.Ohio Valley Company, Cincinatti, OH. 1898. Available online at http://www.ibiblio.org/herbmed/eclectic/kings/

Findling RL, McNamara NK, O'Riordan MA et al. An Open-Label Pilot Study of St. John's Wort in Juvenile Depression. J Am Acad Child Adolesc Psychiatry. 2003;42:908–914.

Fornal CA, Metzler CW, Mirescu C et al. Effects of standardized extracts of St. John's wort on the single-unit activity of serotonergic dorsal Raphe neurons in awake cats: comparisons with fluoxetine and sertraline. Neuropsychopharmacology. 2001;25:858–870.

Franklin M, Cowen PJ. Researching the antidepressant actions of *Hypericum perforatum* (St. John's wort) in animals and man. Pharmacopsychiatry. 2001;34(Suppl 1):S29–37.

Gibbons S, Ohlendorf B, Johnsen I. The genus Hypericum: a valuable resource of anti-Staphylococcal leads. Fitoterapia. 2002;73:300–304.

Giese AC. Hypericism. Photochem Photobiol Rev. 1980;5:229–255.

Gold JL, Laxer DA, Dergal JM et al. Herbal-drug therapy interactions: a focus on dementia. Curr Opin Clin Nutr Metab Care. 2001;4:29–34.

Gordon JB. SSRIs and St. John's wort: Possible toxicity? Am Fam Phys. 1998;57:950,953.

Gruenwald J. Standardized St. John's wort extract clinical monograph. Quarterly Rev of Natural Medicine. 1997;(Winter):289–299.

Grube B, Walper A, Wheatley D. St. John's Wort extract: efficacy for menopausal symptoms of psychological origin. Adv Ther. 1999;16:177–186.

Gulick RM, McAuliffe V, Holden-Wiltse J et al. Phase I studies of Hypericum, the active compound in St. John's Wort, as an antiretroviral agent in HIV-infected adults. AIDS clinical trials group protocols 150 and 258. Ann Intern Med. 1999 130:510–514.

Guzelcan Y, Scholte WF, Assies J et al. Mania during the use of a combination preparation with St. John's wort (*Hypericum perforatum*). Ned Tijdschr Geneeskd. 2001;145:1943–1945.

Hanrahan JR, Chebib M, Davucheron NL et al. Semisynthetic preparation of amentoflavone: A negative modulator at GABA(A) receptors Bioorg Med Chem Lett. 2003;13:2281–2284.

Hansgen KD, Vesper J, Ploch M. Multicenter double–blind study examining the antidepressant effectiveness of the hypericum extract LI 160. J Ger Psychiatry Neurol. 1994;7(Suppl1):S15–S18.

Harrer G, Schmidt U, Kuhn U et al. Comparison of equivalence between the St. John's Wort extract LoHyp-57 and fluoxetine. Arzneimittelforschung. 1999;4:289–296.

Hostanska K, Reichling J, Bommer S et al. Hyperforin a constituent of St John's wort (*Hypericum perforatum L.*) extract induces apoptosis by triggering activation of caspases and with hypericin synergistically exerts cytotoxicity towards human malignant cell lines. Eur J Pharm Biopharm. 2003;56: 121–132.

Hubner WD, Lande S, Podzuweit H. Hypericum treatment of mild depressions with somatic symptoms. J Ger Psychiatry Neurol. 1994;7(Suppl 1):S12–S14.

Hubner WD, Kirste T. Experience with St.John's Wort (*Hypericum perforatum*) in children under 12 years with symptoms of depression and psychovegetative disturbances. Phytother Res. 2001;15:367–370.

Ioannides C. Pharmacokinetic interactions between herbal remedies and medicinal drugs. Xenobiotica. 2002 Jun;32(6):451-78.

Johne A, Schmider J, Brockmoller J et al. Decreased plasma levels of amitriptyline and its metabolites on comedication with an extract from St. John's wort (*Hypericum perforatum*). J Clin Psychopharmacol. 2002;22:46–54.

Jurgenliemk G, Nahrstedt A. Phenolic compounds from *Hypericum perforatum*. Planta Med. 2002;68: 88–91.

Kaehler ST, Sinner C, Chatterjee SS et al. Hyperforin enhances the extracellular concentrations of catecholamines, serotonin and glutamate in the rat locus coeruleus. Neurosci Lett. 1999;262:199–202.

Kako MD, al-Sultan II, Saleem AN. Studies of sheep experimentally poisoned with *Hypericum perforatum*. Vet Hum Toxicol. 1993;35:298–300.

Kamuhabwa AA, Cosserat-Gerardin I, Didelon J et al. Biodistribution of hypericin in orthotopic transitional cell carcinoma bladder tumors: implication for whole bladder wall photodynamic therapy. Int J Cancer. 2002;97:253–260.

Kasper S. Treatment of seasonal affective disorder (SAD) with hypericum extract. Pharmacopsychiatry. 1997;30(Suppl 2):89–93.

Kassu A, Dagne E, Abate D et al. Ethnomedical aspects of the commonly used toothbrush sticks in Ethiopia. East Afr Med J. 1999;76:651–653.

Kleber E, Obry T, Hippeli, Schneider W et al. Biochemical activities of extracts from *Hypericum perforatum*. 1st communication: Inhibition of dopamine-beta-hydroxylase. Arzneimittelforschung. 1999;49:106–109.

Klier CM, Schafer MR, Schmid-Siegel B et al. St. John's wort (*Hypericum perforatum*): is it safe during breastfeeding? Pharmacopsychiatry. 2002;35:29–30.

Kopleman SH, NguyenPho A, Zito WS et al. Selected physical and chemical properties of commercial *Hypericum perforatum* extracts relevant for formulated product quality and performance. AAPS PharmSci. 2001;3:E26.

Kraus GA, Pratt D, Tossberg J et al. Antiretroviral activity of synthetic hypericin and related analogs. Biochem Biophys Res Commun. 1990;149-153.

Lal S, Iskandar H. Antidepressants may cause psychosis in schizophrenic patients. St. John's wort and schizophrenia. CMAJ. 2000;163:262–263.

Lantz MS, Buchalter E, Giambanco V. St. John's Wort and antidepressant drug interactions in the elderly. J Geriatr Psychiat Neurol. 1999;2:7–10.

Lavie G, Valentine F, Levin B et al. Studies of the mechanisms of action of the antiretroviral agents hypericin and pseudohypericin. Proc Natl Acad Sci USA. 1989;86:5963–5967.

Lavie G, Mazur Y, Lavie D et al. Hypericin as an inactivator of infectious viruses in blood components. Transfusion. 1995;35:392–400.

Lavie G, Meruelo D, Aroyo K et al. Inhibition of the CD8+ T cell-mediated cytotoxicity reaction by hypericin: potential for treatment of T cell-mediated diseases. Int Immunol 2000;12:479–486.

Lecrubier Y, Clerc G, Didi R et al. Efficacy of St. John's wort extract WS 5570 in major depression: a double-blind, placebo-controlled trial. Am J Psychiatry. 2002;159:1361–1366.

Lenoir S, Degenring FH, Saller R. A double-blind randomised trial to investigate three different concentrations of a standardised fresh plant extract obtained from the shoot tips of *Hypericum perforatum* L. Phytomedicine. 1999;6:141–146.

Linde K, Ramirez CD, Mulrow A et al. St. John's Wort for depression: An overview and meta-analysis of randomized clinical trials. Br Med J. 1996;313:253–258.

Lopez-Bazzocchi I, Hudson JB, Towers GHN. Antiviral activity of the photoactive plant pigment hypericin. Photochem Photobiol. 1991;54:95-98.

Mai I, Stormer E, Bauer S et al. Impact of St. John's wort treatment on the pharmacokinetics of tacrolimus and mycophenolic acid in renal transplant patients. Nephrol Dial Transplant. 2003;18:819–822.

Maisenbacher P, Kovar KA. Analysis and stability of *Hyperici oleum*. Planta Med. 1992;58:351–354.

Means C. Selected herbal hazards. Vet Clin Small Anim Pract. 2002;32:367–382.

Meruelo D, Lavie G, Lavie D. Therapeutic agents with dramatic antiretroviral activity and little toxicity at effective doses: aromatic polycyclic diones hypericin and pseudohypericin. Proc Natl Acad Sci USA. 1988;85:5230–5234.

Miller LG. Selected clinical considerations focusing on known or potential drug-herb interactions. Arch Intern Med. 1998;158:2200–2211.

Mills S, Bone K. Principles and Practice of Phytotherapy. Churchill Livingstone, Philadelphia, PA. 2000;542–552.

Moraleda G, Wu TT, Jilbert AR et al. Inhibition of duck hepatitis B virus replication by hypericin. Antiviral Res. 1993;20:235–247.

Moses EL, Mallinger AG. St. John's Wort: three cases of possible mania induction. J Clin Psychopharmacol. 2000;20:115–7

Muller WE, Schafer C. Johanniskraut In-vitro-Studie uber Hypericum-Extrakt, Hypericin und Kampferol. DAZ 1996;136:1015–1022.

Muller WE, Singer A, Wonnemann M et al. Hyperforin represents the neurotransmitter reuptake inhibiting constituent of Hypericum extract. Pharmacopschiatry. 1998;31(Suppl 1):16–21.

Nahrstedt A, Butterweck V. Biologically active and other chemical constituents of the herb *Hypericum perforatum*. Pharmacopsychiatry. 1997;30(Suppl 2):129–134.

Nathan PJ. *Hypericum perforatum* (St John's Wort): a non-selective reuptake inhibitor? A review of the recent advances in its pharmacology. J Psychopharmacol. 2001;15:47–54.

Nebel A, Schneider BJ, Baker R et al. Potential metabolic interaction between St. John's wort and theophylline. Ann Pharmacother. 1999;33:502.

Nemeroff CB. The neurobiology of depression. Sci Am. 1998;278:42–49.

Nierenberg AA, Burt T, Mathews J, Weiss AP. Mania associated with St. John's wort. Biol Psychiatry. 1999;46:1707–1708.

Noldner M, Schotz K. Rutin is essential for the antidepressant activity of *Hypericum perforatum* extracts in the forced swimming test. Planta Med. 2002;68:577–580.

Nuller WE, Rolli M, Schafer C et al. Effects of hypericum extract (LI 160) in biochemical models of antidepressant activity. Pharmacopsychiatry. 1997;30(Suppl 2):102–107.

Okpanyi SN, Lidzba H, Scholl BG et al. Genotoxicity of a standardized Hypericum extract. Arzneim Forsch. 1990;40:851–855.

Okpanyi SN, Weischer ML Animal experiments on the psychotropic action of a Hypericum extract. Arzneim-Forsch. 1987;37:10–13.

Ondrizek RR, Chan PJ, Patton WC et al. An alternative medicine study of herbal effects on the penetration of zona-free hamster oocytes and the integrity of sperm deoxyribonucleic acid. Fertil Steril. 1999;71:517–522.

Ondrizek RR, Chan PJ, Patton WC et al. Inhibition of human sperm motility by specific herbs used in alternative medicine. J Assist Reprod Genet. 1999;16:87–91.

Orellane C. St. John's wort helps to fight bladder cancer. Lancet Oncol. 2001;2:399.

Orth HC, Rentel C, Schmidt PC. Isolation, purity analysis and stability of hyperforin as a standard material from *Hypericum perforatum*. J Pharm Pharmacol. 1999;51:193–200.

Pabuccuoglu A, Konyalioglu S, Bas M et al. The in vitro effects of Hypericum species on human leukocyte myeloperoxidase activity. J Ethnopharmacol. 2003;87:89–92.

Patel S, Robinson R, Burk M. Hypertensive crisis associated with St. John's Wort. Am J Med. 2002; 112:507–508.

PDR for Herbal Medicines. (2nd ed) Medical Economics Company Inc., Montvale, NJ. 2000;443–446.

Perfumi M, Panocka I, Ciccocioppo R et al. Effects of a methanolic extract and a hyperforin-enriched CO2 extract of *Hypericum perforatum* on alcohol intake in rats. Alcohol Alcohol. 2001;36:199–206.

Rayburn WF, Gonzalez CL, Christensen HD et al. Impact of hypericum (St.-John's-wort) given prenatally on cognition of mice offspring. Neurotoxicol Teratol. 2001;23:629–637.

Rabanal RM, Arias A, Prado B et al. Antimicrobial studies on three species of Hypericum from the Canary Islands. J Ethnopharmacol. 2002;81:287–292.

Re L, Corneli C, Sturani E et al. Effects of Hypericum extract on the acetylcholine release: a loose patch clamp approach. Pharmacol Res. 2003;48:55–60.

Rezvani AH, Overstreet DH, Yang Y et al. Attenuation of alcohol intake by extract of *Hypericum perforatum* (St. John's Wort) in two different strains of alcohol-preferring rats. Alcohol Alcohol. 1999;34: 699–705.

Roz N, Mazur Y, Hirshfeld A, Rehavi M. Inhibition of vesicular uptake of monoamines by hyperforin. Life Sci. 2002;71:2227–2237.

Ruschitzka F, Meier PJ, Turina M et al. Acute heart transplant rejection due to St. John's Wort. Lancet. 2000;355:548–549.

Schellenberg R, Sauer S, Dimpfel W. Pharmacodynamic effects of two different hypericum extracts in healthy volunteers measured by quantitative EEG. Pharmacopsychiatry. 1998;31(Suppl 1):44–53.

Schempp CM, Pelz K, Wittmer A et al. antibacterial activity of hyperforin from St. John's Wort, against multiresistant Staphylococcus aureus and gram-positive bacteria. Lancet. 1999;353:2129.

Schneck C. St. John's wort and hypomania. J Clin Psychiatry. 1998;59:689.

Schwarz UI, Buschel B, Kirch W. Unwanted pregnancy on self-medication with St John's wort despite hormonal contraception. Br J Clin Pharmacol. 2003;55:112–113.

Siepmann M, Krause S, Joraschky P et al. The effects of St John's wort extract on heart rate variability, cognitive function and quantitative EEG: a comparison with amitriptyline and placebo in healthy men. Br J Clin Pharmacol. 2002;54:277–282.

Sommer H, Harrer G. Placebo-controlled double-blind study examining the effectiveness of an hypericum preparation in 105 mildly depressed patients. J Ger Psychiatry Neurol. 1994;7(Suppl 1): S9–S11.

Southwell IA, Bourke CA. Seasonal variation in hypericin content of *Hypericum perforatum L.* (St. John's Wort). Phytochemistry. 2001;56:437–441.

Southwell IA, Campbell MH. Hypericin content variation in *Hypericum perforatum* in Australia. Phytochemistry 1991;30:475–478.

Spinella M. Herbal Medicines and Epilepsy: The Potential for Benefit and Adverse Effects. Epilepsy Behav. 2001;2:524–532.

Stevinson C, Ernst E. A pilot study of *Hypericum perforatum* for the treatment of premenstrual syndrome. BJOG. 2000;107:870–876.

Suzuki O, Katsumata M, Oya S et al. Inhibition of monoamine oxidase by hypericin. Planta Med. 1984;50:272–274.

Taylor LH, Kobak KA. An open-label trial of St. John's Wort (*Hypericum perforatum*) in obsessive-compulsive disorder. J Clin Psychiatry. 2000;61:575–578.

Thiede HM, Walper A. Inhibition of MAO and COMT by Hypericum extracts and hypericin. J Ger Psychiat Neurol. 1994;7(Suppl 1):S54–S56.

Thiele B, Brink I, Ploch M. Modulation of cytokine expression by hypericum extract. J Ger Psychiat Neurol. 1994;7(Suppl 1):S60–S62.

Volz HP. Controled clinical trials of hypericum extracts in depressed patients, an overview. Pharmacopsychiatry. 1997;30 (Suppl 2):72–76.

Vorbach EU, Arnold KH, Hubner WD. Efficacy and tolerability of St. John's Wort extract Hypericum extract LI 160 in patients with severe depressive incidents according ICD-10. Pharmacopsychiatry. 1997;30(Suppl 1):S81–S85.

Vorbach EU, Arnoldt KH, Wolpert E. St John's wort: a potential therapy for elderly depressed patients? Drugs Aging. 2000;16:189–197.

Vorbach EU, Hubner WD, Arnoldt KH. Effectiveness and tolerance of the Hypericum extract LI 160 in comparison with imipramine: randomized double-blind study with 135 outpatients. J Geriatr Psychiatry Neurol. 1994;7(Suppl 1):S19–23.

Wen J, Chowdhury P, Wills J et al. Toward the molecular flashlight: preparation, properties, and photophysics of a hypericin-luciferin tethered molecule. Photochem Photobiol. 2002;76:153–157.

Wheatley D. Hypericum extract: Potential in the treatment of depression. CNS Drugs. 1998;9:431–440.

Wheatley D. LI 160, an extract of St. John's wort, versus amitriptyline in mildly to moderately depressed outpatients—A controlled 6-week clinical trial. Pharmacopsychiatry. 1997;30 (Suppl 2):77–80.

Williamson EM. Synergy and other interactions in phytomedicines. Phytomedicine. 2001;8:401–409.

Woelk H, Burkard G, Grunwald J. Beefits and risks of the Hypericum extract LI 160: drug monitoring study with 3250 patients. J Geriatric Psychiatry Neurol. 1994;7(Suppl 1):3438.

Wills NJ, Park J, Wen J et al. Tumor cell toxicity of hypericin and related analogs. Photochem Photobiol. 2001;74:216–220.

Winkelmann K, Heilmann J, Zerbe O et al. New phloroglucinol derivatives from *Hypericum papuanum*. J Nat Prod. 2000;63:104–108.

Wong ML, O'Kirwan F, Hannestad JP et al. St. John's wort and imipramine-induced gene expression profiles identify cellular functions relevant to antidepressant action and novel pharmacogenetic candidates for the phenotype of antidepressant treatment response. Mol Psychiatry. 2004;9: 237–251.

Lactuca virosa

Lactuca virosa (Wild Lettuce, Lettuce Opium, Prickly Lettuce and Poison Lettuce, Lactucarium; family *Compositae*) is a biennial native European plant that is said to have a tranquilizing, analgesic, antitussive, and antispasmodic effect (PDR 2000; Mills, Bone 2000). The pale yellow pyramidal shaped flowers are androgynous and grow atop stems that may reach as high as 1 m. Leaves are generally oblong and the underside of the midrib has thorns. Medicinal parts of *L. virosa* are the dried leaves and the milky latex contained in the plant. The ground herb is often prepared as an alcoholic extract (PDR 2000; Felter, Lloyd 1898).

Historical Perspective

The plant's milky secretion was known as Lactucarium by nineteenth-century physicians; it was medicinally prescribed for its sedative properties. Lactucarium was noted to induce sleep in dogs, although intravenous injection of the plant's juice was fatal (Felter, Lloyd 1898).

L. virosa has been used to treat respiratory illness (e.g., whooping cough, asthma, laryngitis, tracheitis), urinary tract disorders, and liver disease (PDR 2000; Mills, Bone 2000). Several *Lactuca* species were known to Native Americans and used for many of the same ailments (Moerman 2002). In particular, the Cherokee used an infusion of *L. canadensis* for both sedative and stimulant effects.

Ingredients

Components include sesquiterpene lactones (e.g., lactucin, lactucopicirin) and triterpenes (e.g., taraxasterol, betamyrin) (PDR 2000).

Adverse Effects

Plant poisoning can occur from consuming fresh leaves or overdosage. Signs of toxicity include tachycardia, tachypnea, mydriasis, tinnitus, dizziness, visual disturbances, drowsiness or excitation, and sweating. Treatment consists of gastric lavage and activated charcoal following induced vomiting (PDR 2000).

Clinical Application in Veterinary Behavior Medicine

Currently, there is no evidence to support its psychoactive properties or its clinical use.

References

Felter HW, Lloyd JU. King's American Dispensatory.Ohio Valley Company, Cincinatti, OH. 1898. Available online at http://www.ibiblio.org/herbmed/eclectic/kings/

Mills S, Bone K. Principles and Practice of Phytotherapy. Churchill Livingstone, Philadelphia, PA. 2000;210,232.

Moerman DE. Native American Ethnobotany. Timber Press, Portland, OR. 2002;294.

PDR for Herbal Medicines. (2nd ed) Medical Economics Company Inc., Montvale, NJ. 2000;453–454.

Lavandula angustifolia

Lavandula angustifolia (English Lavender, French Lavender, Lavande, Lavendelfluten, True Lavender, Lavandula vera, *Lavandula officinalis*) is a small, densely branched shrub. A member of the mint family (*Lamiaceae*), this Mediterranean native can grow as tall as 60 cm and is a favorite of gardeners in Europe and North America. The thin, lanceolate leaves have a characteristic gray-green color (see color plate 1-2). When touched, the leaves emit an aromatic, pleasant fragrance. However, the plant is best known for the fresh fragrance of its flowers, which bloom with 6 to 10 blossoms on terminal spikes (Fig. 1-5). *Lavandula* is probably a reference to its use as an alternative to bathing; *angustifolia* means "narrow

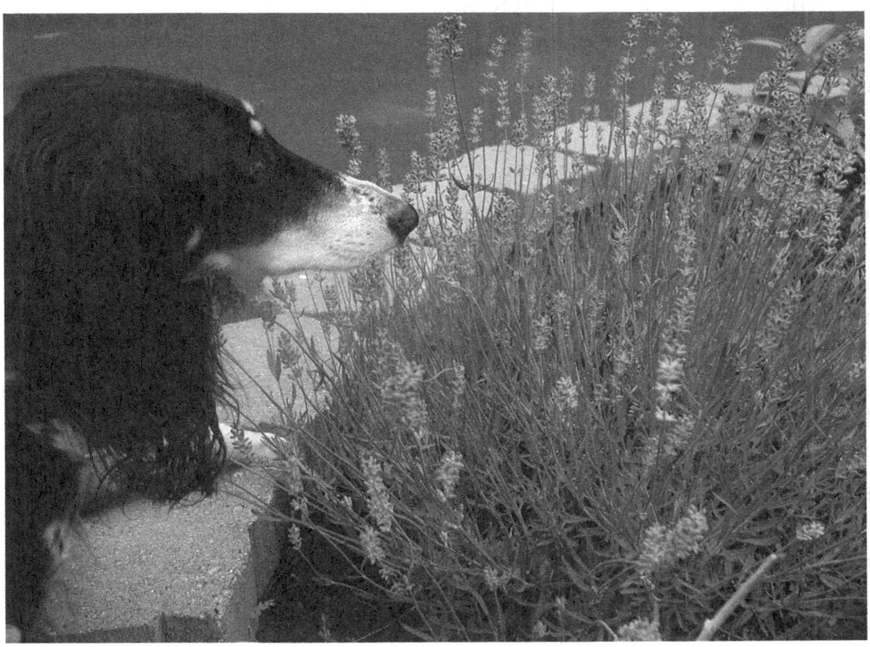

FIGURE 1-5. Aliya, one of the author's two dogs, investigates *Lavandula angustifolia* in her garden. (Photo courtesy of Daniel Wallace)

leaf." Cosmetic and therapeutic applications of lavender date back at least to the time of the ancient Greeks (Russo 2001; PDR 2000).

L. angustifolia has been used for the treatment of digestive complaints, circulatory disorders, wounds, rheumatism, bronchial asthma, insomnia, and nervousness. During the 1800s, physicians prescribed it primarily as a pediatric stimulant (Felter, Lloyd 18981). Today, however, *L. angustifolia* is of clinical interest as a soporific agent, for its anxiolytic and sedative property, and potentially for the treatment of certain types of addiction and withdrawal effects (Cavanagh, Wilkinson 2002; Russo 2001; PDR 2000).

Ingredients

Lavender oil (1–3%) is the medicinal essential oil extracted from the fresh or dried flowers. Primary bioactive compounds studied to date include linalool (20–50%) and linalyl acetate (30–40%). Lavender oil also contains hydroxycoumarins, tannins, and caffeic acid derivatives (e.g., rosmaric acid) (PDR 2000). Essential oils are extracted from plants by a process called steam distillation whereby steam is flushed through the plant material. The essential oil is then collected from the condensed steam (Mills, Bone 2000). Recently, at least 85 components have been identified in lavender oil (Shellie, Mondello, Marriott et al. 2002). The mechanism of action of *L. angustifolia* and its components has not received attention until recently and remains to be determined although the mechanism does appear to be centrally mediated (Nagai, Wad, Usui et al. 2000; Saeki 2000).

CNS Effects

In rodent studies, lavender oil at therapeutic dosage has been shown to prolong the effects of barbiturate and alcohol, and to blunt the stimulation of amphetamine (Atanassova-Shopova, Roussinov 1970) and caffeine (Buchbauer, Jirovetz, Jager et al. 1991); to exert anti-anxiety and sedative effects (Guillemain, Rousseau, Delaveau 1989); to control seizure activity (Yamada, Mimaki, Sashida 1994); and to induce sleep (Hardy, Kirk-Smith, Stretch 1995). Inhalation of lavender oil and its individual components, linalool and linalyl acetate, have shown similar psychoactive properties although a synergistic effect of the compounds in lavender oil has been suggested (Buchbauer, Jirovetz, Jager et al. 1991, 1993).

Clinical studies have focused on the therapeutic benefit of lavender aromatherapy. For example, hemodialysis patents were less anxious during treatment (Itai, Amayasu, Kuribayashi et al. 2000). In an Australian study of 313 patients undergoing radiation therapy, lavender oil aromatherapy was not effective in alleviating anxiety (Graham, Browne, Cox et al. 2003). Nonetheless, the same change was seen in association with water humidification as a control. In Britain, a placebo controlled study of agitated patients with severe dementia concluded that lavender oil aromatherapy produced modest improvement (Holmes, Hopkins, Hensford et al. 2002). In the United States, 17 cancer hospice patients showed an improvement in blood pressure, pain, anxiety, and depression (Louis, Kowalski 2002).

Electroencephalographic studies of the effects of inhaled lavender oil have revealed that lavender oil vapor significantly attenuated alpha-1 EEG activity in the parietal and posterior temporal regions, coinciding with subjective descriptions of feeling comfortable and cheerful, among others (Masago, Matsuda, Kikuchi et al. 2000). In another study (Diego, Jones, Field et al. 1998), lavender aromatherapy increased beta activity, which is associated with drowsiness. Subjects reported feeling more relaxed and showed improved performance in mathematical computations. This may be consistent with some reports that suggest *L. angustifolia* increases arousal in addition to improving mood (Motomura, Sakurai, Yotsuya 2001). Finally, in another EEG study, adults and newborn infants showed similar left frontal EEG activation, which is consistent with less depressed mood and greater approach behavior (Sanders, Diego, Fernandez et al. 2002).

In a recent Iranian study of 45 adults with mild to moderate depression (Akhondzadeh, Kashani, Fotouhi et al. 2003), lavender tincture caused headaches and was not more effective than imipramine. However, a mixture of imipramine and lavender tincture was more effective than imipramine drops alone.

Miscellaneous Effects

Preliminary studies suggest that *L. angustifolia* may have clinical application as an anti-inflammatory and neuroprotective agent. *L. angustifolia* has shown potent inhibition of cutaneous anaphylaxis, inhibition of histamine release from mast cells, and inhibition of mast cell degranulation and tumor necrosis factor-alpha secretion (Kim, Cho 1999). Aqueous extract of *L. angustifolia* exhibited significant protection of cerebellar neurons against glutamate-induced neurotoxicity in rat pups (Buyukokuroglu, Gepdiremen, Hacimuftuoglu et al. 2003).

In a randomized crossover controlled study of Japanese women, autonomic nervous system changes associated with relaxation were evident during foot soaks in water treated with lavender oil (Saeki 2000). In an innovative study, the inhalation of preferred botanical essential oils, including lavender, appears to reduce diastolic blood pressure by a CNS mechanism higher than the midbrain (Nagai, Wad, Usui et al. 2000).

An antibacterial property has been determined and supports the use of lavender baths to heal wounds (PDR 2000). Recently, vapor of lavender oil was shown to exert fungistatic action on the growth of *Aspergillus fumigatus* (Inouye, Tusruoka, Watanabe et al. 2000) and fungicidal activity against *Trichophyton mentagrophytes* and *T. rubrum* (Inouye, Uchida, Yamaguchi 2001).

In a study of guinea pig ileum, lavender oil had a spasmolytic activity that was attributed to cAMP mediation (Lis-Balchin, Hart 1999). This resembles the action of peppermint oil (*Mentha piperita, M. viridis*) and seems to support its traditional application to treat gastrointestinal symptoms.

Adverse Effects

Although reports of adverse effects are few, *L. angustifolia* can trigger hypersensitivity reactions in susceptible individuals. In one case, facial dermatitis was attributed to an allergic reaction to lavender oil (Coulson, Khan 1999). In fact, the resurgence of popularity in cosmetic and medicinal lavender based products has led to an increase in positive patch test reactions in Japan (Sugiura, Hayakawa, Kato et al. 2000). In this island nation, *L. angustifolia* has become extremely popular for aromatherapy and sachets of dried herbs are placed in pillows, drawers, and elsewhere.

L. angustifolia may be ingested as an herbal tea in its dried form (1 to 2 teaspoons/cup of dried herb) or as lavender oil (4 to 5 drops) on a sugar cube. Lavender baths (20 to 100 g of dried herb) and herbal pillows help to relax tension and promote restful sleep (Morris 2002; Russo 2001; PDR 2000).

In a study of stress and cortisol responses in 10-day-old and 15-day-old Japanese macaques, exposure to the scent of lavender had a positive effect. This is consistent with similar studies on human newborns (Kawakami, Tomonaga, Suzuki 2002). In another study of stress and travel sickness in domestic pigs, test subjects were transported in vehicles with bedding of either wheat straw or lavender straw. Pigs traveling with lavender straw showed fewer signs of travel sickness; however, their overall stress level as measured by salivary cortisol levels was unaffected (Bradshaw, Marchant, Meredith et al. 1998).

Clinical Application in Veterinary Behavior Medicine

The use of *L. angustifolia* essential oil in veterinary behavior practice warrants further attention. It might be helpful, for example, to treat carsickness in pets by placing a few drops of lavender oil in the vehicle or in the pet carrier. It could be considered as an adjunct to the treatment of irritable bowel syndrome associated with anxiety. The scent of lavender might help to soothe pets during their introduction to a new home or new housemate. It might be beneficial as an adjunct to treatment of Separation Anxiety Syndrome; it could enhance clinical benefits combined with another psychotropic herb or conventional tricyclic antidepressant therapy. Finally, its calming and neuroprotective effect may prove useful in slowing the effects of free-radical damage associated with Feline and Canine Cognitive Dysfunction Syndromes.

References

Akhondzadeh S, Kashani L, Fotouhi A et al. Comparison of Lavandula angustifolia tincture and imipramine in the treatment of mild to moderate depression in a double-blind, randomized trial. Prog Neuropsychopharmacol Biol Psychiatry. 2003:27:123–127.

Atanassova-Shopova S, Roussinov KS. On certain central neurotropic effects of lavender essential oil. Bull Inst Physiol Bulg Acad Sci. 1970;13:69–76.

Bradshaw RH, Marchant JN, Meredith MJ et al. Effects of lavender straw on stress and travel sickness in pigs. J Altern Complement Med. 1998;4:271–275.

Buchbauer G, Jirovetz L, Jager W et al. Aromatherapy: evidence for sedative effects of the essential oil of lavender after inhalation. Z Naturforsch. 1991;46:1067–1072.

Buchbauer G, Jirovetz L, Jager W et al. Fragrance compounds and essential oils with sedative effects upon inhalation. J Pharm Sci. 1993;82:660–664.

Buyukokuroglu ME, Gepdiremen A, Hacimuftuoglu A et al. The effects of aqueous extract of *Lavandula angustifolia* flowers in glutamate-induced neurotoxicity of cerebellar granular cell culture of rat pups. J Ethnopharmacol. 2003;84:91–94.

Cavanagh HM, Wilkinson JM. Biological activities of lavender essential oil. Phytother Res. 2002;16: 301–308.

Coulson IH, Khan AS. Facial "pillow" dermatitis due to lavender oil allergy. Contact Dermatitis. 1999; 41:111.

Diego MA, Jones NA, Field T et al. Aromatherapy positively affects mood, EEG patterns of alertness and math computations. Int J Neurosci. 1998:96:217–224.

Felter HW, Lloyd JU. King's American Dispensatory.Ohio Valley Company, Cincinatti OH. 1898. Available online at http://www.ibiblio.org/herbmed/eclectic/kings/

Graham PH, Browne L, Cox H et al. Inhalation aromatherapy during radiotherapy: results of a placebo-controlled double-blind randomized trial. J Clin Oncol. 2003;21:2372–2376.

Guillemain J, Rousseau A, Delaveau P. Neurodepressive effects of the essential oil of *Lavandula angustifolia* (French). Ann Pharm Francaises 1980;47:337–343.

Hardy M, Kirk-Smith MD, Sretch DD. Replacement of drug treatment for insomnia by ambient odour. The Lancet. 1995;346:701.

Holmes C, Hopkins V, Hensford C et al. Lavender oil as a treatment for agitated behaviour in severe dementia: a placebo controlled study. Int J Geriatr Psychiatry. 2002;17:305–308.

Inouye S, Tsuruoka T, Watanabe M et al. Inhibitory effect of essential oils on apical growth of *Aspergillus fumigatus* by vapour contact. Mycoses. 2000;43:17–23.

Inouye S, Uchida K, Yamaguchi H. In-vitro and in-vivo anti-Trichophyton activity of essential oils by vapour contact. Mycoses. 2001;44:99–107.

Itai T, Amayasu H, Kuribayashi M et al. Psychological effects of aromatherapy on chronic hemodialysis patients. Psychiatry Clin Neurosc. 2000;54:393–397.

Kawakami K, Tomonaga M, Suzuki J. The calming effect of stimuli presentation on infant Japanese Macaques (*Macaca fuscata*) under stress situation: a preliminary study. Primates. 2002;43:73–85.

Kim HM, Cho SH. Lavender oil inhibits immediate-type allergic reaction in mice and rats. J Pharm Pharmacol. 1999;51:221–226.

Lis-Balchin M, Hart S. Studies on the mode of action of the essential oil of lavender (*Lavandula angustifolia*). Phytother Res. 1999:13:540–542.

Louis M, Kowalski SD. Use of aromatherapy with hospice patients to decrease pain, anxiety, and depression and to promote an increased sense of well-being. Am J Hosp Palliat Care. 2002;19: 381–386.

Masago R, Matsuda T, Kikuchi Y et al. Effects of inhalation of essential oils on EEG activity and sensory evaluation. J Physiol Anthropol Appl Human Sci. 2000:19:35–42.

Mills S, Bone K. Principles and Practice of Phytotherapy. Churchill Livingstone, Philadelphia, PA. 2000;27–30.

Morris N. The effects of lavender (*Lavendula angustifolia*) baths on psychological well-being: two exploratory randomized control trials. Complement Ther Med. 2002;10:223–228.

Motomura N, Sakurai A, Yotsuya Y. Reduction of mental stress with lavender odorant. Percept Mot Skills. 2001;93:713–718.

Nagai M, Wad M, Usui N et al. Pleasant odors attenuate the blood pressure increase during rhythmic handgrip in humans. Neurosci Lett. 2000;289:227–229.

PDR for Herbal Medicines (2nd ed) Medical Economics Company Inc., Montvale, NJ. 2000;277–278.

Russo E. Handbook of Psychotropic Herbs: A Scientific Analysis of Herbal Remedies for Psychiatric Conditions. The Haworth Press, Binghamton, NY. 2001;204–213.

Saeki Y. The effect of foot-bath with or without the essential oil of lavender on the autonomic nervous system: a randomized trial. Complement Ther Med. 2000;8:2–7.
Sanders C, Diego M, Fernandez M et al. EEG asymmetry responses to lavender and rosemary aromas in adults and infants. Int J Neurosci. 2002:112:1305–1320.
Shellie R, Mondello L, Marriott P et al. Characterisation of lavender essential oils by using gas chromatography-mass spectrometry with correlation of linear retention indices and comparison with comprehensive two-dimensional gas chromatography. J Chromatogr A. 2002;970:225–234.
Sugiura M, Hayakawa R, Kato Y et al. Results of patch testing with lavender oil in Japan. Contact Dermatitis. 2000;43:157–160.
Yamada K, Mimaki Y, Sashida Y. Anticonvulsive effects of inhaling lavender oil vapour. Biol Pharm Bull. 1994;17:359–360.

Matricaria chamomilla

Matricaria chamomilla (*Matricaria recutita*, German Chamomile, True chamomile, Chamomile, Fleur de camomile, Kamillenbluten) is an annual member of the daisy family (*Compositae* or *Asteraceae*) that grows as high as 60 cm high (Fig. 1-6). Indigenous to Europe and northwest Asia, *M. chamomilla* has naturalized elsewhere, including North America. The flower has white petals with a yellow center resembling the daisy and is the medicinal part of the plant (Russo 2001; Summer 2000; PDR 2000). When the plant is brushed or injured, it releases an apple scent. "Chamomile" derives from the Greek for "apple (melos) of the ground (chamos)" (Russo 2001).

A close relative of *M. chamomilla* is *Chamaemelum nobile* (also known as English

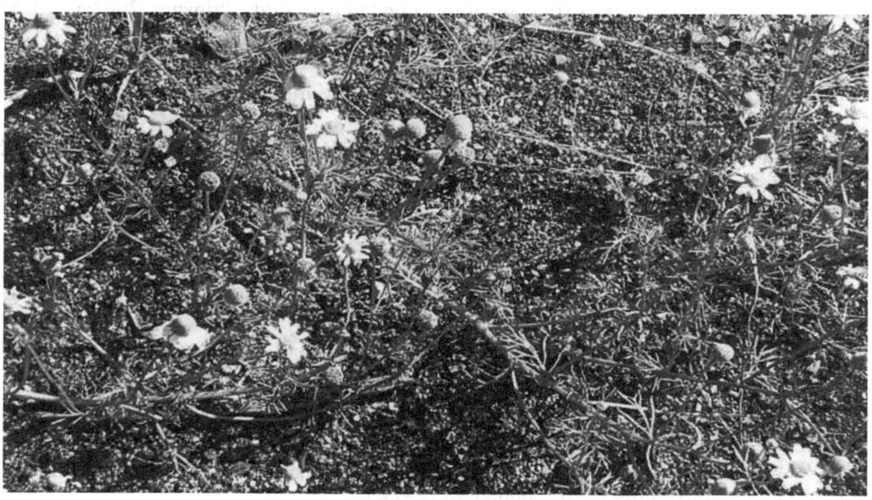

FIGURE 1-6. Daisy-like flowers of *Matricaria chamomilla* (chamomile). (Photo courtesy of Dr. Susan Wynn)

Chamomile, Roman Chamomile, Sweet chamomile, Romische lamillenbluten, *Anthemis nobilis*). Indigenous to southern Europe and northern Africa, *C. nobile* has naturalized to other regions. It has been used almost interchangeably with *M. chamomilla* despite the fact that studies of *C. nobile* are few. Although allergic and anaphylactic reactions similar to those occasionally seen with *M. chamomilla* are likely, there is little to substantiate its effects (Paulsen 2002; Russo 2001; PDR 2000; Mills, Bone 2000).

Historical Perspective

M. chamomilla has been traditionally used to treat hemorrhoids, furuncles, dysmenorrhea, and other anal or genital inflammatory ailments as well as digestive complaints including diarrhea in children and adults. Historically, physicians also prescribed it for nervous irritability, for example, in cases of irritable, cranky children who could be "appeased only when continually carried." It was recommended to relieve a variety of physical and psychological complaints ranging from toothache to impatience. Small doses were thought to be more effective than larger doses, although both were considered to be safe (Mills, Bone 2000; PDR 2000; Felter, Lloyd 1898).

Ingredients

M. chamomilla contains volatile oil (e.g., bisabolol oxide, chamazulene), flavonoids (e.g., apigenin, quercetin, chrysospenol), hydroxycoumarins, and mucilages (PDR 2000; Maday, Szoke, Muskath et al. 1999) (Fig. 1-7).

CNS Effects

In a study of rats under stressful conditions, chamomile oil vapor reduced stress-induced elevations of plasma ACTH. This effect was blocked by flumazenil, implying a GABAergic mechanism similar to that seen in benzodiazepines (Yamada K, Miura T, Mimaki Y et al. 1996). Inhaled *M. chamomilla* vapor also improved overall mood in human subjects compared to placebo (Roberts, Williams 1992).

One of *M. chamomilla*'s traditional uses has been as a sedative tea. Apigenin has

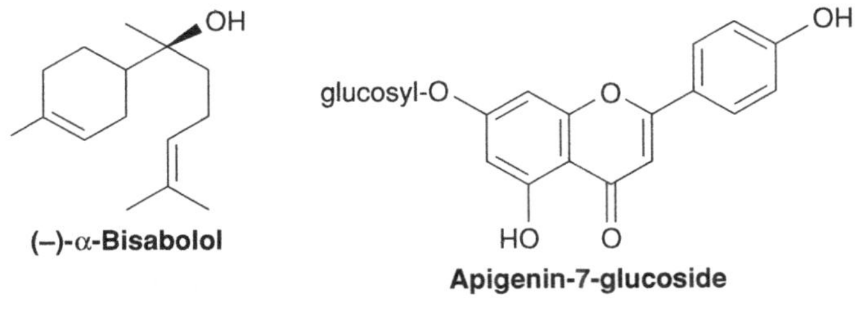

FIGURE 1-7. Active compounds of *Matricaria chamomilla* (Mills, Bone 2000).

anxiolytic and slight sedative effects (PDR 2000; Gyllenhaal, Merritt, Peterson et al. 2000; Viola, Wasowski, Levi de Stein et al. 1995). It competitively inhibited the binding of flunitrazepam and exerted a clear anxiolytic effect, and thus can be considered a ligand for central benzodiazepine receptors. Apigenin had no effect at alpha adrenoceptors, muscarinic receptors, or on $GABA_A$ receptors. However, an anticonvulsant or myorelaxant property was not evident (Viola, Wasowski, Levi de Stein et al. 1995). In another study, anticonvulsant and myorelaxant effects were associated with herniarin, another component of *M. chamomilla* (Ahmad, Misra 1997). Apigenin extracted from dried *M. chamomilla* flowers exhibited a dose-dependent inhibitory effect on GABA and activation of Cl^- channels, Results suggest that apigenin's anxiolytic effect cannot be attributed to interaction with a $GABA_A$-benzodiazepine receptor because it was not blocked by a specific benzodiazepine receptor antagonist (Avallone, Zanoli, Puia et al. 2000; Zanoli, Avallone, Baraldi 2000).

M. chamomilla may potentiate the effects of alcohol and benzodiazepines (PDR 2000). *M. chamomilla* and other herbal sedatives may potentiate the effects of anticonvulsant drugs (Spinella 2001). In a recent study, significant alpha 1 EEG reductions in the parietal and posterior temporal regions of 13 healthy female subjects occurred after inhalation of *M. chamomilla* (Masago, Matsuda, Kikuchi et al. 2000).

Miscellaneous Effects

Bisabolol compounds have a protective effect on the digestive tract against pepsin and acetylsalicylic acid. This would support its traditional use for gastrointestinal spasm, gingivitis and pharyngitis. Bisabolol has also been shown to promote tissue regeneration and granulation (Mills, Bone 2000). Chamazulene (formed from matricine) has antioxidant and anti-inflammatory effects (Fig. 1-8). Apigenin (5,7, 4'-trihydroxyflavone), which is also present in parsley for example, has been shown to inhibit cutaneous papilloma and also has a topical antitumor effect (PDR 2000; Janssen, Mensink, Cox et al. 1998). Topical chamomile extract (Kamillosan®) has

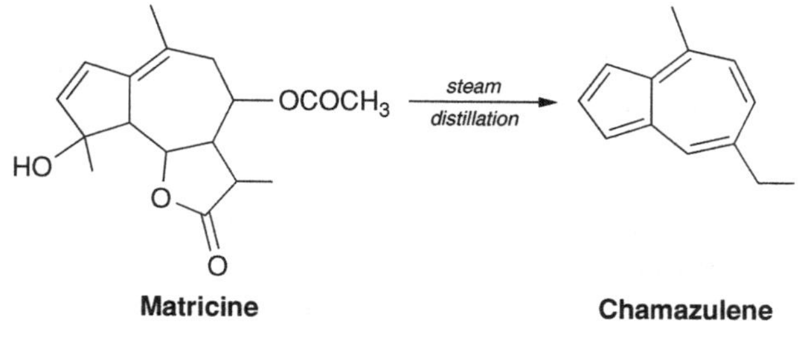

FIGURE 1-8. Active compounds of *Matricaria chamomilla* (Mills, Bone 2000).

been shown to be slightly more effective than 5% hydrocortisone cream in the treatment of atopic eczema (Patzelt-Wenczler, Ponce-Poschl 2000).

Apigenin may have anticancer properties for other types of tumors as well, and has been shown to be a potent inhibitor of COX-2 (cyclooxygenase) and iNOS (inducible nitric oxide synthase) (Hernandez-Ceruelos, Madrigal-Bujaidar, de la Cruz 2002; Reiners, Clift, Mathieu 1999; Liang, Huang, Tsai et al. 1999).

Chamomile oil possesses antibacterial properties against *Staphylococcus aureus, Bacillus spp, E. coli, Streptococcus spp., Leptospira icterohaemorrhagiae* and *Candida albicans* (PDR 2000; Mills, Bone 2000).

Apigenin has been shown to increase atrial rate. This effect has been attributed to a reduction in noradrenaline and monoamine oxidase activity (PDR 2000). The risk of cardiovascular disease is inversely associated with dietary consumption of flavonoids, although this effect does not appear to be due to the inhibition of platelet aggregation (Janssen, Mensink, Cox et al. 1998).

One of the components of *C. nobile*, a flavonoid glucoside called chamaemeloside, has shown hypoglycemic properties (Konig, Wright, Keller et al. 1998). This might be of clinical value, but further research is required.

Adverse Effects

Reports of side effects associated with *M. chamomilla* include allergic reactions such as recurrent facial dermatitis from chamomile tea (Rycroft 2003). Individuals with a known allergy to yarrow, feverfew, and artemisia and other members of the *Compositae* family should avoid chamomile (PDR 2000; Paulsen, Andersen, Hausen 1993). Cross-reactivity with sensitivity to mugwort and birch pollen has been identified (Reider, Sepp, Fritsch et al. 2000). A high degree of cross-reactivity between the common weed *Artemisia vulgaris* and *M. chamomilla* has also been reported (de la Torre Morin, Sanchez Machin, Garcia Robaina et al. 2001).

Coumarin anticoagulants may be potentiated by chamomile because of its hydroxycoumarin contents. Therefore, concomitant use of *M. chamomilla* with antithrombotic compounds should be avoided (PDR 2000).

A recent investigation has identified the risk of microbial contamination of commercial products of *M. chamomilla*. This, of course, is not exclusive to *M. chamomilla* preparations. *Bacillus cereus, Clostridium perfringens*, and *Cryptococcus laurentii* were identified in chamomile products, highlighting the lack of effective sanitary control in the manufacture of this and other herbal products (Martins, Martins, Dias et al. 2001).

Despite the adverse effects noted, *M. chamomilla* preparations are generally regarded as safe (Russo 2001); long-term administration in rats, rabbits, and guinea pigs has not been associated with toxicity (Mills, Bone 2000). In cats, ingestion of *M. chamomilla* has been associated with signs of vomiting, diarrhea, and lethargy. Two cats also exhibited epistaxis and one developed hematomata, consistent with the plant's antithrombotic activity. In dogs, side effects of vomiting and hypersalivation may be more common (Means 2002).

Availability

A recent survey determined that *M. chamomilla* was used by almost 21% of women between the ages of 40 and 60 years, making it the third most popular herbal dietary supplement in those surveyed (Mahady, Parrot, Lee et al. 2003).

M. chamomilla is available in capsule (125 mg, 350 mg), liquid, and oil preparations. Chamomile tea for medicinal uses is prepared as an infusion with boiling water poured over 3 teaspoons of dried or fresh chamomile (PDR 2000; Maliakal, Wanwimolruk 2001).

Clinical Application in Veterinary Behavior Medicine

M. chamomilla may be useful in veterinary behavior medicine because of growing evidence for its sedative and anxiolytic properties. Introduced as a vapor or orally administered, it may help to ease the introduction of new housemates, relocation to a new home, placement with new owners, and other mildly to moderately stressful situations.

References

Ahmad A, Misra LN. Isolation of herniarin and other constituents from *Matricaria chamomilla* flowers. Int J Pharmacognosy. 1997;35:121–125.

Avallone R, Zanoli P, Puia G et al. Pharmacological profile of apigenin, a flavonoid isolated from *Matricaria chamomilla*. Biochem Pharmacol. 2000;59:1387–1394.

De la Torre Morin F, Sanchez Machin I, Garcia Robaina JC et al. Clinical cross-reactivity between *Artemisia vulgaris* and *Matricaria chamomilla* (chamomile). J Investig Allergol Clin Immunol. 2001;11:118–122.

Felter HW, Lloyd JU. King's American Dispensatory.Ohio Valley Company, Cincinatti, OH. 1898. Available online at http://www.ibiblio.org/herbmed/eclectic/kings/

Gyllenhaal C, Merritt SL, Peterson SD et al. Efficacy and safety of herbal stimulants and sedatives in sleep disorders. Sleep Med Rev. 2000;4:229–251.

Hernandez-Ceruelos A, Madrigal-Bujaidar E, de la Cruz C. Inhibitory effect of chamomile essential oil on the sister chromatid exchanges induced by daunorubicin and methyl-methanesulfonate in mouse bone marrow. Toxicol Lett. 2002;135:103–110.

Kagawa D, Jokura H, Ochiai R et al. The sedative effects and mechanism of action of cedrol inhalation with behavioral pharmacological evaluation. Planta Med. 2003;69:637–641.

Konig GM, Wright AD, Keller WJ et al. Hypoglycaemic activity of an HMG-containing flavonoid glucoside, chamaemeloside, from *Chamaemelum nobile*. Planta Med. 1998;64:612–614.

Janssen K, Mensink RP, Cox FJ et al. Effects of the flavonoids quercetin and apigenin on hemostasis in healthy volunteers: results from an in vitro and a dietary supplement study. Am J Clin Nutr. 1998;67: 255–262.

Liang YC, Huang YT, Tsai SH et al. Suppression of inducible cyclooxygenase and inducible nitric oxide synthase by apigenin and related flavonoids in mouse macrophages. Carcinogenesis. 1999;20: 1945–1952.

Maday E, Szoke E, Muskath Z et al. A study of the production of essential oils in chamomile hairy root cultures. Eur J Drug Metab Pharmacokinet. 1999;24:303–308.

Mahady GB, Parrot J, Lee C et al. Botanical dietary supplement use in peri- and postmenopausal women. Menopause. 2003;10:65–72.

Maliakal PP, Wanwimolruk S. Effect of herbal teas on hepatic drug metabolizing enzyme in rats. J Pharm Pharmacol. 2001;53:1323–1329.
Martins HM, Martins ML, Dias MI et al. Evaluation of microbiological quality of medicinal plants used in natural infusions. Int J Food Microbiol. 2001;68:149–153.
Masago R, Matsuda T, Kikuchi Y et al. Effects of inhalation of essential oils on EEG activity and sensory evaluation. J Physiol anthropol Appl Human Sci. 2000;19:35–42.
Means C. Selected herbal hazards. Vet Clin Small Anim Pract. 2002;32:367–382.
Mills S, Bone K. Principles and Practice of Phytotherapy. Churchill Livingstone, Philadelphia, PA. 2000;319–327.
Patzelt-Wenczler R, Ponce-Poschl E. Proof of efficacy of Kamillosan® cream in atopic eczema. Eur J Med Res. 2000;5:171–175.
Paulsen E. Contact sensitization from Compositae-containing herbal remedies and cosmetics. Contact Dermatitis. 2002;47:189–198.
Paulsen E, Andersen KE, Hausen BM. Compositae dermatitis in a Danish dermatology department in one year (I). Results of routine patch testing with the sesquiterpene lactone mix supplemented with aimed patch testing with extracts and sesquiterpene lactones of Compositae plants. Contact Dermatitis. 1993;29:6–10.
PDR for Herbal Medicines (2nd ed) Medical Economics Company Inc., Montvale, NJ. 2000;331–335.
Reider N, Sepp N, Fritsch P et al. Anaphylaxis to chamomile: clinical features and allergen cross-reactivity. Clin Exp Allergy. 2000;30:1436–1443.
Reiners JJ, Clift R, Mathieu P. Suppression of cell cycle progression by flavonoids: dependence on the aryl hydrocarbon receptor. Carcinogenesis. 1999:20:1561–1566.
Roberts A, Williams JM. The effect of olfactory stimulation on fluency, vividness of imagery and associated mood: a preliminary study. Br J Med Psychol. 1992;65:197–199.
Russo E. Handbook of Psychotropic Herbs: A Scientific Analysis of Herbal Remedies for Psychiatric Conditions. The Haworth Press, Binghamton, NY. 2001;115–120.
Rycroft RJ. Recurrent facial dermatitis from chamomile tea. Contact Dermatitis. 2003;48:229.
Spinella M. Herbal medicines and epilepsy: the potential for benefit and adverse effects. Epilepsy Behav. 2001;2:524–532.
Sumner J. The natural history of medicinal plants. Timber Press, Portland, OR. 2000;84.
Viola H, Wasowski C, Levi de Stein M et al. Apigenin, a component of *Matricaria recutita* flowers, is a central benzodiazepine receptors-ligand with anxiolytic effects. Planta Med. 1995;61:213–216.
Yamada K, Miura T, Mimaki Y et al. Effect of inhalation of chamomile oil vapour on plasma ACTH level in ovariectomized-rat under restriction stress. Biol Pharm Bull. 1996;19:1244–1246.
Zanoli P, Avallone R, Baraldi M. Behavioral characterization of the flavonoids apigenin and chrysin. Fitoterapia. 2000;71(Suppl 1):S117–123.

Melissa officinalis

Melissa officinalis (Melissa, Balm, Lemon Balm, Melissenblatter, Feuilles de Melisse, Honey Plant, Sweet Mary, Dropsy Plant) is a perennial member of the mint family *Lamiaceae* and native to the Mediterranean and parts of Asia. Now naturalized to parts of North America, it can grow as high as 90 cm and bears small white flowers atop its uppermost leaves (Fig. 1-9). Prior to flowering, the leaves have a lemony fragrance. Leaves are harvested before blooms appear and quickly dried. Medicinal parts of the plant include the leaves and stem (Russo 2001; PDR 2000; Moerman 2002).

Melissa is the Greek word for bee; *officinalis* implies its use as a medicinal. Its

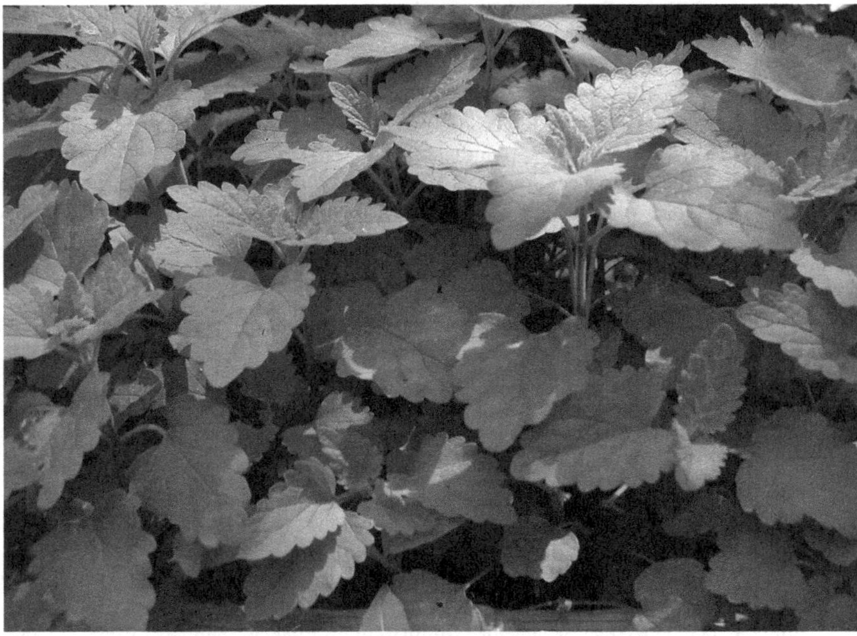

FIGURE 1-9. *Melissa officinalis* (Lemon balm). (Photo courtesy of Daniel Wallace)

common name derives from "balsam," which refers to a fragrant substance. The fragrance of *M. officinalis* is particularly attractive to bees because of a similarity to bee pheromone (Russo 2001; Tyler 1993).

Historical Perspective

Traditionally, *M. officinalis* was used for the treatment of nervousness, insomnia, headache, joint disease, and a variety of abdominal ailments. Its medicinal use has been described by herbalists of the sixteenth and seventeenth centuries as a cure for "melancholy" and "anxious imaginations." Physicians of the nineteenth century appreciated its antispasmodic and diaphoretic properties and prescribed it for dysmenorrhea and fevers. Cherokee Indians used Lemon Balm to treat chills and fevers and as a stimulant, whereas the Costanoan used it for infants with colic (Moerman 2002; Felter, Lloyd 1898).

Ingredients

Primary compounds of *M. officinalis* include the volatile oil (including geranial, neral, citronellal, linalool); glycosides; caffeic acid derivatives; flavonoids (e.g., cosmosiin, cynaroside, isoquercitrin); and triterpene acids (e.g., ursolic acid) (PDR 2000). Traditionally, the essential oil was thought to be most effective; however, evidence now suggests that the leaves contain the bioactive fraction (Russo 2001; Soulimani, Younos, Jarmouni et al. 1991).

Miscellaneous Effects

Proven effects of *M. officinalis* include antiviral (e.g., herpes and HIV inhibitory effects) (Koytchev, Alken, Dundarov 1999; Yamasaki, Nakano, Kawahata et al. 1998; Dimitrova, Dimov, Manolova et al. 1993); antibacterial (Iauk, Lo Bue, Milazzoet al. 2003; Larrondo, Agut, Calvo-Torras 1995), anti-inflammatory (Hohmann, Zupko, Redei et al. 1999); anti-hormonal (Auf'mkolk, Kohrle, Gumbinger et al. 1984), spasmolytic; carminative; and mild sedative properties (PDR 2000; Mills, Bone 2000; Chlabicz, Galasinski 1986). Recent evidence compares the anti-ulcerogenic efficacy of *M. officinalis* and other herbal extracts to that of cimetidene (Khayyal, el-Ghazaly, Kenawy et al. 2001). This effect may be attributed to their flavonoid components and to recognized antioxidant properties.

M. officinalis might be of interest as an herbal treatment for mild cases of hyperthyroidism in cats. It has been shown to possess extra-thyroidal antihormone components in rats (Auf'mkolk, Kohrle, Gumbinger et al. 1984) that deserve further investigation.

CNS Effects

In mice, *M. officinalis* proved to have sedative effects at low doses and induced a peripheral analgesia at higher doses. It also prolonged pentobarbital-induced sleep (Soulimani, Fleurentin, Mortier et al. 1991). However, in a more recent murine study, *M. officinalis* did not show significant anti-anxiety effects (Coleta, Campos, Cotrim et al. 2001).

Recently, *M. officinalis* has been attracting interest because of possible memory-improving properties (Perry, Pickering, Wang 1999). In a recent study of human patients with severe dementia in the United Kingdom, aromatherapy with *M. officinalis* essential oil improved agitation in 60% of subjects, compared with 14% of the placebo group. Melissa treatment also significantly improved quality of life scores (Ballard, O'Brien, Reichelt et al. 2002). In another study of the effects of a commercial *M. officinalis* extract on healthy, young people, a dose of 600 mg was effective in improving mood (more calm) and cognitive performance (Kennedy, Scholey, Tildesley et al. 2002). Previously, it had been suggested that cognitive effects might be due to cholinergic-binding properties observed *in vitro*; however, both nicotinic and muscarinic binding were low in this study. These results were confirmed in a follow-up study, although no cholinesterase inhibitory properties were detected. It was suggested that *M. officinalis* could be of use as an adjunct to traditional treatment of Alzheimer's patients (Kennedy, Wake, Savelev et al. 2003). In a study of Alzheimer's patients in Iran, *M. officinalis* extract improved agitation and cognitive scores compared to control group (Akhondzadeh, Noroozian, Mohammadi et al. 2003).

Despite the scarcity of clinical investigation of the effectiveness and mechanism of *M. officinalis*, ESCOP lists its use for the treatment of irritability, tension, and restlessness, and the German Commission E recommends it as a sleep inducer (Russo 2001). To date, clinical studies of *M. officinalis* have not been carefully designed and have used a range of commercially prepared extracts, making it difficult to interpret data.

Availability

M. officinalis can be prepared as an herbal powder, in liquid or solid form for external application, or in extract or dried forms in infusions. Most commonly, it is taken as Lemon Balm tea and prepared with 1.5 to 4.5 gm of the herb. It is also combined with other herbs in commercial products. *M. officinalis* must be carefully sealed and protected from light and moisture, particularly if it is intended for use as a sedative. The herb's shelf life is limited because bioactive components degrade within six months (Russo 2001; PDR 2000).

Clinical Application in Veterinary Behavior Medicine

M. officinalis could be valuable in the prevention of normal senile cognitive decline as well as pathological changes associated with Cognitive Disorder Syndromes in pets. Based on preliminary evidence, *M. officinalis* may be of interest in treating Feline and Canine Cognitive Disorder Syndrome, principally as an adjunct to medication with other herbs with recognized cognitive-enhancing properties or the synthetic drug selegiline.

M. officinalis might also be helpful for the treatment of psychogenic grooming in pets based upon its anti-inflammatory and sedative properties.

References

Akhondzadeh S, Noroozian M, Mohammadi M et al. *Melissa officinalis* extract in the treatment of patients with mild to moderate Alzheimer's disease: a double blind, randomized, placebo controlled trial. J Neurol Neurosurg Psychiatry. 2003;74:863–866.

Auf'mkolk M, Kohrle J, Gumbinger H et al. Antihormonal effects of plant extracts: iodothyronine deiodinase of rat liver is inhibited by extracts and secondary metabolites of plants. Horm Metab Res. 1984;16:188–192.

Ballard CG, O'Brien JT, Reichelt K et al. Aromatherapy as a safe and effective treatment for the management of agitation in severe dementia: the results of a double-blind, placebo-controlled trial with Melissa. J Clin Psychiatry. 2002;63:553–558.

Chlabicz J, Galasinski W. The components of *Melissa officinalis* that influence protein biosynthesis in-vitro. J Pharm Pharmacol. 1986;38:791–794.

Coleta M, Campos MG, Cotrim MD et al. Comparative evaluation of *Melissa officinalis, Tilia europaea, Passiflora edulis* and *Hypericum perforatum* in the elevated plus maze anxiety test. Pharmacopsyhciatry. 2001;34(Suppl 1):S20–S21.

Dimitrova Z, Dimov B, Manolova N et al. Antiherpes effect of *Melissa officinalis* extracts. Acta Microbial Bulg. 1993;29:65–72.

Felter HW, Lloyd JU. King's American Dispensatory.Ohio Valley Company, Cincinatti OH. 1898. Available online at http://www.ibiblio.org/herbmed/eclectic/kings/

Hohmann J, Zupko I, Redei D et al. Protective effects of the aerial parts of *Salvia officinalis*, *Melissa officinalis* and *Lavandula angustifolia* and their constituents against enzyme-dependent and enzyme-independent lipid peroxidation. Planta Med. 1999;65:576–578.
Iauk L, Lo Bue AM, Milazzo I et al. Antibacterial activity of medicinal plant extracts against periodontopathic bacteria. Phytother Res. 2003;17:599–604.
Kennedy DO, Scholey AB, Tildesley NT et al. Modulation of mood and cognitive performance following acute administration of *Melissa officinalis* (lemon balm). Pharmacol Biochem Behav. 2002;72: 953–964.
Kennedy DO, Wake G, Savelev S et al. Modulation of mood and cognitive performance following acute administration of single doses of *Melissa officinalis* (Lemon Balm) with human CNS nicotinic and muscarinic receptor-binding properties. Neuropsychopharmacology. 203;28:1871–1881.
Khayyal MT, el-Ghazaly MA, Kenawy SA et al. Antiulcerogenic effect of some gastrointestinally acting plant extracts and their combination. Arzneimittelforschung. 2001;51:545–553.
Koytchev R, Alken RG, Dundarov S. Balm mint extract (Lo-701) for topical treatment of recurring herpes labialis. Phytomedicine. 1999;6:225–230.
Larrondo JV, Agut M, Calvo-Torras MA. Antimicrobial activity of essences from labiates. Microbios. 1995;82:171–172.
Mills S, Bone K. Principles and Practice of Phytotherapy. Churchill Livingstone, Philadelphia, PA. 2000;142,172.
Moerman DE. Native American Ethnobotany. Timber Press, Portland, OR. 2002;338.
PDR for Herbal Medicines. (2nd ed) Medical Economics Company Inc., Montvale, NJ. 2000;461–463.
Perry EK, Pickering AT, Want WW et al. Medicinal plants and Alzheimer's disease: from ethnobotany to phytotherapy. J Pharm Pharmacol. 1999;51:527–534.
Russo E. Handbook of Psychotropic Herbs: A Scientific Analysis of Herbal Remedies for Psychiatric Conditions. The Haworth Press, Binghamton, NY. 2001;125–129.
Tyler VE. Phytomedicines in Western Europe: Potential impact on herbal medicine in the Unites States. In: Human medicinal agents from plants. (Kinghorn AD, Balandrin MF, eds.) American Chemical Society, Washington, DC. 1993;33–34.
Soulimani R, Fleurentin J, Mortier F et al. Neurotropic action of the hydroacloholic extract of *Melissa officinalis* in the mouse. Planta Medica. 1991;57:105–109.
Yamasaki K, Nakano M, Kawahata T et al. Anti-HIV-1 activity of herbs in *Labiatae*. Biol Pharm Bull. 1998;21:829–833.

Nepeta cataria

Nepeta cataria (Catnip) is a perennial member of the mint family (*Lamiaceae*) that is native to Europe and naturalized in the United States. The erect, branched stems may grow as long as 1 m. The grayish green leaves are between 2 and 8 cm and have a mint-like aromatic scent (see color plate 1-3). Inflorescences are spike-like and carry small individual flowers on short pedicles. Catnip is the aerial, medicinal part of the perennial catmint plant *N. cataria* (PDR 2000). As are other *Nepeta spp., N. cataria* is classified as a catmint; however, only *N. cataria* is catnip.

Historical Perspective

N. cataria was traditionally used for its antipyretic, antispasmodic, diaphoretic, and sedative effects. Catnip tea possesses a diuretic effect and promotes activity of the gallbladder. Before the introduction of tea to Europe, it was also used as a stimulating drink. Catnip preparations also have a calming effect and have been used for the treatment of migraine, gynecological complaints, and nervous disorders (PDR 2000). It was introduced to the American colonies from Europe as a sedative tea. During the nineteenth century, catnip infusion was used to relieve gastric discomfort such as colic in children. A fluid extract mixture of *N. cataria, Valeriana officinalis,* and *Scutellaria spp.* was considered "an excellent agent for the cure of *nervous headache,* restlessness, and many other nervous symptoms" (Felter, Lloyd 1898). Today, it is taken as an herbal remedy for sleep disorders (Cauffield, Forbes 1999).

In the form of a hot tea, it is also recommended to manage fever in children or adults suffering from symptoms of the common cold or influenza (Mills, Bone 2000). This is consistent with Cherokee and other Native American tribal practices that included its use as a cough and cold syrup when mixed with honey. The Iroquois, for example, also used it to treat children with diarrhea, fever, and colic, and as an antihelminthic (Moerman 2002). They also prepared an infusion of the plant tips for restless babies and as a pediatric soporific (Moerman 2002; Herrick 1977). Catnip infusion was also used by the Cherokee to treat hysteria and as a stimulant (Moerman 2002).

Ingredients

Nepetalic acid and nepetalactone comprise 43% and 40% respectively of the volatile oil, which also includes camphor and thymol. Its active components also include tannins (PDR 2000; Harney, Barofsky, Leary 1978) (Fig. 1-10).

CNS Effects

Essential oils of a related Nepeta species (*N. caesarea*) possessed significant analgesic and sedative activity. An opioid mechanism is suspected because the effect was blocked by naloxone. It was concluded that nepetalactone has a specific opioid receptor subtype agonistic activity (Aydin, Beis, Ozturk et al. 1998). Psychedelic effects of smoking dried catnip leaves have been described as similar to marijuana and reported in a number of respectable publications including the *Journal of the American Medical Association* and the *Wall Street Journal.* However,

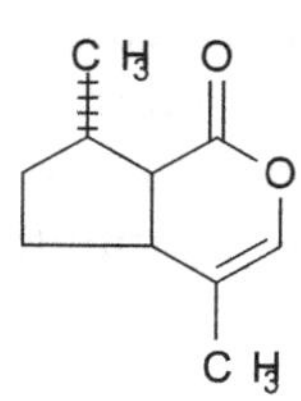

FIGURE 1-10. Chemical structure of nepetalactone, the primary active compound of *Nepeta cataria* (Mills, Bone 2000).

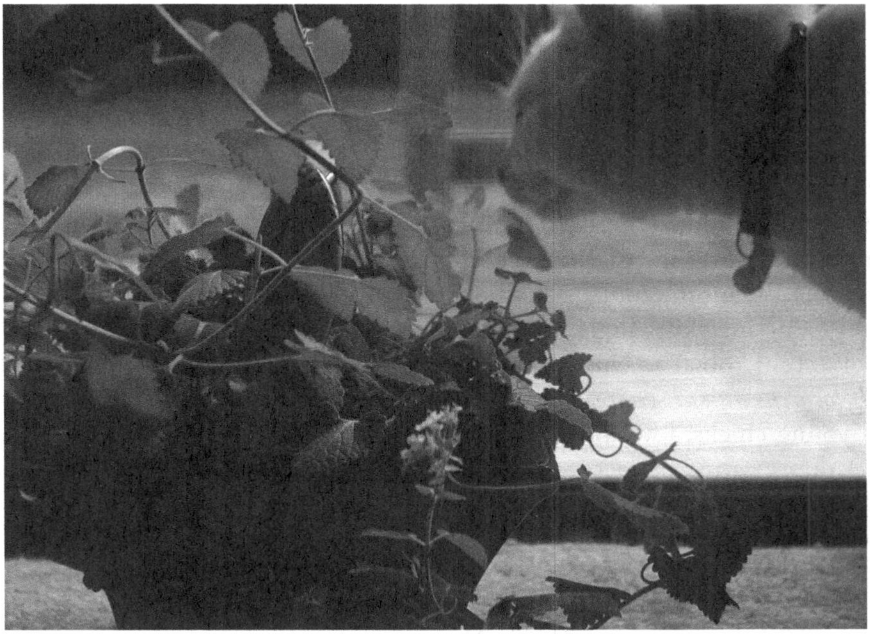

FIGURE 1-11. *Nepeta cataria* (catnip), grown indoors for feline entertainment, attracts Angelica, one of the author's five cats. (Photo courtesy of Dr. Stefanie Schwartz)

its hallucinogenic and toxicological effects have not been studied. Volatile oils of *N. cataria* appear to exert cholinergic effects that may contribute to a psychoactive property. In addition, cis-trans-nepetalactone and valeric acid are structurally similar; the valepotriates have recognized sedative effects (see *Valerian spp.*; Osterhoudt, Lee, Callahan et al. 1997).

Cats show a unique response to fresh and dried catnip (Fig. 1-11). The *catnip effect (catnip response)* is mediated through the main olfactory system (it is not precluded by obliteration of the vomeronasal organ) and includes sequences of sniffing, chewing, rolling, rubbing, swatting, and kicking at the source of catnip (Hart, Leedy 1985). Elements of the catnip effect resemble sexual behavior, although it may more closely mimic playful and predatory patterns (Schwartz 1993). It has no known physiological or histological effects in the cat and is excreted in the urine primarily as nepetalinic acid, although some nepetalactone is eliminated unchanged (Waller, Price, Mitchell 1969).

The LD50 of nepetalactone in mice is 1550 mg/kg. Nepetalic acid and nepetalactone were found to prolong barbiturate anesthesia in mice. Rats initially showed a decrease in performance but developed behavioral tolerance after daily injections of *N. cataria* oil (Harney, Barofsky, Leary 1978). Mice fed *N. cataria* as

10% of their normal diet displayed an increase in stereotypic behavior and a lowered seizure threshold (induced by picrotoxin and strychnine). Short-term effects were compared to an amphetamine-like effect; however, long-term effects were more associated with adaptation to the herb (Massaco, Silva, Gorniak et al. 1995).

Miscellaneous Effects

N. cataria's traditional application as an antispasmodic to treat colic, flatulence, gastritis, nervous dyspepsia, and irritable bowel disease may be explained in part by reports of antimicrobial activity against *Helibacter pylori* by other Nepeta species (Kalpoutzakis, Aligiannis, Mentis et al. 2001). Catmint extract has also shown antimicrobial activity against fungi and Gram-positive bacteria, as well as *Staphylococcus aureus* strains (Nostro, Cannatelli, Crisafi et al. 2001).

In young chicks, low and moderate doses of catnip extract induced sleep. At higher doses, catnip extract lost some of its soporific effect, suggesting a biphasic effect on behavior (Sherry, Hunter 1979). This might explain why catmint has been used traditionally as both a stimulant and a sedative.

Most recently, nepetalactone has been identified as the basis of the aphid sex pheromone. This discovery is now helping to improve new aphid pest control strategies (Birkett, Pickett 2003). Nepetalactone proved more effective than DEET (N,NA-diethyl-3-methylbenzamide) in repelling German cockroaches (Peterson, Nemetz, Jones et al. 2002).

Availability

N. cataria is available in ground and dried forms, as capsules (380 mg) or liquid preparations. However, it is perhaps best taken as an infusion to preserve its more volatile constituents (PDR 2000). It is available dried and fresh from pet supply stores, and dried catnip is sold in the pet sections of grocery stores.

Adverse Effects

There are no known side effects when used according to therapeutic recommendations, although it is not advised during pregnancy (PDR 2000). However, a report of prolonged CNS depression lasting almost three days in a toddler was attributed to consumption of catnip (Osterhoudt, Lee, Callahan et al. 1997).

Clinical Application in Veterinary Behavior Medicine

Although *N. cataria* has not been studied for its psychoactive effects in pets, there is evidence for a sedative effect and indications that it might exacerbate or even trigger compulsive behaviors in susceptible individuals. This suggests it should not be offered to cats with compulsive behavior patterns such as psychogenic licking. Inappropriate urine marking can also become compulsive in some individuals and it would be interesting to study whether catnip might exacerbate these symptoms.

Until *N. cataria* has been better investigated, it should be offered on an occasional basis to catnip-sensitive cats that seem to enjoy its brief psychomotor effects. It may also be added to the treatment programs of indoor pet cats in need of additional intellectual and physical stimulation, and it might be helpful in reintroducing housemates who have been separated due to hospitalization or territorial conflict. Fresh herb can be grown easily as a houseplant and may be used fresh, or growth can be harvested for drying. Placed within easy reach to catnip-sensitive cats, it may redirect destructiveness away from other ornamental houseplants.

References

Aydin S, Beis R, Ozturk Y et al. Nepetalactone: a new opioid analgesic from *Nepeta caesarea Boiss.* J Pharm Pharmacol. 1998;50:813–817.

Birkett MA, Pickett JA. Aphid sex pheromones: from discovery to commercial production. Phytochemistry. 2003;62:651–656.

Cauffield JS, Forbes HJ. Dietary supplements used in the treatment of depression, anxiety, and sleep disorders. Lippincotts Prim Care Pract. 1999;3:290–304.

Felter HW, Lloyd JU. King's American Dispensatory.Ohio Valley Company, Cincinatti, OH. 1898. Available online at http://www.ibiblio.org/herbmed/eclectic/kings/

Harney JW, Barofsky IM, Leary JD. Behavioral and toxicological studies of cyclopentanoid monoterpenes from *Nepeta cataria*. Lloydia. 1978;41:367–374.

Hart BL, Leedy MG. Analysis of the catnip reaction: mediation by olfactory system, not vomeronasal organ. Behav Neural Biol. 1985;44:38–46.

Herrick JW. Iroquois Medical Botany. PhD Thesis. State University of New York, Albany, NY. 1977;423.

Kalpoutzakis E, Aligiannis N, Mentis A et al. Composition of the essential oil of two Nepeta species and in vitro evaluation of their activity against *Helicobacter pylori*. Planta Med. 2001;67:880–883.

Massoco CO, Silva MR, Gorniak SL et al. Behavioral effects of acute and long-term administration of catnip (*Nepeta cataria*) in mice. Vet Hum Toxicol. 1995;37:530–533.

Moerman DE. Native American Ethnobotany. Timber Press, Portland, OR. 2002;353–354.

Nostro A, Cannatelli MA, Crisafi G et al. The effect of *Nepeta cataria* extract on adherence and enzyme production of *Staphylococcus aureus*. Int J Antimicrob Agents. 2001;18:583–585.

Osterhoudt KC, Lee SK, Callahan JM et al. Catnip and the alteration of human consciousness. Vet Hum Toxicol. 1997;39:373–375.

PDR for Herbal Medicines. (2nd ed) Medical Economics Company Inc., Montvale, NJ. 2000;104–105.

Peterson CJ, Nemetz LT, Jones LM et al. Behavioral activity of catnip (*Lamiaceae*) essential oil components to the German cockroach (Blattodea: Blattellidae). J Econ Entomol. 2002;95:377–380.

Schwartz S. On the clinical significance of catnip. Anim Behav Consult Newsletter. 1993;10:1.

Sherry CJ, Hunter PS. The effect of an ethanol extract of catnip (*Nepeta cataria*) on the behavior of the young chick. Experientia. 1979;35:237–238.

Waller GR, Price GH, Mitchell ED. Feline Attractant, cis, trans-nepetalactone: metabolism in the domestic cat. Science. 1969;164:1281–1282.

Papaver somniferum

Papaver somniferum (Opium Poppy, Poppyseed, Mawseed, Oriental Poppy, *Ying su qiao*) is a native annual plant of the Middle East that has naturalized throughout Asia, North Africa, Europe, and even into Mexico. A member of the *Papaveraceae* family, *P. somniferum* is a cultivated crop in India, China, Vietnam,

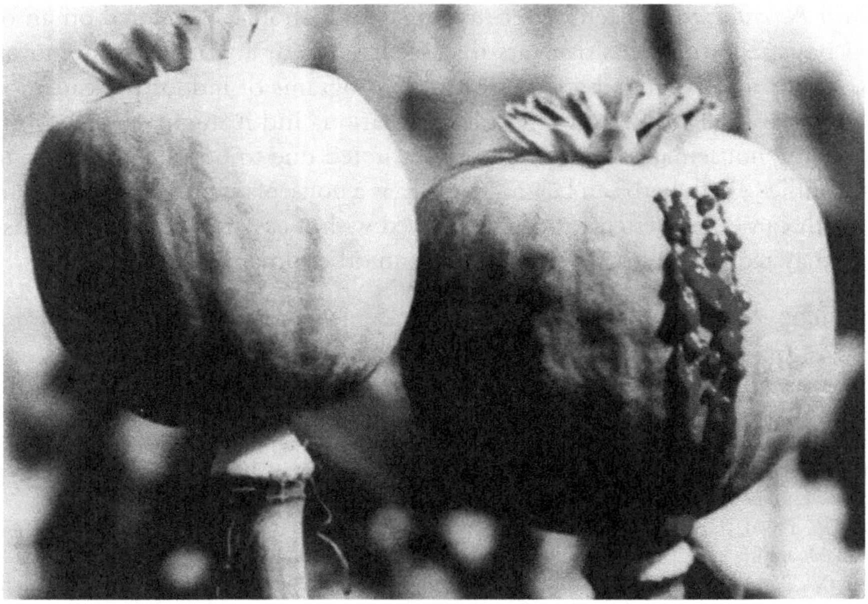

FIGURE 1-12. *Papaver somniferum* capsules showing exudate of raw opium. (Photo courtesy of Dr. Jayvir Anjaria)

Thailand, Indonesia, Turkey and other countries. The Latin *somniferum* means "bringer of sleep"; the origin of *papaver* is unknown. The term "opium" is derived from the Greek for sap. In Sanskrit, *ahiphena* (poppy) suggests a derogatory view of the plant: *ahi* means snake and *phena* means foam or froth (Russo 2001; PDR 2000; Summer 2000).

The flower of *P. somniferum* rises between 30 and 150 cm on an erect stem that bears serrated leaves. The flower is composed of broad sepals that are either white or red (see color plate 1-4). Raw opium, the dried latex collected from the capsules, is used to produce the semi-synthetic heroin (Russo 2001; PDR 2000; Summer 2000) (Fig. 1-12). Poppy seeds are commonly used in baking and in Indian cuisine but are not medicinal, although one study suggests that poppy seeds possess an anticancer effect (Aruna, Sivaramakrishnan 1992).

Historical Perspective

P. somniferum has a long tradition in folk medicine and in TCM and Ayurvedic medicine (Shin, Jang, Chang et al. 2003; PDR 2000). Archeological evidence suggests that *P. somniferum* was used for its medicinal and psychoactive properties in Europe during the Neolithic and Bronze Ages (Summer 2000). The ancient Egyptians may have used opium to calm babies (although this has been disputed);

the Greeks boiled the plant to produce a sleeping potion; and the Romans may have used it in their religious rituals. Today, the seed capsule of immature flowers is incised to collect the medicinal latex using an ancient technique first described by the Greek Dioscorides during the first century (Summer 2000; Nencini 1997; Bisset, Bruhn, Curto et al. 1994).

Until recently, paregoric was a mixture containing opium that was used as a remedy for teething pain in children. The Chinese first used opium mixed with wine as a surgical anesthetic, but it was not until the fourteenth century that Paracelsus combined opium with pure alcohol to prepare the tincture of opium known as laudanum. The cultivation of *P. somniferum* across Arab lands may have followed the spread of Islam; the Koran forbids wine but does not mention the use of drugs such as Cannabis and Papaver (Summer 2000).

P. somniferum has been used to control pain, fever, and spasm and as a sedative in cases of intestinal ulcers, diarrhea, dysentery, gallstones, peritonitis, and cough. It has also been used to treat depression, as well as "nervous irritability, morbid vigilance restlessness" and hysteria (PDR 2000; Felter, Lloyd 1898).

Opium was an essential ingredient in many medicinal preparations but is perhaps most infamous for its addictive potential. Wars have been fought over the lucrative opium trade. The British fought over the rights to import Indian-grown opium into China in two military campaigns (Summer 2000). During the American Civil War, morphine use was so common that addiction to it was referred to as the "soldier's disease." By then, it was also known to the Native Americans and used by the Cherokee as an analgesic and anticonvulsant. The Cherokee also used it for its psychoactive effects as a sedative to soothe and tranquilize (Moerman 2002).

Today, less than 5% of *P. somniferum* crops are destined for pharmaceutical use; the remainder of the opium finds its way into the illegal drug market (Summer 2000). Before the Taliban came to power, Afghanistan was the major producer of illicit crops; Southeast Asia is now the leader. Poppy cultivation in Afghanistan has resumed since the fall of the Taliban, and its profits may be used to fund international terrorism (United Nations News Service 2003; The United States Mission to the European Union 2003; Seibert 2001).

Ingredients

Components of *P. somniferum* include rubber (5–10%); resins; phthalide isochinolines (e.g., narcotine); and benzyl isoquinolines (e.g., papaverine). The isoquinoline alkaloids (20–30%) include morphine (3–23%), codeine (0.2–3.5%), laudanine, narcotine and papaverine (Calixto, Beirith, Ferreira et al. 2000; PDR 2000).

Clinical Effects

Morphine, the primary alkaloid of *P. somniferum*, remains the most important antinociceptive drug (Calixto, Beirith, Ferreira et al. 2000). It causes euphoria, sedation, and narcotic sleep even in small quantities. Codeine is a well-known antitussive. Papaverine is a spasmolytic and vasodilator (PDR 2000; Decker, Wanner, Zenk et al. 2000). Berberine, another poppy alkaloid, has antibiotic, antifungal, and antiprotozoal effects (Summer 2000; Facchini, Penzes, Johnson et al. 1996) as well as potential antitumor activity (Iwasa, Moriyasu, Yamori T et al. 2001).

Recent research has attempted to produce alkaloids by *in vitro* cell culture of two Papaver species, *P. somniferum* and *P. bracteatum*. Researchers were successful in producing a number of major alkaloids, including morphine (Alkhimova, Kyrylenko, Vagyn et al. 2001). In another study of cloned *P. somniferum*, researchers collected codeine (Yoshimatsu, Shimomura 2001). It has recently been suggested that *P. somniferum* produces morphine as a mechanism of self-defense in response to mechanical injury such as that used to collect raw opium (Morimoto, Suemori, Taura et al. 2003; Morimoto, Suemori, Moriwaki et al. 2001). This is not unlike the effect of the opioid pathways production of endorphins and enkephalins including endogenous morphine.

First isolated in 1806, morphine was the first plant alkaloid to be recognized for its medicinal value (Russo 2001). The use and abuse of morphine led to the discovery of the endogenous opioids in circulation and as neurotransmitters. Morphine remained an important antidepressant, along with cannabis and other botanical preparations, until the introduction of imipramine, the first tricyclic antidepressant, in 1957. Since then, the antidepressant drug list has grown to include amitriptyline (Elavil), fluoxetine (Prozac), sertraline (Zoloft), paroxetine (Paxil), bupropion hydrochloride (Wellbutrin), and citalopram (Celexa) (Russo 2001). However, the importance of the opioid receptors in mood disorders is far from forgotten. They remain central to the mystery of CNS balance that, along with other neurotransmitter systems, acts to preserve emotional health and normal function.

Adverse Effects

Side effects associated with *P. somniferum* include constipation, dizziness, headache, pruritus, rash, hyperthermia, clonic twitching, and trembling hands. Morphine also causes constipation and urine retention and depresses respiration. Overdosage can result in bradycardia, respiratory failure, intestinal atonia, and death (PDR 2000; Odendaal 1986). Allergic reactions have also been reported (Moneo, Alday, Ramos et al. 1993). Papaverine is thought to be the main allergen in cases of allergic sensitivity (Decker, Wanner, Zenk et al. 2000). Naloxone is the opioid antagonist used to combat overdose, along with appropriate supportive treatment (PDR 2000).

Clinical Application in Veterinary Behavior Medicine

Derivatives of *P. somniferum* such as morphine and codeine remain in widespread use in conventional medicines and treatment. Despite traditional use in the treatment of depression, *P. somniferum* and its components are considered essentially obsolete for the purposes of application to veterinary behavior medicine. With so many other interesting and safer herbs, the use of a controlled substance with high abuse potential does not seem worthwhile. Still, it is important to include *P. somniferum* in this book because of its rich history, traditional use for its psychoactive properties, and ongoing medical significance.

References

Alkhimova OG, Kyrylenko TK, Vagyn YV, Heslop-Harrison JS. Alkaloid biosynthesis in *Papaver sp.* cells in culture and during organogenesis. Ukr Biokhim Zh. 2001;73:141–146.

Aruna K, Sivaramakrishnan VM. Anticarcinogenic effects of some Indian plant products. Food Chem Toxicol. 1992;30:953–956.

Bisset NG, Bruhn JG, Curto S et al. Was opium known in 18th dynasty ancient Egypt? An examination of materials from the tomb of the chief royal architect Kha. J Ethnopharmacol. 1994;41:99–114.

Calixto JB, Beirith A, Ferreira J et al. Naturally occurring antinociceptive substances from plants. Phytother Res. 2000; 14:401–418.

Decker G, Wanner G, Zenk MH et al. Characterization of proteins in latex of the opium poppy (Papaver somniferum) using two-dimensional gel electrophoresis and microsequencing. Electrophoresis. 2000; 21:3500–3516.

Facchini PJ, Penzes C, Johnson AG et al. Molecular characterization of berberine bridge enzyme genes from opium poppy. Plant Physiol. 1996;112:1669–1677.

Felter HW, Lloyd JU. King's American Dispensatory. Ohio Valley Company, Cincinatti OH. 1898. Available online at http://www.ibiblio.org/herbmed/eclectic/kings/

Frank T. Sharp rise in Afghan poppy grow. Newday. January 9, 2003.

Iwasa K, Moriyasu M, Yamori T et al. In vitro cytotoxicity of the protoberberine-type alkaloids. J Nat Prod. 2001;64:896–898.

Moerman DE. Native American Ethnobotany. Timber Press, Portland, OR. 2002;377.

Moneo I, Alday E, Ramos C et al. Occupational asthma caused by *Papaver somniferum.* Allergol Immunopathol (Madr). 1993;21:145–148.

Morimoto S, Suemori K, Moriwaki J et al. Morphine metabolism in the opium poppy and its possible physiological function. Biochemical characterization of the morphine metabolite, bismorphine. J Biol Chem. 2001;276:38179–38184.

Morimoto S, Suemori K, Taura F et al. New dimeric morphine from opium poppy (*Papaver somniferum*) and its physiological function. J Nat Prod. 2003;66:987–989.

Nencini P.The rules of drug taking: wine and poppy derivatives in the ancient world. VII. A ritual use of poppy derivatives? Subst Use Misuse. 1997;32:1405–1415.

Odendaal JS. Suspected opium poisoning in two young dogs. J S Afr Vet Assoc. 1986;57:113–114.

PDR for Herbal Medicines (2nd ed) Medical Economics Company Inc., Montvale, NJ. 2000;609–610.

Russo E. Handbook of Psychotropic Herbs: A Scientific Analysis of Herbal Remedies for Psychiatric Conditions. The Haworth Press, Binghamton, NY. 2001;8,55.

Seibert T. Afghan poppy growers back in business. Denver Post. December 4, 2001.

Shin MC, Jang MH, Chang HK et al. Modulation of Chelidonii herba on glycine-activated and glutamate-activated ion currents in rat periaqueductal gray neurons. Clin Chim Acta. 2003;337:93–101.

Sumner J. The natural history of medicinal plants. Timber Press, Portland, OR. 2000;126–129.

The United States Mission to the European Union, Brussels, Belgium. U.S. Supports Opium Poppy Cultivation Ban in Afghanistan. April 5, 2002. http://www.usue.be

United Nations News Service, June 17, 2003. Faced with insecurity and drugs, Afghanistan needs beefed up help—UN officials. http://www.globalsecurity.org/military/library/news/2003/06/mil-030617-unnews05.htm

Yoshimatsu K, Shimomura K. Isoquinoline alkaloid production by transformed cultures of *Papaver somniferum.* Kokuritsu Iyakuhin Shokuhin Eisei Kenkyusho Hokoku. 2001;119:52–56.

Passiflora incarnata

Passiflora incarnata (Passion Flower, Passionflower, Maypop, Passion vine, Apricot vine, Granadilla, Passionsblumenkraut, herbe de passiflore; family *Passifloraceae*) is a perennial vine that is native to the southeast United States, Caribbean, and parts of South America. It is a favorite of gardeners in North America and Europe for its exotic-looking white and purple flowers that bloom on a woody vine that can grow as long as 10 m (Russo 2001; PDR 2000). Missionaries projected a religious significance onto its botanical features and gave the flowering vine its name (Russo 2001). *P. edulis* produces edible apple-sized "berries"; however, the aerial leaves and stems of *P. incarnata* are most valued for their medicinal properties (Dhawan, Kumar, Kumar et al. 2001).

Historical Perspective

The first record of its medicinal use appears in the 1800s; however, it may have been used earlier in Brazil to treat fever. Physicians of the nineteenth century valued *P. incarnata* as a treatment for insomnia, pain, and spasm. It was also prescribed to relieve nervousness associated with debility, chronic illness, and various gynecological complaints (Russo 2001; PDR 2000; Felter, Lloyd 1898). Although use by Native Americans was limited, the Cherokee used the plant to minimize the stress of weaning infants and as a social beverage (Moerman 2002). It was in common use by American physicians until the mid twentieth century and has since fallen out of mainstream medical practice, although it remains popular in Europe and in homeopathic practice (Russo 2001).

Ingredients

The dried herb contains cyanogenic glycosides and flavonoids. Important flavones include vitexin, isovitexin, saponarin, schaftoside, isoschaftoside, orientin and isoorientin. Its essential oil contains more than one hundred components that deserve further study. *P. incarnata* flowers are often harvested twice yearly to maximize the content of flavonoids in the flowering shoot (Russo 2001; PDR 2000). The leaves, stems, flowers, and whole plant possess anxiolytic compounds; however, the roots were not effective anxiolytics (Dhawan, Kumar, Sharma 2001c). A recent attempt to identify the primary bioactive constituent of *Passiflora incarnata* suggests a compound with a benzoflavone nucleus (Dhawan, Kumar, Sharma 2001b).

CNS Effects

P. incarnata extract showed high affinity to $GABA_{A,B}$ and Cl^- ion channel receptors, among others (Cott 1995). A murine study found anxiolytic effects with an aqueous extract at 400 mg/kg and sedative effects with another (Soulimani,

Younos, Jarmouni et al. 1997). Anxiolytic action of *P. incarnata* extract has been demonstrated at 100 mg/kg, 125 mg/kg, 200 mg/kg, 300 mg/kg, and 400 m/kg (Dhawan, Kumar, Sharma 2001a, 2002b).

In a recent study (Akhondzadeh, Naghavi, Vazirian et al. 2001), 36 people with generalized anxiety disorder (GAD as defined by DSM IV criteria) were treated with either oxazepam (30 mg/day PO) or *P. incarnata* extract (45 drops/day). Both patient groups improved without observable differences except that the herbal extract caused significantly less job impairment than the benzodiazepine.

Some cultivars of *P. incarnata* may contain trace amounts of beta-carboline alkaloids, which are monoamine oxidase inhibitors; this may provide a partial explanation for any reputed psychoactive properties. The plant also contains trace amounts of maltol, which may have sedative effects in mice. Chrysin, another flavonoid compound isolated from *P. coerulea*, may possess anxiolytic effects without sedative or muscle relaxant action (Wolfman, Viola, Paladini et al. 1994) that may be due to activation of GABA receptors (Zanoli, Avallone, Baraldi 2000). However, none of these components adequately explains the effects of the plant even if any were present in higher concentration (Russo 2001).

P. incarnata components may be effective in minimizing anxiety associated with alcohol withdrawal (Dhawan, Kumar, Sharma 2002a), opiate withdrawal (Akhondzadeh, Kashani, Mobaseri et al. 2001), and nicotine (Dhawan, Dhawan, Chhabra 2003). *P. incarnata* extract does not trigger withdrawal symptoms even after abrupt cessation and is not thought to be addictive at this time (Dhawan, Dhawan, Chhabra 2003). Preparations of *P. incarnata* potentiated the effect of pentobarbital in laboratory mice (Soulimani, Younos, Jarmouni et al. 1997).

Miscellaneous Effects

The glycoside content in *P. incarnata* has been shown to exert a hypotensive effect and stimulate respiration. It may be beneficial in treating insomnia in some people (PDR 2000).

Adverse Effects

Given the lack of clinical investigation into its side effects, toxicity, drug interactions, and therapeutic use, *P. incarnata* preparations should not be used in females who are pregnant or lactating, or in combination with other anesthetic, sedative, or psychoactive drugs.

Availability

Available in capsules (400 mg), liquid extract, it is often used at bedtime as a tea infusion with 1 teaspoon (2 gm) of the dried herb consumed to treat insomnia. It is also added to prepare a sedative bath (PDR 2000). Anecdotally, it has been suggested as an alternative to marijuana cigarettes and may be a mild stimulant when smoked (Russo 2001).

Clinical Application in Veterinary Behavior Medicine

P. incarnata, in combination with other herbal ingredients, has been advocated for the treatment of Feline Hyperesthesia Syndrome (Wynn, Marsden 2003). This poorly understood condition is likely the product of multiple etiologies, some of which may well respond to *P. incarnata*. In most cases, however, a more potent anxiolytic and anticonvulsant medication would be required to manage hyperesthetic cats. Controlled clinical study would be important to prescribe *P. incarnata* with confidence, for use alone or in combination with another psychoactive substance, for treating any behavioral diagnosis. Nonetheless, *P. incarnata* has promise for the treatment of a variety of agitated and anxious mood disorders in people and in pets.

References

Akhondzadeh S, Naghavi HR, Vazirian M et al. Passionflower in the treatment of generalized anxiety: a pilot double-blind randomized controlled trial with oxazepam. J Clin Pharm Ther. 2001;26: 363–367.

Akhondzadeh S, Kashani L, Mobaseri M et al. Passionflower in the treatment of opiates withdrawal: a double-blind randomized controlled trial. J Clin Pharm Ther. 2001;26:369–373.

Cott J. Medicinal plants and dietary supplements: Sources for innovative treatment or adjuncts? Psychopharm Bulletin. 1995;31:131–137.

Dhawan K, Dhawan S, Chhabra S. Attenuation of benzodiazepine dependence in mice by a tri-substituted benzoflavone moiety of *Passiflora incarnata Linneaus*: a non-habit forming anxiolytic. J Pharm Pharm Sci. 2003;6:215–222.

Dhawan K, Kumar R, Kumar S et al. Correct identification of *Passiflora incarnata L.*, a promising herbal anxiolytic and sedative. J Med Food. 2001;4:137–144.

Dhawan K, Kumar S, Sharma A. Comparative biological activity study on *Passiflora incarnata* and *P. edulis*. Fitoterapia. 2001a;72:698–702.

——. Anti-anxiety studies on extracts of *Passiflora incarnata* Linneaus. J Ethnopharmacol. 2001b;78: 165–170.

——. Anxiolytic activity of aerial and underground parts of *Passiflora incarnata*. Fitoterapia. 2001c;72: 922–926.

Dhawan K, Kumar S, Sharma A. Suppression of alcohol-cessation-oriented hyperanxiety of the benzoflavone moiety of *Passiflora incarnata* L. in mice. J Ethnopharmacol. 2002a;81:239–244.

——. Comparative anxiolytic activity profile of various preparations of *Passiflora incarnata* L.: a comment on medicinal plants' standardization. J Altern Complement Med. 2002b:8:283–291.

Felter HW, Lloyd JU. King's American Dispensatory. Ohio Valley Company, Cincinatti, OH. 1898. Available online at http://www.ibiblio.org/herbmed/eclectic/kings/

Mills S, Bone K. Principles and Practice of Phytotherapy. Churchill Livingstone, Philadelphia, PA. 2000;231–234.

Moerman DE. Native American Ethnobotany. Timber Press, Portland, OR 2002;379.

PDR for Herbal Medicines (2nd ed) Medical Economics Company Inc., Montvale, NJ. 2000;573–575.

Russo E. Handbook of Psychotropic Herbs: A Scientific Analysis of Herbal Remedies for Psychiatric Conditions. The Haworth Press, Binghamton, NY. 2001;106–115.

Soulimani R, Younos C, Jarmouni S et al. Behavioral effects of *Passiflora incarnata* and its indole alkaloid and flavonoid derivatives and maltol in the mouse. J Ethnopharmacol. 1997;57:11–20.

Wolfman C, Viola H, Paladini A et al. Possible anxiolytic effects of chrysin, a central benzodiazepine receptor ligand isolated from *Passiflora coerulea*. Pharmacol Biochem Behav. 1994;47:1–4.

Wynn SG, Marsden S. Manual of Natural Veterinary Medicine: Science and Tradition. Mosby Inc, Philadelphia, PA. 2003;459–464.
Zanoli P, Avallone R, Baraldi M. Behavioral characterization of the flavonoids apigenin and chrysin. Fitoterapia.2000;71 (Suppl 1):S117–S123.

Pausinystalia yohimbe

Pausinystalia yohimbe (Yohimbe) is an evergreen tree that is native to the jungles of Cameroon, Congo, West Africa, and Gabon. It grows as high as 30 m. The medicinal part of the tree is the bark of the trunk or branches, which is traditionally dried (PDR 2000).

Traditionally, it has been used in Africa as an aphrodisiac in male virility ceremonies, and as a stimulant to counteract exhaustion (PDR 2000; Mills, Bone 2000). In veterinary medicine, it is a well-known anesthetic reversal agent (Williams, Levy, Robertson 2002). It is also used in the treatment of amitraz toxicity (Andrade, Sakate 2003).

Ingredients

Compounds isolated from yohimbe bark include tannins and indole alkaloids. The alkaloids comprise 2.7–5.9% of its ingredients and include yohimbine, alpha-yohimbine (rauwolscine) and other yohimbine stereoisomers, and corynanthine, among others (PDR 2000).

Sexual Effects

In a study of sexually exhausted rats, yohimbe successfully reversed satiety, indicating that serotonergic mechanisms are partly responsible for sexual inhibition after *ad libitum* copulation in rats (Fernandez-Guasti, Rodriguez-Manzo 2003; Carro-Juareza, Rodriguez-Manzo 2003).

Yohimbine has been used for the treatment of human erectile dysfunction and has been successful in patients whose impotence was attributed to psychogenic, vascular, or diabetic causes. Other FDA approved indications include its use as a sympatholytic and mydriatic agent. Yohimbine has a modest therapeutic benefit compared to placebo and may be particularly useful for erectile disorders that have psychogenic causes (Riley 1994). Other plant derivatives being studied for their potential in treating male impotence include citrulline, berberine, forskolin, and pyrano-isoflavones (Drewes, George, Khan 2003).

Anti-Anxiety Effects

Animal studies of alpha(2)-adrenoceptor antagonists have yielded inconsistent results, with effects ranging from anxiogenesis to anxiolysis. In one murine study, the effects of yohimbine on maze behavior indicated significant anxiolytic-like effects on standard spatiotemporal measures at 2.0–4.0 mg/kg (Cole, Burroughs, Laverty et al. 1995). Yohimbine, an alpha(2)-adrenoceptor antagonist, seems to exert an antagonizing and hyperpolarizing effect on presynaptic rather than post-synaptic alpha(2)receptors (Kovacs, Hernadi 2003).

In an earlier study, nervous Pointer dogs were considered as a model for human anxiety. Treatment with yohimbine to study alpha(2)-adrenergic binding did not reveal significant differences between normal and nervous dogs (Klein, Lenox, Uhde 1988).

The alpha(2)-agonist clonidine reduced separation-triggered vocalization in squirrel monkeys. This effect was reversed by yohimbine, but not by the alpha(1)-antagonist prazosin, implying usefulness for drugs that act directly on alpha(2)-receptors in the treatment of separation anxiety in primates (Harris, Newman 1987).

Yohimbine was associated with a dose-related decrease in access to sweetened milk during competition between dominant rats. This result was consistent with a previous study that showed that access to the sweetened milk by subordinate animals was increased after administration of anxiolytic drugs. These findings support the hypothesis that levels of social competition were associated with different levels of fear (Joly, Sanger 1992). In another report, platelet alpha(2)-adrenergic receptor binding to 3H-yohimbine was studied in respect to several personality variables in 58 adult males in a campus community. Low affinity correlated with psychopathological dependence and paranoia, whereas high affinity correlated with dominance, autonomy and playfulness (Shekim, Bylund, Frankel et al. 1990).

Miscellaneous Effects

Yohimbine causes hypertension in patients with preexisting blood pressure problems (Musso, Vergassola, Pende et al. 1995), but this effect has been used to advantage to treat patients with a variety of hypotensive disorders (Jordan, Shannon, Biaggioni 1998; Mosqueda-Garcia, Fernandez-Violante, Tank et al. 1998). Yohimbine may interfere with clonidine, shortening its duration (Liu 1993). Clonidine, an alpha(2)-adrenoceptor agonist, decreased systolic and diastolic blood pressure, salivation, and subjectively rated alertness, and tended to decrease pupil diameter. In comparison, yohimbine increased systolic and diastolic blood pressure, salivation, subjective alertness, and pupil diameter (Phillips, Szabadi, Bradshaw 2000).

P. yohimbe enhances the analgesic effect of morphine (Gear 1995), potentiates the side effects of naltrexone (Rosen, Kosten, Kreek 1999; Liu, Bonnet, Delaunay et al. 1993) and enhances the effects of ethanol intoxication (McDougle, Krystal, Price et al. 1995). Based upon the close relation between opioid and alpha(2)-adrenoceptor mechanisms, the contribution of both systems to antinociception in rats was investigated (Herradon, Morales, Perez-Garcia et al. 2003). Yohimbine provoked a higher hyperalgesic effect in Lewis rats and decreased morphine antinociception in both strains. In another study, yohimbine caused acute symptoms of opioid withdrawal and elevated craving for opioid drugs in methadone patients. Medications such as yohimbine that increase synaptic noradrenaline are contraindicated in opioid-dependent patients (Stine, Southwick, Petrakis et al. 2002).

P. yohimbe may have potential benefits in weight control management. It may have a boosting effect on lipolysis if administered prior to exercise (McCarty 2002); however, its detrimental effects on insulin may limit its usefulness in some individuals.

Recently, alpha(2)-adrenoceptor agonists were shown to induce interleukin-12 production in mouse macrophages, suggesting a novel way to enhance cell-mediated immune responses (Kang, Lee, Kim 2003).

Anxiogenic Effects

Although there is evidence that supports its anxiolytic properties, there is also evidence that *P. yohimbe* can trigger anxiety. For example, yohimbine was shown to exacerbate anxiety in a study of children with a variety of anxiety disorders (Sallee, Sethuraman, Sine et al. 2000). This apparent conflict has led to suggestions that experimental design and instruction may impact the expectation of human subjects and modify the anxiogenic effects of yohimbine (Albus, Zahn, Breier 1992). However, other explanations have been offered.

Yohimbine's anxiogenic effect may be attributed to activity on both the noradrenergic and dopaminergic systems (Johnston, File 1989). Genetic, epidemiological, biological, and pharmacological evidence suggests that phobic and panic disorders are distinguished by central autonomic dysfunction, which may cause excessive release of norepinephrine from the locus ceruleus. Stimulation of the locus ceruleus by yohimbine can trigger feelings of panic and anxiety in normal controls as well as in patients with panic disorder (Jann, Kurtz 1987; Charney, Woods, Goodman et al. 1987; Rasmussen, Jacobs 1986).

Yohimbine has been shown to induce panic attack in susceptible individuals (Gurguis, Vitton, Uhde 1997). Heightened post-synaptic adrenoreceptor sensitivity may explain the noradrenergic dysregulation associated with panic disorder. Studies suggest that panic disorder is related to a hypersensitivity in the alpha(2)-adrenergic regulation of the noradrenergic system and that depression is related to a reduced sensitivity of the serotonergic system. The pharmacologic treatment response in panic disorder and depression is similar in that both conditions respond to tricyclic antidepressants and monoamine oxidase inhibitors (MAOIs), but different in that panic disorder, in contrast to depression, does respond to benzodiazepines (Heninger, Charney, Price 1988).

A recent study in rats and anxiety in a maze test supports a modulation of the anxiety response to stress by a balance between noradrenergic and peptidergic neurotransmission. Yohimbine was shown to induce anxiety in stressed rats; however, pretreatment with yohimbine prior to stress caused a paradoxical anxiolytic response, which was attributed to release of the neuropeptide galanin (Khoshbouei, Cecchi, Dove et al. 2002). Chronic psychosocial stress in rats caused impaired adaptation to a novel environment, increased anxiety, and elevated sensitivity to yohimbine (Park, Campbell, Diamond 2001). Yohimbine significantly increased the binding potential of the benzodiazepine antagonist flumazenil to benzodiazepine receptors in the hippocampus of rhesus monkeys, lending further support to findings that the presence of an anxiety state potentiates the effect of anxiolytics (Matsunaga, Tsukada, Nishiyama et al. 2001).

In a rodent study, yohimbine (5.0 mg kg-1, IP) increased maximally the extracellular levels of 5-HT in the rat frontal cortex by approximately 230% of the basal levels. However, this effect was prevented by pretreatment with clonidine (Cheng, Costall, Ge et al. 1993). Study of the rat brain has shown that stress increases noradrenaline release in several brain regions, specifically in the hypothalamus, amygdala, and locus coeruleus. This could be closely related to the provocation of negative emotions such as anxiety and/or fear. Yohimbine caused a marked increase in noradrenaline release in the several brain regions and had an anxiolytic action in the conditioned defensive burying test and the modified forced swim test (Tanaka, Yoshida, Emoto et al. 2000).

P. yohimbe has been shown to increase core symptoms of post-traumatic stress disorder (PTSD) in combat veterans (Rasmusson, Hauger, Morgan et al. 2000; Southwick, Paige, Morgan et al. 1999; Bremner, Krystal, Southwick et al. 1996). Abnormal binding of yohimbine to platelet alpha(2)-adrenoceptors has been identified in women with post-partum depression (Best, Wiley, Stump et al. 1988).

Cognitive Effects

Yohimbine causes an increase in plasma norepinephrine from sympathetic nerves as well as the release of epinephrine from the adrenals (Murburg, Villacres, Ko 1991). Yohimbine may enhance recall and emotional recognition by its stimulating effect on central noradrenergic pathways (O'Carroll, Drysdale, Cahill et al. 1999). Yohimbine appeared to facilitate learning despite or because of its anxiogenic effects in mice (Schroeder, Schiltz, Kelley 2003).

CNS noradrenergic responsiveness to yohimbine is enhanced in normal older subjects and in patients with Alzheimer's disease (Peskind, Wingerson, Murray et al. 1995). Yohimbine, an alpha(2)-adrenergic receptor antagonist, inhibited noradrenaline consolidation of memory in the basal ganglia, although its effect was dependent on the timing of noradrenergic stimulation (Gibbs, Summers 2003). This might indicate memory dysfunction as a possible side effect in elevated and prolonged use of yohimbe extract. In a trial on monkeys, yohimbine introduced into the prefrontal cortex interfered with a conditioned response to red or green lights, suggesting that alpha(2)-adrenoceptors are involved in the response inhibition (Ma, Qi, Peng et al. 2003).

Central alpha(2) adrenoceptors appear to be key to cataplexy, a major symptom of narcolepsy. Treatment with yohimbine (1.5-96.0 micrograms/kg IV) of genetically narcoleptic Doberman Pinschers successfully suppressed cataplexy (Nishino, Haak, Shepherd et al. 1990; Aldrich, Prokopowicz, Ockert et al. 1994; Riehl, Nishino, Cederberg et al. 1998).

Adverse Effects

Recognized side effects include anxiety, hypertension, nausea, vomiting, tachycardia, tremor, and insomnia (PDR 2000). Yohimbine is known to exacerbate or trigger panic attacks in patients with agoraphobia or Parkinson's disease and has been associated with heightened anxiety or panic in patients with posttraumatic stress disorder (PSTD) (PDR 2000; Richard, Szegethy, Lichter et al. 1999; Southwick, Morgan Charney et al. 1999; Gurguis, Vitton, Uhde 1997).

A case was reported of a 42-year-old man who developed progressive renal failure, generalized erythrodermic skin eruption, and a lupus-like syndrome that was attributed to treatment with yohimbine for impotence (Sandler, Aronson 1993). In another case, a 62-year-old male ingested one hundred 2.0 mg tablets of yohimbine. Reports of adverse effects were limited to tachycardia, hypertension, and anxiety of brief duration that resolved without treatment (Friesen, Palatnick, Tenenbein 1993).

Availability

Yohimbe is available in capsule (500 mg), liquid (1000 mg/ml), and tablet (5.4 g, 800 mg) form. The recommended dosage for psychogenic impotence in men is 10 mg TID (PDR 2000). Analysis and comparison of commercial preparations of yohimbine (Betz, White, der Marderosian 1995) determined that they range widely in yohimbine content. In addition, the possible presence of undeclared diluents in the products was noted.

Clinical Application in Veterinary Behavior Medicine

The use of anxiogenic substances such as yohimbine may prove useful as a novel treatment of dominance behavior in pets on the basis of the suggestion that social competition may be related to varying levels of fear. It might be of use in the treatment of sexual dysfunction in pets of significant breeding value. To limit anxiogenic effects yet still take advantage of its cognitive enhancing property, yohimbine could be used in conjunction with other cognitive-enhancing agents in the treatment of senile cognitive changes. However, the unpredictability of its anxiogenic or anxiolytic properties limits its usefulness or suggests caution with its use. Nevertheless, it could be of particular value for the treatment of narcoleptic dogs. Further investigation is warranted.

References

Albus M, Zahn TP, Breier A. Anxiogenic properties of yohimbine. II. Influence of experimental set and setting. Eur Arch Psychiatry Clin Neurosci. 1992;241:345–351.

Aldrich MS, Prokopowicz G, Ockert K et al. Neurochemical studies of human narcolepsy: alpha-adrenergic receptor autoradiography of human narcoleptic brain and brainstem. Sleep. 1994;17:598–608.

Andrade SF, Sakate M. The comparative efficacy of yohimbine and atipamezole to treat amitraz intoxication in dogs. Vet Hum Toxicol. 2003;45:124–127.

Best NR, Wiley M, Stump K et al. Binding of tritiated yohimbine to platelets in women with maternity blues. Psychol Med. 1988;18:837–842.

Betz JM, White KD, der Marderosian AH. Gas chromatographic determination of yohimbine in commercial yohimbe products. J AOAC Int. 1995:78:1189–1194.

Bremner JD, Krystal JH, Southwick SM et al. Noradrenergic mechanisms in stress and anxiety: II. Clinical studies. Synapse. 1996;23:39–51.

Carro-Juareza M, Rodriguez-Manzo G. Yohimbine reverses the exhaustion of the coital reflex in spinal male rats. Behav Brain Res. 2003;141:43–50.

Charney DS, Woods SW, Goodman WK et al. Neurobiological mechanisms of panic anxiety: biochemical and behavioral correlates of yohimbine-induced panic attacks. Am J Psychiatry. 1987;144: 1030–1036.

Cheng CH, Costall B, Ge J et al. The profiles of interaction of yohimbine with anxiolytic and putative anxiolytic agents to modify 5-HT release in the frontal cortex of freely-moving rats. Br J Pharmacol. 1993;110:1079–1084.

Cole JC, Burroughs GJ, Laverty CR et al. Anxiolytic-like effects of yohimbine in the murine plus-maze: strain independence and evidence against alpha 2-adrenoceptor mediation. Psychopharmacology (Berl). 1995;118:425–436.

Drewes SE, George J, Khan F. Recent findings on natural products with erectile-dysfunction activity. Phytochemistry. 2003;62:1019–1025.

Fernandez-Guasti A, Rodriguez-Manzo G. Pharmacological and physiological aspects of sexual exhaustion in male rats. Scand J Psychol. 2003;44:257–263.

Friesen K, Palatnick W, Tenenbein M. Benign course after massive ingestion of yohimbine. J Emerg Med. 1993;11:287–288.

Fugh-Berman A. Herb-drug interactions. Lancet. 2000;355:134–138. [Erratum in: Lancet 2000;355: 1020].

Gibbs ME, Summers RJ. Alpha(2)-adrenoceptors in the basal ganglia have a role in memory consolidation and reinforcement. Neuropharmacology. 2003;45:355–367.

Gurguis GN, Vitton BJ, Uhde TW. Behavioral, sympathetic and adrenocortical responses to yohimbine in panic disorder patients and normal controls. Psychiatry Res. 1997;71:27–39.

Harris JC, Newman JD. Mediation of separation distress by alpha 2-adrenergic mechanisms in a non-human primate. Brain Res. 1987;410:353–356.

Heninger GR, Charney DS, Price LH. Noradrenergic and serotonergic receptor system function in panic disorder and depression. Acta Psychiatr Scand Suppl. 1988;341:138–150.

Herradon G, Morales L, Perez-Garcia C et al. The contribution of alpha2-adrenoceptor and opioid receptor mechanisms to antinociception differs in Lewis and Fischer 344 rats. Eur J Pharmacol. 2003;465:251–256.

Jann MW, Kurtz NM. Treatment of panic and phobic disorders. Clin Pharm. 1987;6:947–962.

Johnston AL, File SE. Yohimbine's anxiogenic action: evidence for noradrenergic and dopaminergic sites. Pharmacol Biochem Behav. 1989;32:151–156.

Joly D, Sanger DJ. Social competition in dominant rats can be attenuated by anxiogenic drugs. Behav Pharmacol. 1992;3:83–88.

Jordan J, Shannon JR, Biaggioni I et al. Contrasting actions of pressor agents in severe autonomic failure. Am J Med. 1998;105:116–124.

Kang BY, Lee SW, Kim TS. Stimulation of interleukin-12 production in mouse macrophages via activation of p38 mitogen-activated protein kinase by alpha(2)-adrenoceptor agonists. Eur J Pharmacol. 2003;467:223–231.

Khoshbouei H, Cecchi M, Dove S et al. Behavioral reactivity to stress: amplification of stress-induced noradrenergic activation elicits a galanin-mediated anxiolytic effect in central amygdala. Pharmacol Biochem Behav. 2002;71:407–417.

Klein E, Lenox RH, Uhde TW. Alpha-2 adrenergic receptor binding in platelets and brains of nervous and normal pointer dogs. J Psychiatr Res. 1988;22:241–247.

Kovacs P, Hernadi I. Alpha2 antagonist yohimbine suppresses maintained firing of rat prefrontal neurons in vivo. Neuroreport. 2003;14:833–836.

Liu N, Bonnet F, Delaunay L et al. Partial reversal of the effects of extradural clonidine by oral yohimbine in postoperative patients. Br J Anaesth. 1993;70:515–518.

Ma CL, Qi XL, Peng JY et al. Selective deficit in no-go performance induced by blockade of prefrontal cortical alpha2-adrenoceptors in monkeys. Neuroreport. 2003;14:1013–1016.

Matsunaga T, Tsukada H, Nishiyama S et al. Yohimbine increases the binding potential for [11C]flumazenil in the monkey brain. J Neural Transm. 2001;108:1375–1382.

McCarty MF. Pre-exercise administration of yohimbine may enhance the efficacy of exercise training as a fat loss strategy by boosting lipolysis. Med Hypotheses. 2002;58:491–495.

McDougle CJ, Krystal JH, Price LH et al. Noradrenergic response to acute ethanol administration in healthy subjects: comparison with intravenous yohimbine. Psychopharmacology (Berl). 1995;118: 127–135.

Mills S, Bone K. Principles and Practice of Phytotherapy. Churchill Livingstone, Philadelphia, PA. 2000;225.

Mosqueda-Garcia R, Fernandez-Violante R, Tank J et al. Yohimbine in neurally mediated syncope: physiological implications. J Clin Invest. 1998;102:1824–1830.

Murburg MM, Villacres EC, Ko GN et al. Effects of yohimbine on human sympathetic nervous system function. J Clin Endocrinol Metab. 1991;73:861–865.

Musso NR, Vergassola C, Pende A et al. Yohimbine effects on blood pressure and plasma catecholamines in human hypertension. Am J Hypertens. 1995;8:565–571.

Nishino S, Haak L, Shepherd H et al. Effects of central alpha-2 adrenergic compounds on canine narcolepsy, a disorder of rapid eye movement sleep. J Pharmacol Exp Ther. 1990;253:1145–1152.

O'Carroll RE, Drysdale E, Cahill L et al. Stimulation of the noradrenergic system enhances and blockade reduces memory for emotional material in man. Psychol Med. 1999;29;1083–1088.

Park CR, Campbell AM, Diamond DM. Chronic psychosocial stress impairs learning and memory and increases sensitivity to yohimbine in adult rats. Biol Psychiatry. 2001;50:994–1004.

PDR for Herbal Medicines (2nd ed) Medical Economics Company Inc., Montvale, NJ. 2000;843–846.

Peskind ER, Wingerson D, Murray S et al. Effects of Alzheimer's disease and normal aging on cerebrospinal fluid norepinephrine responses to yohimbine and clonidine. Arch Gen Psychiatry. 1995;52: 774–782.

Phillips MA, Szabadi E, Bradshaw CM. Comparison of the effects of clonidine and yohimbine on spontaneous pupillary fluctuations in healthy human volunteers. Psychopharmacology (Berl). 2000;150: 85–89.

Rasmusson AM, Hauger RL, Morgan CA et al. Low baseline and yohimbine-stimulated plasma neuropeptide Y (NPY) levels in combat-related PTSD.Biol Psychiatry. 2000;47:526–539.

Rasmussen K, Jacobs BL. Single unit activity of locus coeruleus neurons in the freely moving cat. II. Conditioning and pharmacologic studies. Brain Res. 1986;371:335–344.

Richard IH, Szegethy E, Lichter D et al. Parkinson's disease: a preliminary study of yohimbine challenge in patients with anxiety. Clin Neuropharmacol. 1999;22:172–175.

Riehl J, Nishino S, Cederberg R et al. Development of cataplexy in genetically narcoleptic Dobermans. Exp Neurol. 1998;152:292–302.

Riley AJ. Yohimbine in the treatment of erectile disorder. Br J Clin Pract. 1994;48:133–136.
Rosen MI, Kosten TR, Kreek MJ. The effects of naltrexone maintenance on the response to yohimbine in healthy volunteers. Biol Psychiatry. 1999;45:1636–1645.
Sallee FR, Sethuraman G, Sine L et al. Yohimbine challenge in children with anxiety disorders. Am J Psychiatry. 2000;157:1236–1242.
Sandler B, Aronson P. Yohimbine-induced cutaneous drug eruption, progressive renal failure, and lupus-like syndrome. Urology. 1993;41:343–345.
Schroeder BE, Schiltz CA, Kelley AE. Neural activation profile elicited by cues associated with the anxiogenic drug yohimbine differs from that observed for reward-paired cues. Neuropsychopharmacology. 2003;28:14–21.
Shekim WO, Bylund DB, Frankel F et al. Platelet alpha 2-adrenergic receptor binding to 3H-yohimbine and personality variations in normals. Psychiatry Res. 1990;32:125–134.
Southwick SM, Paige S, Morgan CA et al. Neurotransmitter alterations in PTSD: catecholamines and serotonin. Semin Clin Neuropsychiatry. 1999;4:242–248.
Southwick SM, Morgan CA, Charney DS et al. Yohimbine use in a natural setting: effects on posttraumatic stress disorder. Biol Psychiatry. 1999;46:442–444.
Stine SM, Southwick SM, Petrakis IL et al. Yohimbine-induced withdrawal and anxiety symptoms in opioid-dependent patients. Biol Psychiatry. 2002;51:642–651.
Tanaka M, Yoshida M, Emoto H et al. Noradrenaline systems in the hypothalamus, amygdala and locus coeruleus are involved in the provocation of anxiety: basic studies. Eur J Pharmacol. 2000;405:397–406.
Williams LS, Levy JK, Robertson SA et al. Use of the anesthetic combination of tiletamine, zolazepam, ketamine, and xylazine for neutering feral cats. JAVMA. 2002;220:1491–5.

Piscidia Species

A native of Central America and northern South America, *Piscidia piscipula* (Dogwood, Jamaican Dogwood, Fish Poison Tree) is a small tree that reaches as high as 15 m. Its flowers are blue and white; however, it is the bark that is valued for its medicinal properties. The gray-brown bark is between 3 and 6 mm thick and fissured (PDR 2000).

Historical Perspective

During the 1800s, *P. piscipula* was used to treat pain, insomnia, gastrointestinal disease, rheumatism, and gynecological disorders. Some physicians used it preferentially over opium to control cancer-related pain. It was also prescribed for "hysterical convulsions, delirium tremens and the insomnia of insanity" (Felter, Lloyd 1898).

Ingredients

Compounds of *P. piscipula* include tannins and isoflavonoids (e.g., jamaicine, ichthynone, rotenone) (PDR 2000).

Miscellaneous Effects

Despite some evidence for its sedative and spasmolytic effects, its use as a medicinal substance is currently uncommon (Tillotson, Tillotson, Abel 2001; PDR

2000; Mills, Bone 2000; Della Loggia, Zilli, Del Negro et al. 1988). In an early murine study, *P. erythrina* showed sedative-anxiolytic activity similar to *M. chamomilla* (chamomile) but its effect was weaker compared to Valerian (Della Loggia, Tubaro, Redaelli 1981). The plant's traditional use to treat skin infections is substantiated by a recent report of its antimycotic properties (Caceres, Lopez, Giron et al. 1999).

Clinical Application in Veterinary Behavior Medicine

Evidence does not indicate the clinical usefulness of *Piscidia spp.* at this time.

References

Caceres A, Lopez BR, Giron MA et al. Plants used in Guatemala for the treatment of dermatophytic infections. 1. Screening for antimycotic activity of 44 plant extracts. J Ethnopharmacol. 1991;31: 263–276.

Della Loggia R, Tubaro A, Redaelli C. Evaluation of the activity on the mouse CNS of several plant extracts and a combination of them. Riv Neurol. 1981;51:297–310.

Della Loggia R, Zilli C, Del Negro P et al. Isoflavones as spasmolytic principles of *Piscidia erythrina*. Prog Clin Biol Res. 1988;280:365–368.

Felter HW, Lloyd JU. King's American Dispensatory. Ohio Valley Company, Cincinatti, OH. 1898. Available online at http://www.ibiblio.org/herbmed/eclectic/kings/

Mills S, Bone K. Principles and Practice of Phytotherapy. Churchill Livingstone, Philadelphia, PA. 2000; 232–233.

PDR for Herbal Medicines. (2nd ed) Medical Economics Company Inc., Montvale, NJ. 2000;428–429.

Russo E. Handbook of Psychotropic Herbs: A Scientific Analysis of Herbal Remedies for Psychiatric Conditions. The Haworth Press, Binghamton, NY. 2001;129–131.

Tillotson AK, Tillotson HSH, Abel R. The One Earth Herbal Sourcebook. Kensington Publishing, New York, NY. 2001;444.

Tilia spp.

Tilia cordata (*T. platyphyllos,* Linden tree, Lime tree, Basswood) from the family *Tiliaceae*, is a common deciduous of northern temperate zones. The striking tree is characterized by its towering height (as high as 25 to 30 m) and fissured, dark-gray bark. The Linden leaf has a bluish-green underside with rusty down along the veins (Fig. 1-13). In the spring, the yellowish-white Linden flower (Linn flower, Lime flower, Fleur de tilleul, Lindenbluten) blooms in clusters with a honey-like fragrance. The fruit of *T. cordata* is a thin-shelled, pear-shaped nut that contains a single seed (Russo 2001; PDR 2000; Summer 2000). Silver Linden flowers from *T. tomentosa* are gathered and dried in the shade (PDR 2000; Russo 2001).

The medicinal parts of *T. cordata (T. platyphyllos)* are the fresh or dried flowers (sedative, anxiolytic, anticonvulsive, diuretic, antimicrobial, antitussive, hypotensive, and astringent properties), leaves (diaphoretic effects), wood (antimicrobial, hypotensive, diuretic, choleretic effects) and charcoal (leg ulcers and intestinal ail-

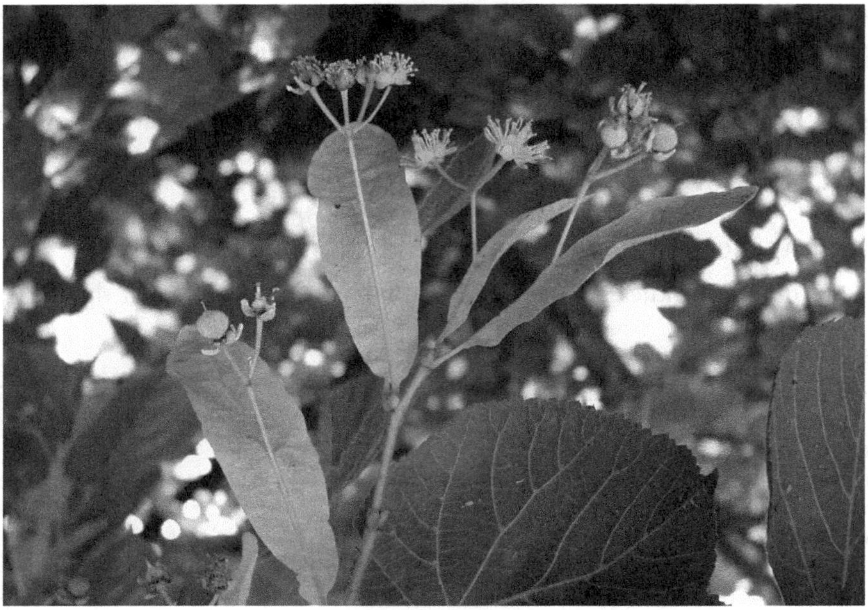

FIGURE 1-13. Leaves and fruit of *Tilia cordata*. (Photo courtesy of Prof. George Ellmore)

ments). Most traditional uses remain unproven although recent research has begun to show proof to substantiate some of these claims (Choi, Choi, Han et al. 2002; Matsuda, Ninomiya, Shimoda et al. 2002; Yildirim, Mavi, Oktay et al. 2000).

Historical Perspective

*T. europa*ea was in common use through the 1800s as a nervine, stimulant, and tonic. It was prepared as an infusion, bath, or enema to relieve restlessness, nervous headaches, and mild hysteria and to promote sleep. Linden flower infusion was used to treat colds (Felter, Lloyd 1898). Native Americans used a variety of Linden (*T. americana*) for many of the same uses prescribed by European herbalists. Among them, the Iroquois prepared an infusion as a stimulant beverage (Moerman 2002; Summer 2000).

Tilia flower tea, alone or in mixture with other herbal ingredients, is a popular sedative drink in Europe and Latin America (PDR 2000; Russo 2001; Viola, Wolfman, Levi de Stein et al. 1994). The floral preparation is usually taken as an herbal tea or infusion (2 gm is just over 1 tsp) (PDR 2000; Mills, Bone 2000).

Ingredients

Silver Linden flowers (*T. argentea)* and Linden flowers (*T. cordata, T. platyphyllos*) contain flavonoids (e.g., tiliroside, quercetrin, isoquercitrinastragalin), hydroxicoumarins, mucilages, caffeic acid derivatives, and essential oil (e.g., citronellal, limonene). Flavonoids include the recognized psychoactive compounds chrysin (also a compound of Passionflower, *Passiflora coerulea*) and apigenin (e.g., identified in Chamomile, *Matricaria chamomilla*) (Russo 2001; Viola, Wolfman, Levi de Stein et al. 1994).

Miscellaneous Effects

Tilia flavonoids may explain its possible sedative and anxiolytic effects. In a recent Portuguese study on mice, however, *T. europaea* failed to induce any significant anxiolytic effect (Coleta, Campos, Cotrim et al. 2001). In a study conducted in Argentina, a bioactive extract of *T. argentea* that produced sedative and anxiolytic effects in mice was demonstrated (Viola, Wolfman, Levi de Stein et al. 1994).

In a Turkish study comparing the flavonoid composition of three Tilia species (*T. platyphyllos, T. rubra, T. argentea*), researchers determined that each species displayed a characteristic profile depending upon the sample source (e.g., flower vs. leaf) and the species (Toker, Aslan, Yesilada et al. 2001). This finding is of significance to the design of future studies investigating Tilia properties. It is possible that the Tilia flower's reported hypotensive property contributes to the calming effect associated with the tea by inhibiting the physiological events associated with anxiety.

Adverse Effects

Although there are no known toxic effects of Tilia preparations, allergy is relatively common and widespread given the distribution of the tree (Weber 2002; Mur, Feo Brito, Lombardero et al. 2001; Picardo, Rovina, Cristaudo et al. 1988).

Clinical Application in Veterinary Behavior Medicine

Tilia spp. and their medicinal preparations deserve further attention in controlled studies to determine their therapeutic value. Reports of a psychoactive property of Tilia flowers are promising, but inconclusive at this time.

References

Choi HR, Choi JS, Han YN et al. Peroxynitrite scavenging activity of herb extracts. Phytother Res. 2002;16:364–367.

Coleta M, Campos MG, Cotrim MD et al. Comparative evaluation of *Melissa officinalis, Tilia europaea, Passiflora edulis* and *Hypericum perforatum* in the elevated plus maze anxiety test. Pharmacopsychiatry. 2001;34(Suppl 1):S20–S21.

Felter HW, Lloyd JU. King's American Dispensatory. Ohio Valley Company, Cincinatti, OH. 1898. Available online at http://www.ibiblio.org/herbmed/eclectic/kings/

Matsuda H, Ninomiya K, Shimoda H et al. Hepatoprotective principles from the flowers of *Tilia argentea* (linden): structure requirements of tiliroside and mechanisms of action. Bioorg Med Chem. 2002;10:707–712.

Mills S, Bone K. Principles and Practice of Phytotherapy. Churchill Livingstone, Philadelphia, PA. 2000;233.

Moerman DE. Native American Ethnobotany. Timber Press, Portland, OR. 2002;562–563.
Mur P, Feo Brito F, Lombardero M et al. Allergy to linden pollen (*Tilia cordata*). Allergy. 2001;56:457–458.
PDR for Herbal Medicines (2nd ed) Medical Economics Company Inc., Montvale, NJ. 2000;477–478.
Picardo M, Rovina R, Cristaudo A et al. Contact urticaria from Tilia (lime). Contact Dermatitis. 1988;19:72–73.
Russo E. Handbook of Psychotropic Herbs: A Scientific Analysis of Herbal Remedies for Psychiatric Conditions. The Haworth Press, Binghamton, NY. 2001;129–131.
Sumner J. The natural history of medicinal plants. Timber Press, Portland, OR. 2000;65,67.
Toker G, Aslan M, Yesilada E et al. Comparative evaluation of the flavonoid content in officinal Tiliae flos and Turkish lime species for quality assessment. J Pharm Biomed Anal. 2001;26:111–121.
Viola H, Wolfman C, Levi de Stein M et al. Isolation of pharmacologically active benzodiazepine receptor ligands from *Tilia tomentosa* (*Tiliaceae*). J Ethnopharmacol. 1994;44:47–53.
Weber RW. American linden, *Tilia americana*. Ann Allergy Asthma Immunol. 2002;88:A4.
Yildirim A, Mavi A, Oktay M et al. Comparison of antioxidant and antimicrobial activities of tilia (*Tilia argentea*), sage (*Salvia triloba*), and black tea (*Camellia sinensis*) extracts. J Agric Food Chem. 2000; 48:5030-5034.

Turnera diffusa

Turnera diffusa var. aphrodisiaca (Damiana, Pastorica, Hierba de la pastora, Venado, Oreganillo, Shepherd's herb, Stag's herb, Damianablatter) is a member of the *Turneraceae* family. This shrub grows as high as 2 m in arid regions of the Caribbean, Mexico, southwestern United States, and southern parts of Africa. The medicinal leaf of *T. diffusa* is smooth, pale green, and between 1 to 2.5 cm long and 6 mm wide. Solitary yellow flowers are 8 to 12 mm long. The aromatic fruit contains many encapsulated seeds (Russo 2001; PDR 2000; Lowry 1984).

Historical Perspective

T. diffusa leaves are harvested during bloom time and are used traditionally for the prevention and treatment of sexual disorders and as an aphrodisiac (PDR 2000). Damiana has been used as a remedy for sexual dysfunction, diabetes, nephritis, and menstrual complaints (Lowry 1984). It has also been used for a slightly euphoric effect to restore balance in emotional states of depression and anxiety (Mills, Bone 2001).

The use of *T. diffusa* was first recorded by a Spanish missionary as early as 1699, although it was already well known to ancient Mexicans, including the Maya, to combat the lethargy due to the effects of alcohol or sexual excess, and other complaints (Lowry 1984). A Mexican liqueur called "Damiana" and marketed as a "liqueur for lovers" contains a small amount of *T. diffusa* and was once sold in a bottle shaped like a woman's torso.

Physicians of the nineteenth century prescribed it for its aphrodisiac (for male impotence and female frigidity), laxative, diuretic, anti-inflammatory, and antidepressant effects although some were not convinced of its effectiveness (Felter, Lloyd 1898).

Ingredients

Chief among the volatile oils are cymene, cineole, pinene, cadinen, and calamene. Hydroquinone glycosides (e.g., arbutin) and cyanogenic glycosides (e.g., barterin) are also identified components (PDR 2000; Lowry 1984). In one study, *T. diffusa* was among the more potent progesterone-receptor binding phytoprogestins (Zava, Dollbaum, Blen 1998).

Clinical Effects

An early publication reported that *T. diffusa* could be smoked to produce a brief state of euphoria (Lowry 1984), although there is no evidence to support this claim (Huang, Kinghorn, Farnsworth 1982).

Until recently, the effectiveness of *T. diffusa* as a sexual stimulant or psychoactive has been almost entirely anecdotal. However, a recent study of sexual function in women supports its effectiveness in combination with other herbal substances (Ito, Trant, Polan 2001). In a study of sexual potency in rats, *T. diffusa* extract improved the performance of sexually impotent male rats without affecting their general level of activity (Arletti, Benelli, Cavazzuti et al. 1999).

Availability

T. diffusa is available in a fluid extract or in capsules of between 380 to 450 mg (PDR 2000) and is also taken as a tea infusion (Lowry 1984).

Clinical Application in Veterinary Behavior Medicine

T. diffusa preparations may be useful to promote sexual performance in breeding animals. For example, it may heighten sexual interest in newly introduced breeding pairs, or to support the libido of breeders in unfamiliar environments. Although side effects have not been reported (PDR 2000), long-term studies and research into its mechanism of action are necessary before *T. diffusa* can be comfortably recommended for any medicinal properties.

References

Arletti R, Benelli A, Cavazzuti E et al. Stimulating property of *Turnera diffusa* and *Pfaffia paniculata* extracts on the sexual-behavior of male rats. Psychopharmacology (Berl). 1999;143:15–19.

Felter HW, Lloyd JU. King's American Dispensatory. Ohio Valley Company, Cincinatti, OH. 1898. Available online at http://www.ibiblio.org/herbmed/eclectic/kings/

Huang ZJ, Kinghorn AD, Farnsworth NR. J Pharm Sci. 1982;71:270–271.

Ito TY, Trant AS, Polan ML. A double-blind placebo-controlled study of ArginMax, a nutritional supplement for enhancement of female sexual function. J Sex Maritzl Ther. 2001;27:541–549.

Lowry TP. Damiana. J Psych Drugs. 1984;16:267–268.

Mills S, Bone K. Principles and Practice of Phytotherapy. Churchill Livingstone, Philadelphia, PA. 2000;234.

PDR for Herbal Medicines. (2nd ed) Medical Economics Company Inc., Montvale, NJ. 2000;244.

Russo E. Handbook of Psychotropic Herbs: A Scientific Analysis of Herbal Remedies for Psychiatric Conditions. The Haworth Press, Binghamton, NY. 2001;199–202.
Zava DT, Dollbaum CM, Blen M. Estrogen and progestin bioactivity of foods, herbs, and spices. Proc Soc Exp Biol Med. 1998;217:369–378.

Valeriana officinalis

The genus *Valerianae* has more than 200 species, many of which are used medicinally around the world. *Valeriana officinalis* (Valerian, Vandal Root, Amantilla, Setwall, Setewale, Heliotrope, Capon's Tail, Phu, Hokkai-Kisso, Baldrianwurzel, Baldrion) is found in Europe and in parts of Asia but is cultivated commercially across Europe, Japan, and the United States (Russo 2001; PDR 2000; Mills, Bone 2000). The plant grows 50 to 100 cm tall, although other subspecies may grow taller; it has an erect, unbranched stem with dentate leaflets on the leaves (Fig. 1-14). The fragrant hermaphrodite flowers are bright pink to white (see color

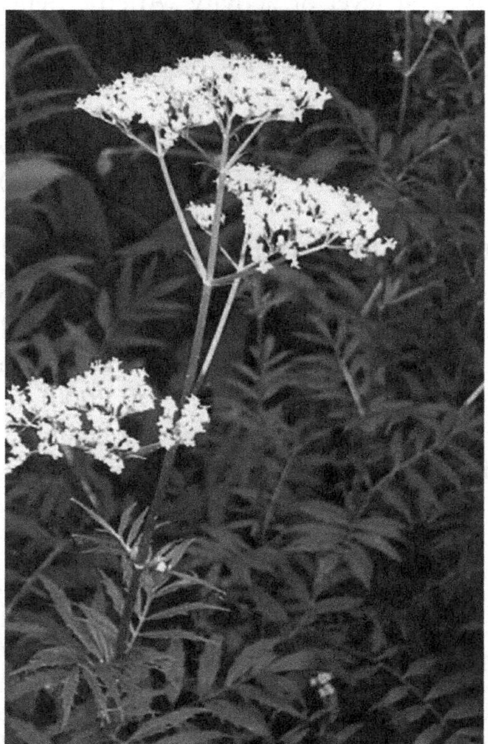

FIGURE 1-14. Flowers and leaves of *Valeriana officinalis.* (Photo courtesy of Dr. Susan Wynn)

Plate 1-5). The medicinal part of the plant is the root (rhizome), which is harvested in September and dried. The rhizome is short and unbranched. The plant prefers sandy, humus soil in low-lying, damp areas (Russo 2001; Mills, Bone 2000; PDR 2000).

The name *Valeriana* may derive from the Latin *valere* (well-being). However, ancient references refer to it as *phu*, which is probably an onomatopoeic reference to the odor of the dried root. The dried root acquires a characteristic, unpleasant odor attributed to isovaleric acid. The characteristic odor has been compared to the smell of sweaty socks and is apparently attractive to cats if not to people (Russo 2001; Foster 1996).

V. officinalis and other subspecies such as *V. wallichii* are well known in Ayurveda (Mills, Bone 2000). Internationally, researchers have been studying local subspecies of Valerianae and reports of biological activity similar to *V. officinalis* will likely reveal new perspectives on the potential of *Valerianae* for medicinal purposes.

Historical Perspective

During the 1800s, Shakers in New Hampshire marketed a preparation of valerian for "nervousness, lowness of spirits, debility . . . hysteria, restlessness . . . and every other disease arising from mental affection and nervous exhaustion" (Sumner 2000). Physicians of this period recommended it as an antispasmodic, anticonvulsant, stimulant, tonic and calmative. It was used to treat hypochondria and depression. They also reported side effects at higher doses that included "headache, mental excitement, visual illusions, giddiness, restlessness, agitation, and even spasmodic movements, and frequently nausea" (Felter, Lloyd 1898).

During World War II, it was recommended as a palliative treatment for stress associated with air raids. By then, barbiturates were gaining popularity and *V. officinalis* was omitted from the National Formulary of the United States and all but forgotten (Russo 2000; Sumner 2000; Wagner, Wagner, Hening 1998).

Ingredients

Plant compounds include iridoids (also known as the valepotriates, including valtrate, isovaltrate; 0.5–2%); volatile oils (e.g., monoterpenes; sesquiterpenes such as the pungent isovalerenic acid; 0.35-1.0%); nonvolatile sesquiterpenes (e.g., valerenic acid); pyridine alkaloids; caffeic acid derivatives (e.g., chlorogenic acid) (Fig. 1-15). Glutamine is also present in high concentrations in the extract (PDR 2000; Mills, Bone 2000; Houghton 1999). Other valerian subspecies contain varying amounts of active compounds. For example, the iridoid content is 3–8% in *V. edulis* (Mexican valerian) and 3–6% in *V. wallichii* (Indian valerian). Some compounds are unique to the subspecies. Valerenic acid, for instance, is characteristic of *V. officinalis*. The valepotriates are transformed into baldrinal and homobaldrinal, which have been shown to exert an antidepressant effect in mice

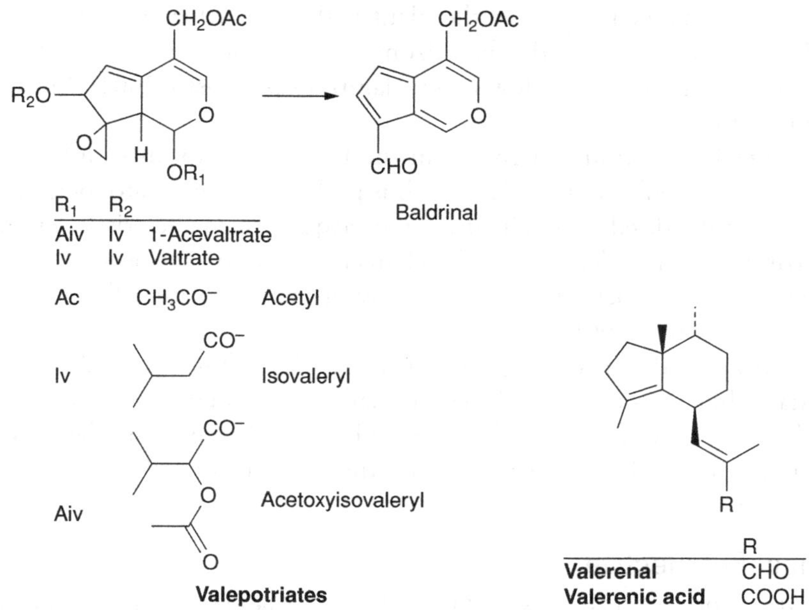

FIGURE 1-15. *Active compounds of Valeriana officinalis* (Mills, Bone 2000)

(Mills, Bone 2000; Houghton 1999; Wagner, Bladt 1996; von der Hude, Scheutwinkel-Reich, Braun 1986). New compounds continue to be discovered in Valeriana species (Marder, Viola, Wasowski et al. 2003; Tang, Liu, Yu 2003; Schumacher, Scholle, Holzl et al. 2002; Dharmaratne, Nanayakkara, Khan 2002). The metabolism of *V. officinalis* is not completely clear at this time (Russo 2000).

Valepotriates are thermolabile and decompose readily in low or high pH and in alcoholic solutions. *In vitro*, some have showed cytotoxicity, but this is not a concern with oral administration; gastric acidity breaks the unstable valepotriates into safer metabolites (Mills, Bone 2000).

In a recent study in Australia, 31 different commercial preparations of *V. officinalis* were analyzed for the concentration of their active ingredients, specifically the valepotriates, valerenic acid, and valerenic acid derivatives. Valepotriates were undetectable in most products. The mean concentration of valerenic acid ranged from 0.8 mg/g to 3.56 mg/g. An important variation in active components existed between products (Shohet, Wills, Stuart 2001). Although commercial herbal preparations should be better standardized and quality-controlled, there are additional complications to consider. The contents of valerenic acid derivatives and valepotriates in roots of different species, varieties, and individuals of *Valeriana spp.* cultivated under the same environmental conditions were analyzed (Gao, Bjork 2000). Content of valerenic acid derivatives (11.65–0.15 mg/g) and valepotriates (1.81–0.03 mg/g) varied markedly between species or varieties of Valerianae. The variation of valerenic acid derivatives (12.34–3.01 mg/g) and valepotriates (3.67–0.92 mg/g) between individuals of one commercial cultivar of *V. officinalis* were also significant (Gao, Bjork 2000). In a Dutch study, seasonal variations of *V. officinalis* components were analyzed (Bos, Woerdenbag, van Putten et al. 1998). Based on their findings, it was recommended to harvest plants in the September after planting when the content of *V. officinalis* root essential oil is highest. Valepotriates peak in March of the spring following planting.

CNS Effects

The pharmacological effects of *V. officinalis* extract and valerenic acid appear to be mediated through modulation of $GABA_A$ receptor function (Yuan, Mehendale, Xiao et al. 2004). Experiments have shown that *V. officinalis* extract, principally valerenic acid, increases the availability of GABA by inhibiting its reuptake by as much as 50%, decreasing its degradation, and increasing its release by induction of Ca++ channels. Glutamine in the extract is more easily transported across the blood-brain barrier and converted directly to GABA. *V. officinalis*' GABAergic effect is therefore both direct and indirect (PDR 2000; Santos, Ferreira, Cunha et al. 1994a,b; Santos, Ferreira, Faro et al. 1994). Elsewhere, four lignans were isolated from *V. officinalis* root and tested for their relative affinities for $5\text{-}HT_{1A}$-, $GABA_A$-, benzodiazepine, and μ-opiate-receptors. Lignans showed affinity for the $5\text{-}HT_{1A}$ and μ-opiate receptors, and one lignan had a particular affinity for the $5\text{-}HT_{1A}$ receptor (Bodesheim, Holzl 1997).

A murine study compared a commercially available *V. officinalis* root extract with diazepam and chlorpromazine. Sedative activity of the extract was moderate and anticonvulsant properties were minimal (Leschner, Muller, Rudmann 1993). However, in a clinical, placebo-controlled study of 121 human insomniacs, subjects positively rated a standardized 70% ethanol extract of *V. officinalis* root containing 0.4–0.6% valerenic acid more than double the rating of placebo at the end of the 28-day trial (Vorbach, Gortelmeyer, Bruning 1996).

In a small, poorly designed study of 12 healthy subjects, electroencephalographic measurements were documented at a low (500 mg *V. officinalis* and 120 mg *Humulus lupulus*) and high dose (1500 mg *V. officinalis* and 360 mg *H. lupulus*) of a mixture of *V. officinalis* and *H. lupulus*, and compared to placebo. The higher dose produced significant increases in delta (slow wave), decreases in alpha and a weak decrease in beta-wave activity (Vonderheid-Guth, Todorova, Brattstrom et al. 2000). It is unfortunate that the herbs were not studied alone or in sequence so that results could be more clearly interpreted.

Miscellaneous Effects

In cats, intravenous injection of 50 mg/kg had a bradycardic and hypotensive effect, although another feline study determined no pharamacologic activity at a dose of 250 mg/kg. Sporadic reports of valerian ingestion in pets were typically not associated with adverse effects, although one cat experienced lethargy and sedation (Means 2002).

Behavioral and Psychological Effects

V. officinalis extract is a CNS depressant, sedative, and anxiolytic (PDR 2000). In studies on mice, extract from a Japanese valerian subspecies demonstrated an antidepressant effect (Oshima, Matsuoka, Ohizumi 1995; Sakamoto, Mitani, Nakajima 1992). In cats, valepotriates had anxiolytic and antiaggressive properties (von Eickstedt, Rahman 1969).

Patients with coexisting signs of depression and anxiety may respond better to a combination of *V. officinalis* with *Hypericum perforatum* (St. John's wort) compared to those treated with *H. perforatum* alone (Muller, Pfeil, von den Driesch 2003). A number of earlier studies indicated that this herbal combination was equivalent to amitriptyline and desipramine (Mills, Bone 2000); however, the mechanism of action is unclear.

The use of *V. officinalis* extract alone or in combination with other herbal sedatives such as *Melissa officinalis* (Lemon Balm) or *Passiflora incarnata* (Passionflower) may facilitate withdrawal from long-term use of benzodiazepines (Mills, Bone 2000; Brown 1994).

The odor of *V. officinalis* oil reduced stress-induced plasma corticosterone levels in the skin of mice subjected to stress, suggesting that odorant inhalation may modify various physiological pathways (Hosoi, Tanida, Tsuchiya 2001). In a placebo-controlled study, 54 subjects were evaluated for physiological signs of stress (heart rate, blood pressure) and subjective ratings of pressure during psychometric testing. *V. officinalis* was slightly more beneficial than *Piper methysticum* (kava) compared to the placebo group, which showed no significant improvement (Cropley, Cave, Ellis et al. 2002).

Hypnotic Effects

In people, *V. officinalis* is used primarily as a hypnotic (PDR 2000). In a recent study, a Mexican subspecies of valerian was shown to possess a significant hypnotic effect comparable to *V. officinalis* (Herrera-Arellano, Luna-Villegas, Cuevas-Uriostegui et al. 2001). Another study focused on pharmacological activity of *V. adscendens* extract harvested in the Andes (Capasso, de Feo, de Simone et al. 1996). Two newly discovered active compounds isolated from *V. wallichii*, hesperidin and 6-methylapigenin, have sleep-enhancing properties that appear to be synergistic. Hesperidin has sedative and sleep-inducing properties; 6-methylapigenin has anxiolytic effects (Marder, Viola, Wasowski et al. 2003). Synergistic mechanisms between compounds within a plant's chemical makeup appear to potentiate the overall effect of herbal extracts, including *Piper methysticum*, *Hypericum perforatum*, and *V. officinalis* (Spinella 2002; Williamson 2001; Russo 2000).

Although some indicate *V. officinalis* may take several weeks to take effect as a hypnotic in people (Russo 2000), other data suggest that its use as a sleep-aid may be more dose dependent. In a meta-analysis of nine sleep trials using *V. officinalis*, results were often contradictory, and inconsistencies between trials in terms of patients, experimental design, and procedures and methodological quality precluded conclusions regarding the hypnotic effect of *V. officinalis* (Stevinson, Ernst 2000). Nonetheless, the hypnotic effect of *V. officinalis* is thought to be promising, although long-term studies with higher numbers of subjects are warranted (Gyllenhaal, Merritt, Peterson et al. 2000).

In a recent study of treatment of insomnia in the elderly, *V. officinalis* (400 and 800 mg) was compared to temazepam and diphenhydramine in 14 elderly volunteers ranging in age from 65 to 89 years old. *V. officinalis* was equivalent to placebo on measures of psychomotor performance and sedation (Glass, Sproule, Herrmann et al. 2003). In contrast, in a clinical study of 202 insomniacs ranging in age from 18 to 73 years, a six-week course of *V. officinalis* extract (600 mg per diem) was equivalent to 10 mg per diem of oxazepam in the treatment of insomnia (Ziegler, Ploch, Miettinen-Baumann et al. 2002).

V. officinalis (600 mg at bedtime) was prescribed for stress-induced insomnia over a six-week period and was reported to be effective. Vivid dreaming was the most commonly reported adverse effect associated with *V. officinalis*, reported in 16% of the subjects tested (Wheatley 2001). In another sleep study, *V. officinalis* was more effective than placebo and showed a significantly lower frequency of side effects (3%) compared to placebo (18%) (Donath, Quispe, Diefenbach 2000).

Triazolam (Halcion®; 0.125 mg tab), a commonly prescribed benzodiazepine sleep-inducer, was compared to a mixture of *V. officinalis* root (160 mg) and *Melissa officinalis* (Lemon Balm) extract (80 mg) in tablet form (Dressing, Reimann, Low et al. 1992). Both treatments were effective sleep inducers; however, the herbal mixture of *V. officinalis* and *M. officinalis* was not associated with sedation or cognitive changes the next day. Unlike the benzodiazepine hypnotics, *V. officinalis* is not associated with addiction, withdrawal, or a morning-after "hangover" (Russo 2000; Brown 1994).

Miscellaneous Effects

V. officinalis has been used to treat menstrual "states," pregnancy, uterine spasticity, menopause, fainting, muscle cramps due to nervousness, and colic. It possesses antispasmodic, muscle relaxant, and anti-ulcer properties (PDR 2000). Its antispasmodic effect has been attributed to relaxation of smooth muscle and not by interaction with autonomic receptors (Hazelhoff, Malingre, Meijer 1982).

Preliminary findings indicate that *V. officinalis* has important antimicrobial activity (Murakami, Ye, Kawanishi et al. 2002; von der Hude, Scheutwinkel-Reich, Braun 1986). The valepotriate metabolites baldrinal and homobaldrinal exhibited genotoxic activity against Salmonella, suggestive of their cytotoxic potential.

However, orally administered valepotriates were innocuous in pregnant rats and their offspring, although some toxic effects were noted with intraperitoneal routes of administration (Tufik, Fujita, De Seabra et al. 1994). Recently, *V. officinalis* root extract has been shown to have a promising inhibitory effect *in vitro* against the HIV virus without injuring host cells (Murakami, Ye, Kawanishi et al. 2002).

Some evidence suggests that attention deficit hyperactivity disorder (ADHD) may respond to *V. officinalis*; however, no controlled or long-term studies have confirmed this (Valpiani 1995; Russo 2000). In a placebo-controlled study of five children with intellectual deficits and varying degrees of hyperactivity, an eight-week trial of *V. officinalis* treatment reduced sleep latency and nocturnal time awake, lengthened total sleep time, and improved sleep quality (Francis, Dempster 2002).

Adverse Effects and Drug Interactions

V. officinalis may potentiate anesthetic sedation and other drugs that target GABA receptors. The potential for drug interaction in presurgical candidates is very real, and patients undergoing surgery must be carefully screened for use of synthetic or natural medicines (Yuan, Mehendale, Xiao et al. 2004). Animal studies have shown that *V. officinalis* extract potentiates the effect of barbiturates and benzodiazepines, a finding that is consistent with its affinity for $GABA_A$-benzodiazepine receptor complexes (Hiller, Zetler 1996; Leuschner, Muller, Rudmann 1993).

In one study (Ortiz, Nieves-Natal, Chavez 1999), *V. officinalis* extract enhanced benzodiazepine binding. Using flunitrazepam, *V. officinalis* displayed a biphasic interaction, potentiating binding at lower doses and inhibiting it at higher concentrations. This biphasic interaction was also demonstrated with the inhibition of GABA reuptake by *V. officinalis* extracts. These results suggest that there are at least two distinct biological activities by *V. officinalis* at benzodiazepine and GABA receptor sites. In some individuals, *V. officinalis* can act as a stimulant and should be avoided (Mills, Bone 2000; Tillotson, Tillotson, Abel 2001; Stevens 1909). This may be partly explained by the biphasic effect on diazepine and GABAergic systems at higher doses, or it could be an idiosyncratic response.

Although adverse effects are rare at the recommended therapeutic dosages, gastrointestinal upset, contact allergy, headache, restlessness, sleeplessness, mydriasis, and cardiac effects have been reported (PDR 2000; Garges, Varia, Doraiswamy 1998). One case of "overdose" was reported following consumption of 20 times the recommended therapeutic dose (estimated 20 g of powdered valerian were ingested by an 18-year-old). Clinical signs of fatigue, lightheadedness, and complaints of abdominal and chest discomfort were considered mild, and laboratory data (hemogram, serum biochemistry, UA, ECG) were unremarkable. Activated charcoal was administered and symptoms resolved within 24 hours (Willey, Mady, Cobaugh 1995). In a poorly documented case report, the possibility of delayed cardiotoxicity in a commercial mixture containing *V. officinalis*, cyproheptadine (H-1 antihistamine with sedative effects), and hyoscine (an atropine derivative) was described (Chan TY, Tang CH, Critchley 1995). This observation is inconclusive because the patient described had preexisting cardiovascular disease and was taking large doses of the herbal cocktail several times a day (Murakami, Ye, Kawanishi et al. 2002). A clinical report of three drug abusers who experimented with an intravenous cocktail of *V. officinalis* and *Lactuca virosa* (Wild Lettuce) describes systematic adverse reactions that included fever, abdominal and back pain, neck stiffness, headache, leucocytosis, and mild liver function abnormalities. All recovered within three days (Mullins, Horowitz 1998).

Although earlier studies have not determined any additive effect between *V. officinalis* and alcohol (Mayer, Springer 1974; Mills, Bone 2000), *V. officinalis* should not be combined with alcohol or the operation of motor vehicles and other machinery without further study (PDR 2000).

Herbal sedatives such as *V. officinalis*, *Piper methysticum*, *Matricaria chamomilla* and *Passiflora incarnata* should not be used concomitantly with antiepileptic medications because of possible potentiation of their sedative and cognitive effects (Spinella 2001).

V. officinalis is approved for use in the United States as a nutritional supplement. In Europe, the only restriction on its use is for children younger than three years of age. ESCOP advises caution by those taking valerian during operation of machinery or motor vehicles. Neither ESCOP nor the German Commission E note any adverse effects or drug interactions (Russo 2000; Mills, Bone 2000). Nonetheless, in the absence of long-term clinical trials, the use of compounds that contain *V. officinalis* is inadvisable during pregnancy or lactation.

Availability

V. officinalis is available for use internally in the form of tincture, extracts, fresh juice, and other preparations. It is also available as a bath additive, although this use has not been validated (Ammer, Melnizky 1999). Capsules are available in 100 mg, 250 mg, 380 mg, 400 mg, 445 mg, 450 mg, 475 mg, 493 mg, 500 mg, 530 mg, 550 mg, and 1000 mg. Tablets are currently marketed in 160 mg and 550 mg. The recommended dosage varies with the preparation and use, ranging between 100 mg to 1800 mg of *V. officinalis* extract (15 g of root powder per diem). The dosage for restlessness is 220 mg of extract TID. The hypnotic dosage is 400 mg to 900 mg of extract 30 minutes before bedtime. Teas are also widely available and the dosage recommended is one cup (150 ml) BID or TID or PRN at bedtime (PDR 2000).

Commercial preparations of *V. officinalis* extract are projected to cost less than a monthly supply of prescription hypnotics, although diphenhydramine is an OTC antihistamine with hypnotic effects and is also quite inexpensive (Russo 2000).

V. officinalis tinctures and extracts should be stored at room temperature in tightly sealed containers. The use of nonplastic containers is not advised. All preparations must be protected from exposure to light (PDR 2000). A minimum of 0.5% volatile oil content is required for medicinal preparations of *V. officinalis* root (ESCOP Monograph 1992).

Clinical Application in Veterinary Behavior Medicine

V. officinalis may be beneficial in cases of feline aggression accompanied by anxiety. This is commonly seen, for example, in cases of social aggression between feline housemates secondary to redirected fear aggression or redirected territorial aggression triggered by another animal approaching the home. It could also be helpful in introducing new house pets to each other. The herbal combination of *V. officinalis* with *Hypericum perforatum* may have effects comparable to amitriptyline, a tricyclic antidepressant commonly used in veterinary behavior practice. This mixture could be effective, for example, in cases of feline house soiling and feline or canine separation anxiety syndrome.

Based upon reports of its hypnotic and stress-relieving effects, *V. officinalis*, used alone or in combination with *Melissa officinalis*, could be applied to cases of inconvenient crepuscular and nocturnal play in young cats, or in pups adjusting to the first nights in a new home.

References

Ammer K, Melnizky P. Medicinal baths for treatment of generalized fibromyalgia. Forsch Komplementarmed. 1999;6:80–85.

Bodesheim U, Holzl J. Isolation and receptor binding properties of alkaloids and lignans from Valeriana officialis Pharmazie. 1997;52:386–391.

Bos R, Woerdenbag HJ, van Putten FMS et al. Seasonal variation of the essential oil, valerenic acid and derivatives, and valepotriates in *Valeriana officinalis* roots and rhizomes, and the selection of plants suitable for phytomedicines. Planta Med. 1998;64:143–147.

Brown DJ. Valerian root: non-addictive alternative for insomnia and anxiety. Quart Rev Nat Med. 1994; 221-224.

Capasso A, de Feo V, de Simone F et al. Pharmacological effects of aqueous extracts from Valeriana adsendens. Phytother Res. 1996;10:309–312.

Chan TY, Tang CH, Critchley JA. Poisoning due to an over-the-counter hypnotic, Sleep-Qik (hyoscine, cyproheptadine, valerian). Postgrad Med J. 1995;71:227–228.

Cropley M, Cave Z, Ellis J et al. Effect of kava and valerian on human physiological and psychological responses to mental stress assessed under laboratory conditions. Phytother Res. 2002;16:23–27.

Dharmaratne HR, Nanayakkara NP, Khan IA. (-)-3 beta,4 beta-epoxyvalerenic acid from *Valeriana officinalis*. Planta Med. 2002;68:661–662.

Donath F, Quispe S, Diefenbach K et al. Critical evaluation of the effect of valerian extract on sleep structure and sleep quality. Pharmacopsychiatry. 2000;33:47–53.

Dressing H, Riemann D, Low H et al. Insomnia: Are valerian/lemon balm combination of equal value to benzodiazepine? Therapiewoche. 1992;42:726–736.

ESCOP (European Scientific Cooperative for Phytotherapy). *Valerianae Radix*. European Monograph, 1992.

Felter HW, Lloyd JU. King's American Dispensatory. Ohio Valley Company, Cincinatti, OH. 1898. Available online at http://www.ibiblio.org/herbmed/eclectic/kings/

Foster S. *Valerian*: *Valeriana officinalis*. Austin, TX: American Botanical Council. 1996.

Francis AJ, Dempster RJ. Effect of valerian, *Valeriana edulis*, on sleep difficulties in children with intellectual deficits: randomised trial. Phytomedicine. 2002;9:273–279.

Gao XQ, Bjork L. Valerenic acid derivatives and valepotriates among individuals, varieties and species of Valeriana. Fitoterapia. 2000;71:19–24.

Garges HP, Varia I, Doraiswamy PM. Cardiac complications and delirium associated with valerian root withdrawal. JAMA. 1998;280:1566–1567.

Glass JR, Sproule BA, Herrmann N et al. Acute pharmacological effects of temazepam, diphenhydramine, and valerian in healthy elderly subjects. J Clin Psychopharmacol. 2003;23:260–268.

Gyllenhaal C, Merritt SL, Peterson SD et al. Efficacy and safety of herbal stimulants and sedatives in sleep disorders. Sleep Med Rev. 2000;4:229–251.

Hazelhoff B, Malingre TM, Meijer DK. Antispasmodic effects of valeriana compounds: an in-vivo and in-vitro study on the guinea-pig ileum. Arch Int Pharmacodyn Ther. 1982;257:274-287.

Herrera-Arellano A, Luna-Villegas G, Cuevas-Uriostegui ML et al. Polysomnographic evaluation of the hypnotic effect of *Valeriana edulis* standardized extract in patients suffering from insomnia. Planta Med. 2001;67:695–699.

Hiller KO, Zetler G. Neuropharmacological studies on ethanol extracts of *Valeriana officinalis*: behavioural, anticonvulsant properties. Phytotherapy Res. 1996;10:145–151.

Hosoi J, Tanida M, Tsuchiya T. Mitigation of stress-induced suppression of contact hypersensitivity by odorant inhalation. Br J Dermatol. 2001;145:716–719.

Houghton PJ. The scientific basis for the reputed activity of Valerian. J Pharm Pharmacol. 1999;51: 505–512.

Leuschner J, Muller J, Rudmann M. Characterisation of the central nervous depressant activity of a commercially available valerian root extract. Arzneimittelforschung. 1993;43:638–641.

Marder M, Viola H, Wasowski C et al. 6-Methylapigenin and hesperidin: new valeriana flavonoids with activity on the CNS. Pharmacol Biochem Behav. 2003;75:537–545.

Mayer B, Springer E. Psychoexperimental studies on the effect of a valepotriate combination as well as the combined effects of valtratum and alcohol. Arzneimittelforschung. 1974;24:2066–2070.

Means C. Selected herbal hazards. Vet Clin Small Anim Pract. 2002;32:367–382.

Mills S, Bone K. Principles and Practice of Phytotherapy. Churchill Livingstone, Philadelphia, PA. 2000;581–589.

Mullins ME, Horowitz BZ. The case of the salad shooters: intravenous injection of wild lettuce extract. Vet Hum Toxicol. 1998;40:290–291.

Muller D, Pfeil T, von den Driesch V. Treating depression comorbid with anxiety: results of an open, practice-oriented study with St John's wort WS 5572 and valerian extract in high doses. Phytomedicine. 2003;10(Suppl 4):25–30.

Murakami N, Ye Y, Kawanishi M et al. New Rev-transport inhibitor with anti-HIV activity from *Valerianae Radix*. Bioorg Med Chem Lett. 2002;12:2807–2810.

Ortiz JG, Nieves-Natal J, Chavez P. Effects of *Valeriana officinalis* extracts on [3H]flunitrazepam binding, synaptosomal [3H]GABA uptake, and hippocampal [3H]GABA release. Neurochem Res. 1999; 24:1373–1378.

Oshima Y, Matsuoka S, Ohizumi Y. Antidepressant principles of Valeriana fauriei roots. Chem Pharm Bull (Tokyo). 1995;43:169–170.

PDR for Herbal Medicines. (2nd ed) Medical Economics Company Inc., Montvale, NJ. 2000;783–786.

Russo E. Handbook of Psychotropic Herbs: A Scientific Analysis of Herbal Remedies for Psychiatric Conditions. The Haworth Press, Binghamton, NY. 2001;95–106.

Santos MS, Ferreira F, Cunha AP et al. Synaptosomal GABA release as influenced by valerian root extract: involvement of the GABA carrier. Arch Int Pharmacodyn Ther. 1994;327:220–231.

Santos MS, Ferreira F, Cunha AP et al. An aqueous extract of valerian influences the transport of GABA in synaptosomes. Planta Med. 1994;60:278–279.

Santos MS, Ferreira F, Faro C et al. The amount of GABA present in aqueous extracts of valerian is sufficient to account for [3H]GABA release in synaptosomes. Planta Med. 1994;60:475–476.

Sakamoto T, Mitani Y, Nakajima K. Psychotropic effects of Japanese valerian root extract. Chem Pharm Bull (Tokyo). 1992;40:758–761.

Schumacher B, Scholle S, Holzl J et al. Lignans isolated from valerian: identification and characterization of a new olivil derivative with partial agonistic activity at A(1) adenosine receptors. J Nat Prod. 2002;65:1479–1485.

Shohet D, Wills RB, Stuart DL. Valepotriates and valerenic acids in commercial preparations of valerian available in Australia. Pharmazie. 2001;56:860–863.

Spinella M. Herbal Medicines and Epilepsy: The Potential for Benefit and Adverse Effects. Epilepsy Behav. 2001;2:524–532.

Spinella M. The importance of pharmacological synergy in psychoactive herbal medicines. Altern Med Rev. 2002;7:130–137.

Stevinson C, Ernst E. Valerian for insomnia: a systematic review of randomized clinical trials. Sleep Med. 2000;1:91–99.

Stevens AA. Modern Materia Medica and Therapeutics. (5th ed) W.B.Saunders Co., Philadelphia, PA. 1909;135–136.

Sumner J. The natural history of medicinal plants. Timber Press, Portland, OR. 2000;176.

Tang Y, Liu X, Yu B. Iridoids from the rhizomes and roots of *Valeriana jatamansi.* J Nat Prod. 2002; 65:1949–1952.

Tillotson AK, Tillotson HS, Abel R. The One Earth Herbal sourcebook. Kensington Publishing, New York, NY 2001;222–223.

Tufik S, Fujita K, de Seabra ML et al. Effects of a prolonged administration of valepotriates in rats on the mothers and their offspring. J Ethnopharmacol. 1994;41:39–44.

Valpiani C. *Valeriana officinalis.* Austral Trad Med Soc J. 1995;1:57–62.

von der Hude W, Scheutwinkel-Reich M, Braun R. Bacterial mutagenicity of the tranquilizing constituents of Valerianaceae roots. Mutat Res. 1986;169:23–27.

von Eickstedt KW, Rahman S. Psychopharmacologic effect of valepotriates. Arzneimittelforschung.1969;19:316–319.

Vonderheid-Guth B, Todorova A, Brattstrom A et al. Pharmacodynamic effects of valerian and hops extract combination (Ze 91019) on the quantitative-topographical EEG in healthy volunteers. Eur J Med Res. 2000;5:139–144.

Vorbach EU, Gortelmeyer R, Bruning J. Therapie von Insomnien. Wirksamkeit und Vertraeglichkeit eine Baldrianpraeparats. Psychopharmakotherapie. 1996;3:109–115.

Wagner H, Bladt S. Plant drug analysis: a thin layer chromatography atlas.(2nd ed) Springer-Verlag, Berlin. 1996:342–344.

Wagner J, Wagner ML, Hening WA. Beyond benzodiazepines: alternative pharmacologic agents for the treatment of insomnia. Ann Pharmacother. 1998;32:680–691.

Wheatley D. Kava and valerian in the treatment of stress-induced insomnia. Phytother Res. 2001;15: 549–551.

Willey LB, Mady SP, Cobaugh DJ. Valerian overdose: a case report. Vet Hum Toxicol. 1995;37:364–365.

Williamson EM. Synergy and other interactions in phytomedicines. Phytomedicine. 2001;8:401–409.

Yuan CS, Mehendale S, Xiao Y et al. The gamma-aminobutyric acidergic effects of valerian and valerenic acid on rat brainstem neuronal activity. Anesth Analg. 2004;98:353–358.

Ziegler G, Plich M, Miettinen-Baumann A et al. Efficacy and tolerability of valerian extract LI 156 compared with oxazepam in the treatment of non-organic insomnia: a randomized, double-blind, comparative clinical study. Eur J Med Res. 2002;7:480–486.

Verbena spp. (V. officinalis, V. hastata)

Verbena officinalis (Enchanter's Plant, Herb of the Cross, Herb of Grace, Juno's Tears, Pigeons' Grass, Pigeonweed, Simpler's Joy, Vervain) is a flowering herb na-

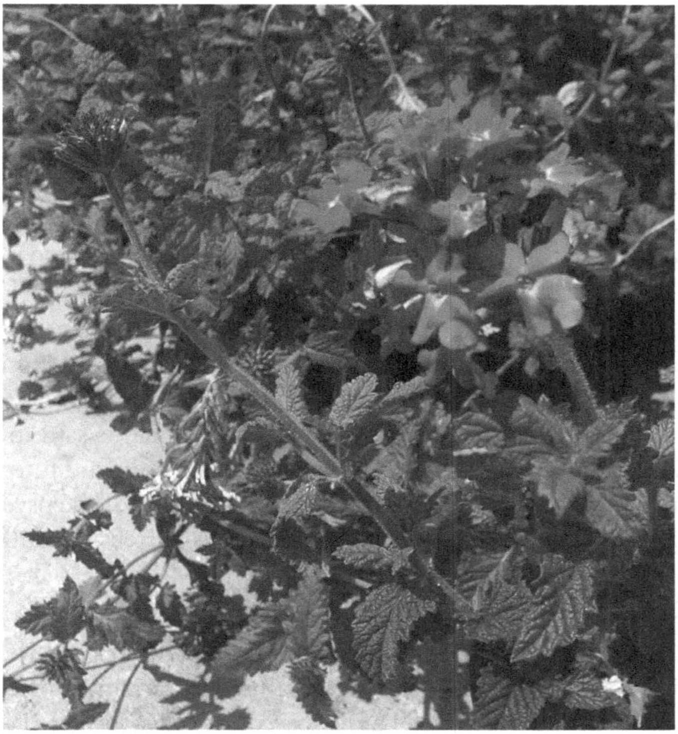

FIGURE 1-16. *Verbena canadensis* hybrid in bloom. (Photo courtesy of Dr. Stefanie Schwartz)

tive to the Mediterranean. It grows wild and is also a favorite among gardeners. Varieties may be annual, biennial, or perennial. Its soft green leaves are wrinkled, oblong in shape, and have bristles (Fig. 1-16). The lavender flowers of *V. officinalis* are small and arranged along the branches. The medicinal parts of *Verbena spp.* consist of the dried aerial parts. The herb is cultivated commercially in Eastern Europe. The plant is harvested during bloom time and hung to dry (PDR 2000). This plant, like *Vitex agnus-castus* (Chaste tree), is a member of the *Verbenaceae* family (del Pozo, Gastaminza, Navarro et al. 1994).

Historical Perspective

Traditionally, *Verbena* has been used for a myriad of medical complaints including digestive (oral, pharyngeal, liver, gallbladder), renal (urinary tract, kidney), dermatological (pruritus, burns), respiratory (coughs, asthma, whooping cough), gynecological (postpartum depression, lactation, dysmenorrhea, irregular menstruation, menopause), orthopedic (rheumatism, gout) and psychological (nervousness, hysteria, anxiety) symptoms. It has been used in the West as well as in traditional Chinese medicine (TCM) (Russo 2001; PDR 2000; Mills, Bone 2000; Grases, Melero, Costa-Bauza et al. 1994; Felter, Lloyd 1898).

Native Americans used several Verbena species. For example, *Verbena hastata* (Blue Vervain, Swamp Verbena) was in widespread use (and for many of the same symptoms noted above) among the Cherokee, Iroquois, Chippewa, Dakota, and Delaware tribes and others (Moerman 2000). Herbalists believe that Verbena restores balance to the nervous system ("nervine tonic") and often prescribe it for anxiety, "hysteria," nervous exhaustion, and depression (Russo 2001; Mills, Bone 2000).

Verbena spp. should not be confused with *Aloysia triphylla* (Lemon Verbena), a native shrub of South America with lemon-scented leaves that is cultivated in the Mediterranean and other warm countries (PDR 2000). The dried leaves and stems are the source of the medicinal oil of vervain, which is said to be antispasmodic and sedative. Bioactive components include apigenin and luteolin (Carnat, Carnat, Chavignon et al. 1995). Published data in support of the psychoactive use of *Aloysia triphylla* in veterinary behavior medicine is currently insufficient.

Ingredients

Identified components include the iridoide monoterpenes (e.g., verbenalin, dihydroverbenalin, hastatoside), flavonoids (e.g., luteolin, artemitin, nepein, scutellarin), and caffeic acid derivatives (e.g., verbascoside, eucovoside) (PDR 2000).

Clinical Effects

Verbenalin has proven use for its antitussive and lactogenic properties. Verbena also has recognized benefits to improve edema and has mild analgesic, cytotoxic, and antitumoral properties (PDR 2000). Verbenalin, hastatoside, and verbascoside were among *V. officinalis* extract components that exhibited anti-inflammatory activity (Deepak, Handa 2000).

V. officinalis appears to have particular binding affinity for estradiol and progesterone as do other popular herbs (Zava, Dollbaum, Blen 1998).

In a recent Japanese study, an aqueous extract of *V. hastata* in rats prolonged the hypnotic effect of pentobarbital and was reversed by flumazenil, substantiating its use as a sedative (Akanum, Honda, Inoue 2002).

Species of Verbena native to India (*V. hybrida* and *V. bonariensis*) were among several plants with promising contraceptive properties in laboratory animals (Prakash 1985).

Adverse Effects

Toxic effects of *Verbena spp.* are few; however, allergic reactions including anaphylaxis triggered by contact hypersensitivity have been reported (Potter, Mather, Lockey et al. 1995; del Pozo, Gastaminza, Navarro et al. 1994).

Availability

Verbena officinalis is available as a powder, liquid extract (2 to 4 ml per diem), and tincture (5–10 ml SID-TID). The dried herb may be consumed as an herbal tea (2 to 4 gm SID-TID) (PDR 2000).

Clinical Application in Veterinary Behavior Medicine

Laboratory evidence is sparse regarding psychoactive properties of *Verbena spp.*, and the absence of clinical studies does not suggest its usefulness in clinical practice at this time. Nevertheless, it might be helpful in controlling urinary incontinence associated with estrogen deficiency in dogs.

References

Akanmu MA, Honda K, Inoue S. Hypnotic effects of total aqueous extracts of Verbain hastate (*Verbenaceae*) in rats. Psychiatry Clin Neurosci. 2002;56:309–310.

Carnat A, Carnat AP, Chavignon O et al. Luteolin 7-diglucuronide, the major flavonoid compound from *Aloysia triphylla* and *Verbena officinalis*. Planta Med. 1995;61:490.

Deepak M, Handa SS. Antiinflammatory activity and chemical composition of extracts of *Verbena officinalis*. Phytother Res. 2000;14:463–465.

del Pozo MD, Gastaminza G, Navarro JA et al. Allergic contact dermatitis from *Verbena officinalis*. Contact Dermatitis. 1994;31:200–201.

Felter HW, Lloyd JU. King's American Dispensatory. Ohio Valley Company, Cincinatti, OH. 1898. Available online at http://www.ibiblio.org/herbmed/eclectic/kings/

Grases F, Melero G, Costa-Bauza A et al. Urolithiasis and phytotherapy. Int Urol Nephrol. 1994;26: 507–511.

Mills S, Bone K. Principles and Practice of Phytotherapy. Churchill Livingstone, Philadelphia, PA. 2000;234, 246.

Moerman DE. Native American Ethnobotany. Timber Press, Portland, OR. 2002;591–592.

PDR for Herbal Medicines. (2nd ed) Medical Economics Company Inc., Montvale, NJ. 2000;788–789.

Potter PC, Mather S, Lockey P et al. Immediate and delayed contact hypersensitivity to verbena plants. Contact Dermatitis. 1995;33:343–346.

Prakash AO. Biological evaluation of some medicinal plant extracts for contraceptive efficacy in females. Contracept Fertil Sex (Paris). 1985;13:649–655.

Russo E. Handbook of Psychotropic Herbs: A Scientific Analysis of Herbal Remedies for Psychiatric Conditions. The Haworth Press, Binghamton, NY. 2001;275–276.

Zava DT, Dollbaum CM, Blen M. Estrogen and progestin bioactivity of foods, herbs, and spices. Proc Soc Exp Biol Med. 1998;217:369–378.

Vitex agnus-castus

Vitex agnus-castus is a small tree that grows as high as 5 to 6 m in height. A member of the verbena family (*Verbenaceae*), it is native to the Mediterranean basin and is found as far as western Asia (Mills, Bone 2000; PDR 2000). Alternative names include the Chaste Tree, Chasteberry, Monk's pepper, agneau chaste, gatillier, and keuschlammfruchte (Mills, Bone 2000). The deciduous leaves are palmate, with lance-like leaflets as long as 10 cm. The violet flowers give way to round black berries measuring about 5 mm. The medicinal parts of *V. agnus-castus* are the fruit and leaves, which are dried (Mills, Bone 2000; PDR 2000).

Traditionally, dried *V. agnus-castus* berries and leaves have been used to treat depression, sleep disorders, gynecological complaints (e.g., dysmenorrhea, endometriosis, PMS, menopause) (Fugh-Berman, Kronenberg 2003; Loch, Selle, Boblitz 2000; Hardy 2000), lactation disorders, anxiety (Kuruuzum-Uz, Stroch, Demirezer et al. 2003), acne, and flatulence. Insufficient milk production remains the most common traditional application. *V. agnus-castus* has also been used to improve libido in both genders and to suppress appetite (PDR 2000; Mills, Bone 2000).

Historical Perspective

Around 400 BC, Hippocrates recommended *V. agnus-castus* for the treatment of various injuries, inflammation, and enlargement of the spleen. Persian texts of the ninth and twelfth centuries mentioned its use for the control of insanity, "madness," and epilepsy. *V. agnus-castus* first appeared in Welsh medical journals after the early thirteenth century (Hobbs 1991). In the Middle Ages, ripe, chaste berries were used to suppress sexual urges and became a symbol of chastity. Monks used the dried fruit to control their libidinal tendencies, and its peppery taste made it useful as a pepper substitute. Its use continued for the treatment of gynecological disorders into the mid-1900s (Mills, Bone 2000). By the end of the eighteenth century, the use of *V. agnus-castus* in England had waned but regained popularity there in the 1800s. Elsewhere in Europe, it retained its popularity. By the 1950s, *V. agnus-castus* drew the interest of the scientific community (Hobbs 1991).

Ingredients

V. agnus-castus extract contains iridoid glycosides (e.g., aucubin, agnoside), monoterpenes, sesquiterpenes (in the essential oil), and flavonoid compounds (PDR 2000; Mills, Bone 2000). Casticin, a methoxylated flavone (Mills, Bone 2000), and cytotoxic flavonoids (Hirobe, Qiao, Takeya et al. 1997) have been identified in *V. agnus-castus* (Fig. 1-17). A Greek study of native *V. agnus-castus* showed that the extraction technique is critical to the quality of essential oil obtained from the plant (Sorensen, Katsiotis 2000).

Vitex Species in Eastern Medicine

V. agnus-castus has not been used in either Traditional Chinese Medicine or in Ayurvedic medicine, however other Asian Vitex species are well-known to Eastern traditions. For example, the Indian native *V. negundo* is discussed at length in the section on Ayurvedic herbs.

V. peduncularis, a species native to Thailand, was also found to possess significant anti-inflammatory properties (Suksamrarn, Kumpun, Kirtikara et al. 2002). Another verbena family member in Brazil is being studied for its potential antivi-

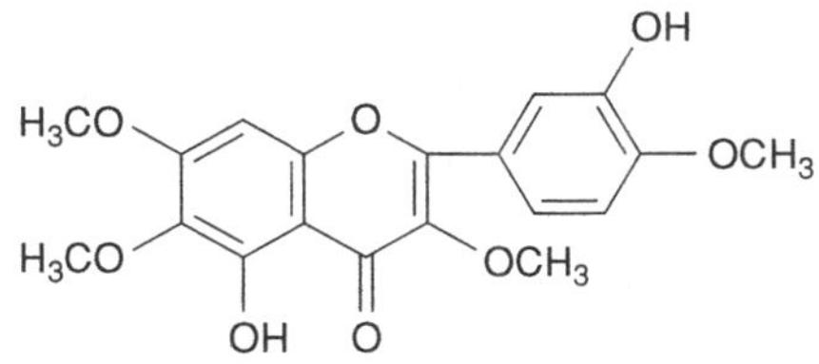

FIGURE 1-17. Active compound of *Vitex agnus-castus* (Mills, Bone 2000).

ral properties in acyclovir-resistant Herpes simplex virus type 1 (Goncalves, Leitao, Monache et al. 2001). In Bangladesh, *V. trifolia* was determined to possess antimicrobial activity (Hossain, Paul, Sohrab 2001) and its traditional application for the treatment of asthma was confirmed in Indonesia (Ikawati, Wahyuono, Maeyama 2001). Finally, Japanese researchers have determined preliminary evidence of anticancer properties of an extract of *V. agnus-catus* from Israel (Ohyama, Akaike, Hirobe et al. 2003).

Neuroendocrine Effects

V. agnus-castus properties include dopamine agonism, prolactin inhibition, progesterogenic effects, and FSH-suppressive properties (PDR 2000; Mills, Bone 2000; Jarry, Leonhardt, Gorkow et al. 1994). *V. agnus-castus* extract exerts a D2-dopaminergic effect (PDR 2000; Jarry, Leonhardt, Gorkow et al. 1994) and shows an affinity for opioid receptors (micro and kappa subtype) (Meier, Berger, Hoberg et al. 2000). Earlier studies showed its ability to reduce cystic and hemorrhagic ovarian follicles. Corpus luteal development is improved via dopaminergic effects on the anterior pituitary, which inhibits prolactin (Mills, Bone 2000). *V. agnus-castus* extract has a proven therapeutic effect on stress-induced hyperprolactin anemia (PDR 2000).

V. agnus-castus possesses prolactin-suppressive dopaminergic compounds that have been clinically proven to improve symptoms of premenstrual syndrome, in particular premenstrual mastalgia (painfully swollen breasts) (Wuttke, Jarry, Christoffel et al. 2003). In early studies on guinea pigs, low doses resulted in lowered estrogen, elevation in progesterone, follicular development, and glandular proliferation of breast tissue. However, at higher doses, inhibition of all gonadotrophic hormones and growth hormones occurred (Mills, Bone 2000). Inhibition of lactation has been associated with aucubin (0.3%) and agnoside (0.6%); these iridoid glycosides comprise the main active ingredients of *V. agnus-castus* extract (PDR 2000; Mills, Bone 2000). Many "bust enhancing" over-the-counter herbal products contain *V. agnus-castus* extract among many other ingredients, although this may be counterproductive (Fugh-Berman 2003).

In a comparative study, 41 women with premenstrual dysphoric disorder (PMDD) were treated with either fluoxetine or *V. agnus-castus* extract. No significant difference was found between the patient groups, suggesting that PMDD may respond well to either fluoxetine or *V. agnus-castus*. Researchers determined, however, that psychological symptoms responded better to fluoxetine whereas the herb more effectively alleviated physical symptoms (Atmaca, Kumru, Tezcan 2003).

In a recent placebo-controlled study of 20 healthy men, subjects ingested various doses of *V. agnus-castus* extract ranging between 120 to 480 mg per diem. Melatonin secretion was increased within the normal circadian rhythm of its production, suggesting a possible application for the treatment of sleep disturbances (Dericks-Tan, Schwinn, Hildt 2003).

Miscellaneous Effects

A newly discovered component of *V. agnus-castus* berries called vitexicarpin has shown promise in the treatment of inflammatory and immunoregulatory disorders such as rheumatoid arthritis and lymphoma (You, Son, Chang et al. 1998).

Availability

Available in whole or powdered form as capsules (40 mg, 100 mg) or liquid extract, the daily dose favored in Europe is 30 to 40 mg of *V. agnus-castus* preparation (PDR 2000). Alternatively, higher doses may be taken (500 mg) once or twice a day, although prolonged use at higher doses should be avoided (Mills, Bone 2000).

Adverse Effects

V. agnus-castus berries have been associated with the eruption of skin rashes in the form of itching and urticaria (Mills, Bone 2000; PDR 2000). Other reported side effects include nausea, short-term headache, as well as gastrointestinal and abdominal complaints (Mills, Bone 2000). Nonetheless, the PDR notes that its use is contraindicated in pregnant and nursing mothers (PDR 2000).

Clinical Application in Veterinary Behavior Medicine

V. agnus-castus has shown promising preliminary effects in its ability to enhance mood when compared to fluoxetine. It could be helpful in a variety of clinical situations in which antidepressants and selective serotonin reuptake inhibitors are prescribed. In addition, evidence for an anti-inflammatory effect in related species suggests it could be of value in the treatment of compulsive disorders in pets. Future investigation will clarify its application and effectiveness.

References

Atmaca M, Kumru S, Tezcan E. Fluoxetine versus *Vitex agnus castus* extract in the treatment of premenstrual dysphoric disorder. Hum Psychopharmacol. 2003;18:191–195.

Dericks-Tan JS, Schwinn P, Hildt C. Dose-dependent stimulation of melatonin secretion after administration of agnus castus. Exp Clin Endocrinol Diabetes. 2003;111:44–46.

Fugh-Berman A. "Bust-enhancing" herbal products. Obstet Gynecol. 2003;101:1345–1349.

Fugh-Berman A, Kronenberg F. Complementary and alternative medicine (CAM) in reproductive-age women: a review of randomized controlled trials. Reprod Toxicol. 2003;17:137–152.

Goncalves JL, Leitao SG, Monache FD et al. In vitro antiviral effect of flavonoid-rich extracts of *Vitex polygama* (*Verbenaceae*) against acyclovir-resistant herpes simplex virus type 1. Phytomedicine. 2001; 8:477–480.

Hardy ML. Herbs of special interest to women. J Am Pharm Assoc (Wash). 2000;40:234–242.

Hirobe C, Qiao ZS, Takeya K et al. Cytotoxic flavonoids from *Vitex agnus-castus*. Phytochemistry. 1997;46:521–524.

Hobbs C. The chaste tree: *Vitex agnus castus*. Pharm Hist. 1991;33:19–24.

Hossain MM, Paul N, Sohrab MH et al. Antibacterial activity of *Vitex trifolia*. Fitoterapia. 2001;72: 695–697.

Ikawati Z, Wahyuono S, Maeyama K. Screening of several Indonesian medicinal plants for their inhibitory effect on histamine release from RBL-2H3 cells. J Ethnopharmacol. 2001;75:249–256.

Jarry H, Leonhardt S, Gorkow C et al. In vitro prolactin but not LH and FSH release is inhibited by compounds in extracts of *Agnus castus*: direct evidence for a dopaminergic principle by the dopamine receptor assay. Exp Clin Endocrinol. 1994;102:448–454.

Kuruuzum-Uz A, Stroch K, Demirezer LO et al. Glucosides from *Vitex agnus-castus*. Phytochemistry. 2003;63:959–964.

Loch EG, Selle H, Boblitz N. Treatment of premenstrual syndrome with a phytopharmaceutical formulation containing *Vitex agnus castus*. J Womens Health Gend Based Med. 2000;9:315–320.

Meier B, Berger D, Hoberg E et al. Pharmacological activities of *Vitex agnus-castus* extracts in vitro. Phytomedicine. 2000;7:373–381.

Mills S, Bone K. Principles and Practice of Phytotherapy. Churchill Livingstone, Philadelphia, PA. 2000;328–334.

Ohyama K, Akaike T, Hirobe C et al. Cytotoxicity and apoptotic inducibility of *Vitex agnus-castus* fruit extract in cultured human normal and cancer cells and effect on growth. Biol Pharm Bull. 2003;26: 10–18.

PDR for Herbal Medicines. (2nd ed) Medical Economics Company Inc., Montvale, NJ. 2000;176–177.

Sorensen JM, Katsiotis ST. Parameters influencing the yield and composition of the essential oil from Cretan *Vitex agnus-castus* fruits. Planta Med. 2000;66:245–250.

Suksamrarn A, Kumpun S, Kirtikara K et al. Iridoids with anti-inflammatory activity from *Vitex peduncularis*. Planta Med. 2002;68:72–73.

Wuttke W, Jarry H, Christoffel V et al. Chaste tree (*Vitex agnus-castus*): pharmacology and clinical indications. Phytomedicine. 2003;10:348–357.

You KM, Son KH, Chang HW et al. Vitexicarpin, a flavonoid from the fruits of *Vitex rotundifolia*, inhibits mouse lymphocyte proliferation and growth of cell lines in vitro. Planta Med. 1998;64: 546–550.

CHAPTER

2

Native American Psychoactive Herbs

> "Indians and animals know better how to live than white man; nobody can be in good health if he does not have all the time fresh air, sunshine, and good water."
> —*Chief Flying Hawk,* Oglala Sioux (1852–1931)

Introduction

By the middle of the nineteenth century, Native American herbal remedies commingled with European plant remedies. Colonial settlers brought along their own plant pharmacopoeia; it was inevitable that botanical collections and their applications would be shared between the indigenous and colonizing populations. For example, *Humulus lupulus* (hop) was used as an hypnotic by Native Americans, and *Leonurus cardiaca* (motherwort) was adopted by the Algonquin for the treatment of gynecological disorders (Sumner 2000).

It is beyond the scope of this book to explore every detail of Native American ethnobotany, or to fully investigate the many plants they used for the alleviation of psychological symptoms. Table 5-1 offers a compilation of the plants used by many tribes for a variety of emotional or behavioral concerns. Among the tabulated species, some were mentioned more consistently for use within the same tribe for different symptoms, or in more than one tribe for the same or similar application. A discussion of these particular plants follows below. Plants such as *Peyote* and *Psilocibe* are not included in this table because the Native Americans did not use them as psychological aids *per se*; however, they are discussed elsewhere in this text because of their psychoactive properties and potential for abuse. Some of the better-studied plants (and perhaps more promising in their potential for clinical use) such as *Lobelia spp.* and *Panax quinquefolius* are presented in greater detail later in this section.

Cypripedium calceolus

Cypripedium calceolus var. pubescens (Yellow Lady's Slipper, Lady's Slipper, American Valerian, Nerve Root, Bleeding Heart, Noah's Ark, Venus Shoe, Moccasin Flower, Monkey Flower; family *Orchidaceae*) is a native perennial of North America and cultivated in Europe. It grows as high as 70 cm in swamps, bogs, and forests. This orchid is increasingly rare and is considered an endangered species in the Northeastern United States. The dried rhizome is valued for its medicinal properties. The "nerve root" itself is used for its sedative and antispasmodic effects, and to treat anxiety, agitation, hysteria, insomnia, and gynecological complaints (PDR 2000).

Several varieties of *C. calceolus* were in common use by Native Americans. *C. acaule* (Pink Lady's Slipper) was used by the Algonquin and Cherokee to relieve stomachaches and for kidney troubles. The Iroquois used it as an analgesic, as did the Cherokee, who also used it as an antihelminthic and antispasmodic. The Penobscot, Chippewa, and Okanagan also used *Cypripedium spp.* (Pink Lady's Slipper, Lesser and Greater Yellow Lady's Slipper) for miscellaneous medicinal properties. However, the Iroquois, Penobscot, and Micmac used the plant for its sedative, anxiolytic effects to treat "fits," "nervousness," and "hysterical affections." In fact, the Meskwaki believed in its usefulness as a love medicine (Moerman 2002; Chandler, Freeman, Hooper 1979; Herrick 1977; Speck 1917).

During the nineteenth century, *Cypripedium spp.* were used medicinally to treat "insomnia, nervous irritability, neuralgia, and delirium, all from atony; menstrual irregularities, with despondency; tendency to dementia at climacteric; mental depression from sexual abuse." An infusion combining *Nepeta cataria*, *Scutellaria lateriflora*, and *Cypripedium pubescens*, for example, was used as a headache remedy (Felter, Lloyd 1898).

Ingredients

Compounds include phenanthrene quinones; volatile oil; and tannins (PDR 2000).

Adverse Effects

C. calceolus is a skin irritant, possibly due to phenanthrene quinone compounds (PDR 2000).

Availability

C. calceolus is available as an alcohol based extract (tincture). The dried form is prepared as a tea infusion of 2 to 4 g (approximately 2 teaspoons) (PDR 2000).

Clinical Application in Veterinary Behavior Medicine

Currently, there are no data to substantiate traditional applications of *C. calceolus*. Furthermore, its regrettably precarious survival precludes its use for any purpose.

References

Chandler FR, Freeman L, Hooper SN. Herbal Remedies of the Maritime Indians. J Ethnopharm. 1979;1:49–68.

Felter HW, Lloyd JU. King's American Dispensatory. Ohio Valley Company, Cincinatti, OH. 1898. Available online at http://www.ibiblio.org/herbmed/eclectic/kings/

Herrick JW. Iroquois Medical Botany. State University of New York, Albany, NY. PhD Thesis. 1977.

Moerman DE. Native American Ethnobotany. Timber Press, Portland, OR. 2002;191–192.

Moerman DE. University of Michigan–Dearborn. Native American Ethnobotany Database, 2003. http://herb.umd.umich.edu/

Northern Prairie Wildlife Research Center, U.S. Department of the Interior, US Geological Survey, 2004. http://www.npwrc.usgs.gov/

PDR for Herbal Medicines (2nd ed) Medical Economics Company Inc., Montvale, NJ. 2000;541.

Speck FG. Medicine Practices of the Northeastern Algonquians. Proceedings of the 19th International Congress of Americanists. 1917;303–321.

Eschscholzia californica

Eschscholzia californica (California Poppy; family *Papaveraceae*), the state flower of California, is a native annual or perennial of southern California and northern Mexico. It is grown in Europe as well and is prized for its bright, yellow-orange flowers. The blooms can be up to 4 cm in diameter and are held atop bluish-green stems that reach as high as 30 to 60 cm (see color plate 2-1). The medicinal part of the plant is the aerial portion, which is harvested and dried during bloom time (Russo 2001; PDR 2000; Mills, Bone 2000).

E. californica was well known to Native Americans in the southwestern United States. The Luiseno and Neeshenam ate the leaves as greens; the Luiseno enjoyed the flowers as a sort of candy (Moerman 2002). However, the Mendocino people valued its analgesic properties for headaches, stomachaches, and toothaches. The Pomo, Kashya, and Mendocino also applied it topically to stop lactation in nursing mothers. The Costanoan used the blossoms to treat head lice but also recognized a sedative and soporific effect. They laid the flowers beneath a child's bed to induce sleep. Nevertheless, the Costanoan cautioned against its use in pregnant or nursing women because they believed the odor was toxic. The Mahuna tribe also considered the plant to be poisonous. The Mendocino also used the root for a narcotic effect.

Preparations of the *E. californica* are advocated for the treatment of anxiety, nervousness, insomnia, depression, mood swings, sensitivity to weather, constitutional weakness of the nervous system, nighttime incontinence in children, vasomotor dysfunction, neurasthenia, and neuropathy, among other conditions (Russo 2001). *E. californica* is popular in France to treat insomnia (PDR 2000).

The plant has drawn some attention as a recreational substitute for smoking marijuana; however, its reputed effect is not deserved (Russo 2001).

Ingredients

E. californica contains cyanogenic glycosides and isoquinoline alkaloids (e.g., californidine; escholzine or eschscholzine; and alpha, beta-allocryptopine) (PDR 2000). Recently, six flavonoid glycosides have been isolated and include quercetin and isorhamnetine (Beck, Haberline 1999).

CNS Effects

Californidine has soporific, anxiolytic, sedative, and spasmolytic properties. There is some evidence that another alkaloid isolated in the crude extract, protopine, was responsible for reduced activity and barbiturate-induced sleep in mice (Vincieri, Celli, Mulinacci et al. 1988). Several years later, another murine study showed a mild anxiolytic effect at 25 mg/kg and a sedative effect between 100 and 200 mg/kg (Rolland, Fleurentin, Lanhers et al. 1991). In a follow-up study in mice, *E. californica* extract again appeared to possess an affinity for benzodiazepine receptors and had sedative and anxiolytic effects (Rolland, Fleurentin, Lanhers et al. 2001). Unfortunately, there have not been any clinical studies of its psychoactive properties in people or in other animals.

Chelerythrine, an alkaloid of *E. californica* well known as a classical protein kinase C inhibitor, is of increasing scientific interest. It produced significant analgesia in one study (Yashpal, Pitcher, Parent et al. 1995) and demonstrated significant affinity for vasopressin receptors and inhibition of vasopressin binding (Granger, Serradeil-le Gal, Augereau et al. 1992). Recently, chelerythrine has also been shown to potentiate the GABA response of opioid-induced analgesia of the periaqueductal gray (Lee, Hahm, Min et al. 2003). In another study, morphine tolerance in mice was completely reversed with low doses of chelerythrine (Bohn, Lefkowitz, Caron 2002).

An alcoholic extract of *E. californica* inhibited dopamine beta-hydroxylase, adrenaline, and MAO_B, resulting in the preservation of elevated catecholamine levels (Kleber, Schneider, Schafer et al. 1995). Protopine was also shown to increase GABA binding comparable to benzodiazepine receptor affinity and to displace flurazepam from diazepine receptors (Schafer, Schafer, Schneider et al. 1995). Support of the *E. californica's* reported analgesic activity was demonstrated by an inhibition of enkephalin (Reimeier, Schneider, Schneider et al. 1995).

Availability

The herb is most often found mixed with other botanical compounds for use as plant sedatives. It is often brewed as an herbal tea using 2 gm per 150 ml of water.

Adverse Effects

Despite the lack of side effects associated with its use (Paul, Maurer 2003; PDR 2000; Mills, Bone 2000) and preliminary evidence of beneficial bioactivity, the

German Commission E does not recommend *E. californica* for any of its claimed uses and cautions against its consumption during pregnancy and lactation (Russo 2001).

Clinical Application in Veterinary Behavior Medicine

E. californica cannot be considered to be of clinical importance at this time because of the paucity of evidence for its psychoactive benefits. Preliminary evidence suggests its components impact on GABAergic and opioid systems, but further research is needed to establish its therapeutic potential.

References

Beck MA, Haberlain H. Flavonol glycosides from Eschscholzia californica. Phytochemistry. 1999;50: 239–332.

Bohn LM, Lefkowitz RJ, Caron MG. Differential mechanisms of morphine antinociceptive tolerance revealed in (beta)arrestin-2 knock-out mice. J Neurosci. 2002;22:10494–10500.

Granger I, serradeil-le Gal C, Augereau JM et al. Benzophenanthridine alkaloids isolated from *Eschscholtzia californica* cell suspension cultures interact with vasopressin (V1) receptors. Planta Medica. 1992;58:35–38.

Kleber E, Schneider W, Schafer HL et al. Modulation of key reactions of the catecholamine metabolism by extracts from *Eschscholtzia californica* and *Corydalis cava*. Arzneimittelforshchung. 1995;45: 127–131.

Lee JJ, Hahm ET, Min BI et al. Roles of protein kinase A and C in the opioid potentiation of the GABAA response in rat periaqueductal gray neuron. Neuropharmacology. 2003;44:573–583.

Mills S, Bone K. Principles and Practice of Phytotherapy. Churchill Livingstone, Philadelphia, PA. 2000; 229–230.

Moerman DE. Native American Ethnobotany. Timber Press, Portland, OR. 2002;228.

Paul LD, Maurer HH. Studies on the metabolism and toxicological detection of the *Eschscholtzia californica* alkaloids californine and protopine in urine using gas chromatography-mass spectrometry. J Chromatogr B Analyt Technol Biomed Life Sci. 2003;789:43–57.

PDR for Herbal Medicines (2nd ed) Medical Economics Company Inc., Montvale, NJ. 2000;140–141.

Reimeier C, Schneider I, Schneider W et al. Effects of ethanolic extracts from *Eschscholtzia californica* and Corydalis cava on dimerization and oxidation of enkephalins. Arzneimittelforschung. 1995;45: 132–136.

Rolland A, Fleurentin J, Lanhers MC et al. Behavioural effects of the American Traditional plant *Eschscholzia californica*: Sedative and anxiolytic properties. Planta Med. 1991;57:212–216.

Rolland A, Fleurentin J, Lanhers MC et al. Neurophysiological effects of an extract of *Eschscholzia californica* (*Papaveraceae*). Phytother Res. 2001;15:377–381.

Russo E. Handbook of Psychotropic Herbs: A Scientific Analysis of Herbal Remedies for Psychiatric Conditions. The Haworth Press, Binghamton, NY. 2001;120–123.

Schafer HL, Schafer H, Schneider W et al. Sedative action of extract combinations of *Eschscholtzia californica* and *Corydalis cava*. Arzneimittelforschung. 1995;45:124–126.

Vincieri FF, Celli S, Mulinacci N et al. an approach to the study of the biological activity of *Eschscholzia californica*. Pharmacol Res Comm. 1988;20 (Suppl 5):41–44.

Yashpal K, Pitcher GM, Parent A et al. Noxious thermal and chemical stimulation induce increases in 3H-phorbol 12,13–dibutyrate binding in spinal cord dorsal horn as well as persistent pain and hyperalgesia, which is reduced by inhibition of protein kinase C. J Neurosci. 1995;15:3263–3272.

Lobelia inflata

Lobelia inflata (Emetic Herb, Emetic Weed, Pukeweed, Gagroot, Vomitwort, Vomitroot, Indian Tobacco, Wild Tobacco, Bladderpod, Eyebright, and Asthma Weed; family *Campanulaceae*) is an annual or biennial herb indigenous to Canada, the northern United States, and Kamchatka. It grows between 30 and 60 cm tall. Yellow-green leaves taste like tobacco when chewed. The flowers are violet-blue with tinges of pale yellow. *L. inflata* seeds are encapsulated in the fruit (Moerman 2002; PDR 2000). Modern herbalists use the fresh or dried aerial parts as well as the seeds for medicinal preparations (PDR 2000); however, Native Americans also used the root for a variety of purposes (Moerman 2002).

Native Americans used *L. inflata* to treat skin, respiratory, and gastrointestinal ailments; it was also used in religious ceremonies. The Iroquois used *L. inflata* as a love potion, an antidote to love potions, to treat ailments caused by "witchcraft," and to help those suffering with grief (Moerman 2003; Moerman 2002). Native Americans also knew other species of Lobelia for their medicinal value. Notably, the Iroquois added *Lobelia cardinalis* to other medicines to strengthen their effects; as a love medicine; and to treat ailments caused by "witchcraft." The Pawnee and Meskwaki people also used its roots in a love medicine (Moerman 2002). The Iroquois used *Lobelia siphilitica* as an antibewitchment infusion; Meskwaki couples with marital problems ate the chopped roots as a love medicine to avert divorce (Moerman 2002). The Iroquois used *Lobelia kalmii* and *Lobelia spicata* as emetic antidotes to love medicines.

The use of Lobelia has been traced back to early settlers; however, during the 1800s it was considered to be the remedy of choice for treating angina pectoris, neuralgia of the heart, pulmonary apoplexy, pleurisy, pleuro-pneumonia, acute and chronic pneumonia, whooping cough, eczema, erisypelas, tetanus, convulsive movements, rigidity of muscular tissues including the uterus, rigid perineum or vaginal walls, nausea, and headache. Its primary use, however, was as an emetic. At least two physicians of this time were tried for the deaths of patients attributed to the medicinal administration of Lobelia preparations (Felter, Lloyd 1898).

Ingredients

Identified compounds include the piperidine alkaloids (e.g., lobeline, lobelanine, lobelanidine). The primary active compound is lobeline, an alkaloid that provokes vomiting. This emetic alkaloid is similar to emetine found in the ipecacuanha root (*Cephaelis ipecacuanha*) from which is derived the well-known pediatric preparation ipecac.

CNS Effects

L. inflata's antispasmodic effect may be accompanied by a feeling of relaxation, and herbalists recommend it for the treatment of irritability, tension headaches, insomnia, anxiety, and restlessness. It appears to inhibit dopamine uptake and promotes dopamine release from storage vesicles within the presynaptic terminal (Dwoskin, Crooks 2002). In Japanese studies on mice, beta-amyrin palmitate was isolated from *L. inflata* leaves and attributed with an antidepressant and sedative activity (Subarnas, Tadano, Nakahata et al. 1993; Subarnas, Tadano, Oshima et al. 1993).

Results of these studies also suggested that beta-amyrin palmitate antagonizes the locomotor stimulation of methamphetamine (Subarnas, Tadano, Oshima et al. 1993). In other research, lobeline inhibited amphetamine-induced release of dopamine but did not show an addictive effect, suggesting its application in the treatment of methamphetamine abuse (Dwoskin, Crooks 2002).

Miscellaneous Effects

Lobeline is structurally similar to nicotine and has been found to possess both agonist and antagonist properties at nicotinic receptors (Subarnas, Tadano, Oshima et al. 1993). It may be helpful to those trying to quit smoking. In fact, the Cherokee smoked it in order to ease withdrawal from tobacco addiction whereas the Iroquois drank the infusion to help those addicted to alcohol or tobacco (Moerman 2002; Herrick 1977).

Adverse Effects

L. inflata's use may be limited by numerous side effects such as nausea, vomiting, diarrhea, headache, respiratory difficulties, cardiac arrhythmias, anxiety, and somnolence. Convulsions and respiratory failure can be fatal following ingestion of 4 gm; further, as little as 0.6 to 1 gm of *L. inflata* leaves can be toxic (PDR 2000).

Availability

Although the herb may be taken as a hot infusion, some suggest it may be more effective as a liquid extract (Mills, Bone 2000b). *L. inflata* is used as an expectorant and respiratory spasmolytic in the treatment of bronchopulmonary congestion, asthma, and nonproductive cough (PDR 2000; Mills, Bone 2000a). It is available as an over-the-counter remedy for the treatment of childhood asthma (Mazur, De Ybarrondo, Miler et al. 2001).

Clinical Application in Veterinary Behavior Medicine

Given the potential toxicity of *L. inflata* and the availability of alternative and safer psychoactive herbs, it is not recommended for use in veterinary behavior practice at this time. Notwithstanding, its psychoactive properties deserve further research.

References

Dwoskin LP, Crooks PA. A novel mechanism of action and potential use for lobelia is a treatment for psychostimulant abuse. Biochem Pharmacol. 2002;63:89–98.

Felter HW, Lloyd JU. King's American Dispensatory. Ohio Valley Company, Cincinatti, OH. 1898. Available online at http://www.ibiblio.org/herbmed/eclectic/kings/
Herrick JW. Iroquois Medical Botany. State University of New York, Albany, NY. PhD Thesis. 1977.
Mazur LJ, De Ybarrondo L, Miler J et al. Use of alternative and complementary therapies for pediatric asthma. Tex Med. 2001;97:64–68.
Mills S, Bone K. Principles and Practice of Phytotherapy. Churchill Livingstone, Philadelphia, PA. 2000a;57,210–213.
___Principles and Practice of Phytotherapy. Churchill Livingstone, Philadelphia, PA. 2000b;57, 233–234.
Moerman DE. Native American Ethnobotany. Timber Press, Portland, OR. 2002; 311–312.
Moerman DE. University of Michigan—Dearborn. Native American Ethnobotany Database, 2003. http://herb.umd.umich.edu/
PDR for Herbal Medicines (2nd ed) Medical Economics Company Inc., Montvale, NJ. 2000;479–480.
Subarnas A, Tadano T, Nakahata N et al. A possible mechanism of antidepressant activity of beta-amyrin palmitate isolated from *Lobelia inflata* leaves in the forced swimming test. Life Sci. 1993;52: 289–296.
Subarnas A, Tadano T, Oshima Y et al. Pharmacological properties of beta-amyrin palmitate, a novel centrally acting compound, isolated from *Lobelia inflata* leaves. J Pharm Pharmacol. 1993;45:545–550.
Teng L, Crooks PA, Dwoskin LP. Lobeline displaces [3H]dihydrotetrabenazine binding and releases [3H]dopamine from rat striatal synaptic vesicles: comparison with d-amphethamine. J Neurochem. 1998;71:258–265.

Lophophora williamsii

Lophophora williamsii (Peyote, Devil's Root, Mescal Button, Dumpling Cactus, Sacred Mushroom, Pellote) is a spineless globular cactus distinguished by 13 vertical ribs that is native to southern Texas and northern Mexico. One rhizome may create a cactus formation as wide as 1.5 meters. It is used illegally for its hallucinogenic effect and in Native American religious ritual (PDR 2000).

Ingredients

The mescaline content (7%) of *L. williamsii* is known to trigger aural, auditory, and visual kinesthetic hallucinations. "Mescal Buttons" are dried, 0.5 cm–thick slices of the sprout, which are between 3 and 4.5 cm in diameter (PDR 2000).

Historical and Cultural Perspective

L. williamsii is used to enhance the religious experience and expression of Native Americans. The Peyote Religion, also known as the Native American Church, has revitalized the religious use of the psychedelic peyote cactus in a number of tribes in the United States. Among the Navajo, it is simply known as "azéé'" which means "medicine." Peyotism has been demonized and criminalized. Yet its use is centuries old. In fact, "Peyote Buttons" have been found in aboriginal archaeological sites that are 5,700 years old (Bruhn, De Smet, El-Seedi et al. 2002). Archaelogical evidence in Mexico and Texas indicate that Native Americans used *L. williamsii* and *Sophora secundiflora* (Mescal Bean), both of which contain mescaline, for their psychotropic properties as far back as 8500 BC (Bruhn, De Smet, El-Seedi et al. 2002). Today, they are used primarily for their psychoactive effects.

The Native American Church emerged from the Ute and Oto Indians and reflects a synthesis of Native and Christian traditions. It was rejected by the Navajo at first, but gradually was embraced by many. In Traditional Navajo spirituality, there are many deities. The NAC focuses on only one (the Creator), although the Peyote itself transcends to become a deity in itself. There are many traditional Navajo rituals and ceremonies; however, for the NAC there is only the all-night Peyote ritual although prayer content will vary (Milne, Howard 2000; Lewton, Bydone 2000). In Traditional Navajo belief, a person's illness is attributed to contact with natural phenomena, but in the Peyote religion, illness results from the individual's misbehavior and urges confession to a greater degree than in Traditional Navajo religious belief.

Just as there is evidence for cultural differences regarding the use of psychoactive drugs, there are differences in indigenous healing practices, including the treatment of psychiatric disorders (Calabrese 1997). In Western healing practices, the "heart" is central to the person's physical body and being. Among the Navajo, emphasis is on knowledge and thinking (Lamphere 2000). The ritual use of *L. williamsii* to enhance self-awareness and gain spiritual insight becomes clear from this perspective. Traditional Navajo healing emphasizes causal agents of disease and not the symptoms the disease produces (Milne, Howard 2000). Disease results from contamination with various natural phenomena, such as animals, ghosts, contact with enemies living or dead, and other natural phenomena. The Navajo believe that they are the embodiments of natural elements as well as certain animals and other figures of the Navajo legends. These sacred elements and entities also have the power to cause illness.

L. williamsii is consumed communally as part of all-night ritual healings during personal or family crises (Calabrese 1997). The Peyote ritual symbolizes death and rebirth, including changes in consciousness that facilitate communication with the Peyote spirit or the Great Spirit (Calabrese 1997). The ritual use of *L. williamsii* is extended to all members of the group, including children. However, *L. williamsii* use is considered to be beneficial, even imparting protection against the use of alcohol.

In a recent and well-publicized case, two Native American Peyotists were dismissed from their jobs as substance-abuse counselors. Peyotists discourage the use of alcohol. From the Native perspective, there was no contradiction. However, the decision to fire them disregarded the traditional use of *L. williamsii*, despite previous Constitutional protection extended to the Peyote religion (Calabrese 1997).

The ritual use of hallucinogens is not limited to North America. Sacramental use of *L. williamsii* has been compared to wine incorporated in Judeo-Christian religious practices. In the African Bwiti religion, for example, iboga root derived from a shrub (*Tabernanthe iboga*) is used ritually for its hallucinogenic component ibogaine. This psychoactive compound has been found useful in the treatment of cocaine addiction (Calabrese 1997). *P. methysticum* (Kava) use in Polynesia is another example of a psychoactive substance in ritual. The Daime Santo and Uniao de Vegetal of the Brazilian Amazon basin are plant-derived religions that use a decoction prepared from the woody parts of the forest liana *Banisteriopsis caapi* (*Aya-huasca*, "vine of the soul" in the Quechua language of the South American Andes) with additional plant ingredients such as leaves from the shrub *Psychotria viridis* (Halpern 2004; Riba, Valle, Urbano et al. 2003).

CNS Effects

Mescaline, the hallucinogenic alkaloid in *L. williamsii*, is absorbed from the intestine and concentrates specifically in the frontal lobe of the right hemisphere (Gilmore 2001). Mescaline affects peripheral nerve function by altering the neuron's permeability to K^+. However, its primary effect is on serotonin, both centrally and peripherally. The initial phase of response involves digestive symptoms such as vomiting and nausea, followed by tremor, mydriasis, and mild tachycardia and hypertension. The sensory effects of visual hallucinations peak within six hours following ingestion; symptoms of intoxication subside within 14 hours in most cases. Occasionally, this phase is accompanied by anxiety and panic attack that may predispose the patient to injury (Gerber 1967).

Adverse Effects

Use of *L. williamsii* by pregnant women is contraindicated, given evidence of a teratogenic effect on fetal hamsters (Gerber 1967).

Clinical Application in Veterinary Behavior Medicine

The harvest of cacti containing mescaline (*Lophophora williamsii; Trichocereus pachanoi, Opuntia cylindrical*) is considered legal only for indigenous ritual and religious purposes (Gilmore 2001).

L. williamsii and other hallucinogenic fungi have been suggested for treating obsessive-compulsive disorder (OCD) (see *Psylocibe spp.*) (Perrine 1999). Safer and legal conventional and herbal remedies are available. There is no basis for the clinical veterinary application of *L. williamsii.*

References

Bruhn JG, De Smet PA, El-Seedi HR et al. Mescaline use for 5700 years. The Lancet. 2002;359:1866.

Calabrese JD. Spiritual healing and human development in the Native American church: toward a cultural psychiatry of peyote. Psychoanal Rev. 1997;84:237–255.

Gerber WF. Congenital malformations induced by mescaline, lysergic acid, diethylamide, and bromlysergic acid in the hamster. Science. 1967;19:265–267.

Gilmore HT. Peyote use during pregnancy. South Dakota J Med. 2001;54:27–29.

Halpern JH. Hallucinogens and dissociative agents naturally growing in the United States.Pharmacol Ther. 2004;102:131–138.

Lamphere L. Comments on the Navajo Healing Project. Med Anthropology Quarterly. 2000;14:598–602.
Lewton EL, Bydone V. Identity and healing in three Navajo religious traditions: sa'ah naaghai bik'eh hozh. Med Anthropol Q. 2000;14:476–497.
Milne D, Howard W. Rethinking the role of diagnosis in Navajo religious healing. Med Anthropology Quarterly. 2000;14:543–570.
PDR for Herbal Medicines (2nd ed) Medical Economics Company Inc., Montvale, NJ. 2000;588–589.
Riba J, Valle M, Urbano G et al. Human pharmacology of ayahuasca: subjective and cardiovascular effects, monoamine metabolite excretion, and pharmacokinetics. J Pharmacol Exp Ther. 2003;306: 73–83.

Panax quinquefolius

Panax quinquefolius (American Ginseng, Canadian ginseng; family Araliaceae) is an obligate shade perennial plant native to eastern North America. Panax means panacea and implies its use as a cure-all; quinquefolius means "five leaves." It grows as tall as 60 cm and bears red fruit in the summer. The medicinal part of the plant is the root, which is harvested in late summer to fall. Demand is highest for mature roots, and plants are generally harvested after five years when active compounds reach peak concentration (Miskell, Parmenter, Eaton-Rye 2003; Russo 2001).

The plant is considered endangered in the wild but is cultivated commercially for export to Asia, where it is known as Xi yang shen and used primarily for the treatment of respiratory complaints. It has a sweeter flavor compared to *Panax ginseng* (Chinese ginseng) and is therefore prized as a yin agent, but is contraindicated in yang debilitation. By TCM standards, it is considered to be a cooling agent that enters the Heart, Lung and Kidney channels (Russo 2001; Zhong, Wiseman, Ellis 1996).

Historical Perspective

The temperate forests of Canada mirror the preferred growth conditions of *P. ginseng* in China. In fact, a Jesuit missionary of the eighteenth century working in China predicted that a species of Panax would likely be found in Canada. Two years later, *Panax quinquefolius* was discovered in 1716 near Montreal, Canada. Exportation of American ginseng began soon after and had become a major industry by the nineteenth century (Russo 2001). Indeed, it was considered to be scarce soon after its exploitation began (Felter, Lloyd 1898). The Cherokee and Chippewa took advantage of the demand and cultivated *P. quinquefolius* as a cash crop for 50 cents a pound at the end of the nineteenth century (Moerman 2002), although it sold to Asian markets for as much as $7.50 per pound (Felter, Lloyd 1898). The plant was valued as a cure for nervous dyspepsia, loss of appetite, mental and nervous exhaustion, asthma and bronchitis, convulsions, and paralysis (Felter, Lloyd 1898). By 1995, sales of wild and cultivated American ginseng were valued at $75 million (Russo 2001).

P. quinquefolius was well known to Native Americans and was taken as an infusion, chewed, carried in a pouch or herb bundle, or topically applied. The Delaware, Oklahoma, Iroquois, Mohegan, and Seminole people used it as a panacea. Its aphrodisiac effects were also recognized. The Meskwaki women used it "to get a husband." The Pawnee men used it as a love medicine. The Seminole men rubbed it on their skin and clothing to win back the affections of a divorced wife (Moerman 2002). The Seminole also used it as a pediatric sedative to help children with bad dreams. The Iroquois used *P. quinquefolius* as a stimulant and the Menominee valued it as a "strengthener of mental powers." The Cherokee used it as an anticonvulsant and to combat "nervous affections." The Cherokee also valued *Panax trifolius* (Dwarf Ginseng) as a remedy for "nervous debility" and other complaints (Moerman 2002). The Iroquois used it as a stimulant and to cure laziness. Finally, the Menominee used it to strengthen mental powers (Smith 1927).

Ingredients

P. ginseng and *P. quinquefolius* contain ginsenosides common to both species, including Rb_{1-3}, Rc, Rd, Re, $Rg_{1,2}$, Ro and F2 (Foster 1996). One study determined that Rf and Rg2 are absent in *P. quinquefolius* (Awang 1998), although Rf has since been identified in both (Ji, Harkey, Henderson et al. 2001). Rb_1 and Re are present in high proportion (Awang 1998; Ma et al. 1996).

Neuroprotective and Antioxidant Effects

Like *P. ginseng, P. quinquefolius* has shown a dose-dependent nicotinic activity on *in vitro* study of the human cerebral cortex (Lewis, Wake, Court et al. 1999). Loss of nicotinic receptor binding is associated with age-related conditions such as dementia. *P. quinquefolius* deserves further attention for its potential in the treatment of cognitive dysfunction in aging people and pets.

P. quinquefolius exhibited potent antioxidant activity by chelation of metal ions as well as by free radical scavenging (Kitts, Wijewickreme, Hu 2000). *P. quinquefolius* extract and ginsenoside Rb1 alone were shown to inhibit Na+ channel activity, which may help to explain their neuroprotective effect during ischemia. Drugs that block Na+ channels are known to provide cytoprotection during cerebral ischemia (Liu, Li, Liu et al. 2001). In a study of the effects of *P. quinquefolius, Ginkgo biloba*, and *Hypericum perforatum* extracts on the survival and regeneration of retinal ganglion cells, herbal extracts used alone were unsuccessful in offering neuroprotection to injured optic cells. However, a mixture of the three herbs significantly extended survival of retinal cells, suggesting their synergism in producing a significant neuroprotective effect (Cheung, So, Lu et al. 2002).

CNS and Behavioral Effects

Behavioral effects have not been as closely studied in this Panax species compared to *P. ginseng* but deserve investigation. Ginsenoside Rb_1 has been shown to reduce aggression and increase learning in murine studies (Awang 1998).

P. quinquefolius extract was shown to behave as a GABA receptor agonist, binding to GABA receptors when applied directly to the rat brainstem. Regulation of GABAergic neurotransmission may be an important part of the mechanism of action of *P. quinquefolius* (Yuan, Attele, Wu et al. 1998), although there may be significant variation in neuronal activity between plants cultivated in different environments (Yuan, Wang, Wu et al. 2001).

Anticancer Effects

In a Harvard Medical School study, *P. quinquefolius* extract was compared to estradiol and induced estrogen-regulated genes in MCF-7 breast cancer cells. However, unlike estradiol, *P. quinquefolius* induced a dose-dependent decrease in cell proliferation and was subsequently found to act synergistically with breast cancer therapeutic agents to suppress cancer cell proliferation *in vitro* (Duda, Zhong, Navas et al. 1999).

In a recent Canadian study, *P. quinquefolius* extract was 45 times more potent than *P. ginseng* extract G115 in inhibiting CYP1A2. Inhibition of cytochrome P450 enzymes is thought to be a mechanism of antitumor activity (Chang, Chen, Benetton 2002).

Miscellaneous Effects

There is preliminary evidence of immunostimulatory activity by *P. quinquefolius* via cytokine stimulation of macrophages (Assinewe, Amason, Aubry et al. 2002). It may also possess a mild analgesic effect (Yang, Pang, Tsang et al. 2001).

Although a hypoglycemic activity has been attributed to *P. quinquefolius* (Vuksan, Sievenpiper, Wong et al. 2001; Vuksan, Sievenpiper, Koo et al. 2000), a more recent Canadian study suggests that the ginsenoside profile of different batches of *P. quinquefolius* may result in a variable postprandial hypoglycemic effect (Sievenpiper, Arnason, Leiter et al. 2003).

Availability

The preparation and dosage of *P. quinquefolius* is the same as for *P. ginseng* (Russo 2001). Available commercial preparations include a wide range of dosages in capsule form (10 mg up to 1250 mg), liquid, tablet, and tea. In people, a dose of 400 mg a day of *P. ginseng* (PDR 2000) has been recommended to improve cognitive function. Based on this information and pending clinical confirmation, an initial dose of 200 mg per diem is recommended for *P. quinquefolius* administration to pets.

Adverse Effects

There have been no reports of adverse effects with *P. quinquefolius*. Nonetheless, much more *in vitro* and clinical data are needed before an appropriate dosage is determined and before the unlikely conclusion is reached that this herb is free of side effects.

Clinical Application in Veterinary Behavior Medicine

P. quinquefolius has not received quite as much scientific attention compared to its more famous relative *P. ginseng* (Chinese Ginseng). However, many of its Native American applications appear to be supported by an accumulating body of evidence that suggests many bioactive properties common to both ginsengs. The antioxidant and neuroprotective properties of *P. quinquefolius* might be helpful for the treatment of debilitated patients recovering or suffering from nonspecific ailments, emotional stress, and degenerative organic brain diseases. Its neuroprotective activity may also be helpful in aging pets or those suffering from mild psychomotor seizures, although *P. quinquefolius* is likely to be best used as an adjunct to other alternative or conventional medications for these conditions.

In veterinary behavior practice, its antiaggressive properties deserve investigation. Its GABAergic effect suggests that it may also be helpful in the treatment of mild to moderate anxiety in cases of noise phobias, transition to a new home, and separation-related misbehavior. Future research and clinical trials will clarify its therapeutic applications.

References

Assinewe VA, Amason JT, Aubry A et al. Extractable polysaccharides of *Panax quinquefolius* (North American ginseng) root stimulate TNFalpha production by alveolar macrophages. Phytomedicine. 2002;9:398–404.

Awang DV. The anti-stress potential of North American ginseng (*Panax quinquefolius*). J Herbs Spices Med Plants. 1998;6:87–91.

Chang TK, Chen J, Benetton SA. In vitro effect of standardized ginseng extracts and individual ginsenosides on the catalytic activity of human CYP1A1, CYP 1A2, and CYP1B1. Drug Metab Dispos. 2002;30:378–384.

Cheung ZH, So KF, Lu Q et al. Enhanced survival and regeneration of axotomized retinal ganglion cells by a mixture of herbal extracts. J Neurotrauma. 2002;19:369–378.

Duda RB, Zhong Y, Navas V et al. American ginseng and breast cancer therapeutic agents synergistically inhibit MCF-7 breast cancer cell growth. J Surg Oncol. 1999;72:230–239.

Felter HW, Lloyd JU. King's American Dispensatory. Ohio Valley Company, Cincinatti, OH. 1898. Available online at http://www.ibiblio.org/herbmed/eclectic/kings/

Foster S. American ginseng: *Panax quinquefolius*. Austin, TX: American Botanical Council. 1996.

Ji QC, Harkey MR, Henderson GL et al. Quantitative determination of ginsenosides by high-performance liquid chromatography-tandem mass spectrometry. Phytochem Anal. 2001;12:320–326.

Kitts DD, Wijewickreme AN, Hu C. Antioxidant properties of a North American ginseng extract. Mol Cell Biochem. 2000;203:1–10.

Lewis R, Wake G, Court G et al. Non-ginsenoside nicotinic activity in ginseng species. Phytother Res. 1999;13:59–64.

Liu D, Li B, Liu Y et al. Voltage-dependent inhibition of brain Na(+) channels by American ginseng. Eur J Pharmacol. 2001;413:47–54.

Miskell JA, Parmenter G, Eaton-Rye JJ. Decreased Hill reaction rates and slow turnover of transitory starch in the obligate shade plant *Panax quinquefolius* L. (American ginseng). Planta. 2002;215: 969–979.

Moerman DE. Native American Ethnobotany. Timber Press, Portland, OR. 2002;376–377.

PDR for Herbal Medicines (2nd ed) Medical Economics Company Inc., Montvale, NJ. 2000; 346–350.

Russo E. Handbook of Psychotropic Herbs: A Scientific Analysis of Herbal Remedies for Psychiatric Conditions. The Haworth Press, Binghamton, NY. 2001;192–195.
Sievenpiper JL, Arnason JT, Leiter LA et al. Variable effects of American ginseng: a batch of American ginseng (*Panax quinquefolius*) with a depressed ginsenoside profile does not affect postprandial glycemia. Eur J Clin Nutr. 2003;57:243–248.
Smith HH. Ethnobotany of the Menomini Indians. Bulletin of the Public Museum of the City of Milwaukee. 1923;4:1–174.
Vuksan, Sievenpiper JL, Koo VY et al. American ginseng (*Panax quinquefolius*) reduces postprandial glycemia in nondiabetic subjects and subjects with type 2 diabetes mellitus. Arch Intern Med. 2000;160:1009–1013.
Vuksan V, Sievenpiper JL, Wong J et al. American ginseng (*Panax quinquefolius*) attenuates postprandial glycemia in a time-dependent but not dose-dependent manner in healthy individuals. Am J Clin Nutr. 2001;73:753–758.
Yang JC, Pang CS, Tsang SF et al. Effect of American ginseng extract (*Panax quinquefolius*) on formalin-induced nociception in mice. Am J Chin Med. 2001;29:149–154.
Yuan CS, Attele AS, Wu JA et al. Modulation of American ginseng on brainstem GABAergic effects in rats. J Ethnopharmacol. 1998;62:215–222.
Yuan CS, Wang X, Wu JA et al. Effects of *Panax quinquefolius* on brainstem neuronal activities: comparison between Wisconsin-cultivated and Illinois-cultivated roots. Phytomedicine. 2001;8:178–183.
Zhong YX, Wiseman N, Ellis A. Fundamentals of Chinese medicine. Paradigm Publications; Brookline, MA. 1996;342.

Piper methysticum

"The man who drinks *awa* is still a man, but the man who drinks liquors becomes a beast." —*Hawaiian proverb* (Russo 2001)

Piper methysticum Forster (Kava, Kava-kava [Polynesian], Awa or Ava [Hawaiian, Tahitian], Yangona/Yanqona [Fijian]) is a perennial, dioecious shrub and member of the pepper family *Piperaceae*. Pale yellowish-green, valentine-shaped leaves grow as long as 28 cm (Fig. 2-1). *P. methysticum* prefers altitudes of 150–300 meters above sea level. It thrives in deep, humus-rich, well-drained soil with a pH between 5.5–6.5. It requires considerable watering (>2,000 mm/yr) and high humidity (over 70%). Depending on the variety of Kava, plants can live between 15 and 30 years. *P. methysticum* grows up to 3 or 4 m high; however, it is often harvested between 2 and 2.5 m. Although male and female plants are identified, *P. methysticum* is a sterile cultivar of the wild *P. wichmannii*; therefore, seed production is not possible and propagation is entirely dependent on people (Russo 2001; Lebot, Merlin, Lindstrom 1992).

More than 2000 species of *P. methysticum* are found throughout the tropics, of which ten have been used traditionally as spices or in medicinal preparations. Examples include *P. nigrum* (black pepper) and the long peppers (*P. officinarum* and *P. longum*) (Piscopo 1997). The northern part of Vanuatu (formerly the New Hebrides) is apparently the origin of dissemination, although New Guinea is the likely source of the wild ancestor *P. wichmannii* (Russo 2001).

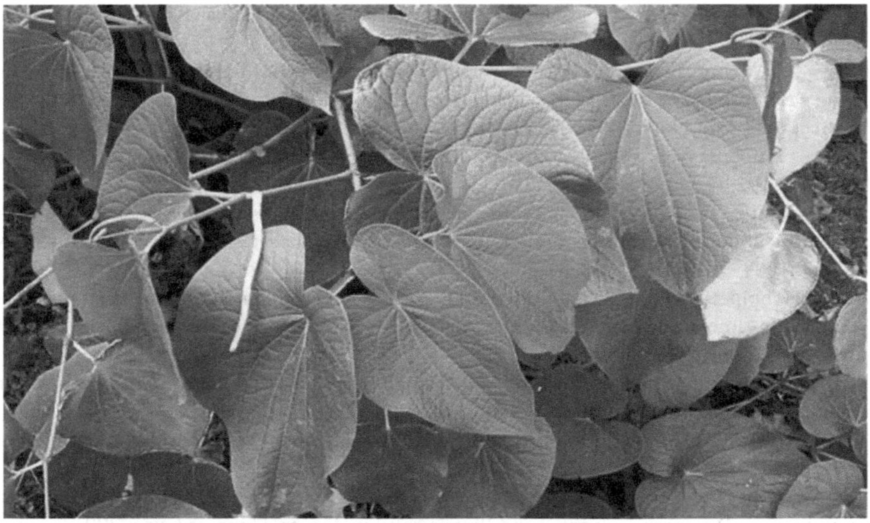

FIGURE 2-1. Heart-shaped leaves of *Piper methysticum* (kava). (Photo courtesy of Dr. Susan Wynn)

P. methysticum is reproduced from cloned plants, selected for continued propagation according to the effects of their prepared roots for ritual practice. At least 122 *P. methysticum* clones from 29 Pacific islands have been identified. Several varieties of *P. methysticum* are cultivated across Melanesia, Micronesia, and Polynesia. Each variety had its own distinct purpose. A common variety, for instance, was used informally whereas a less common variety was reserved for ceremonial use (Piscopo 1997). Different strains are distinguished by external appearance (morphotype), enzyme representation (zymotype) or kavalactones composition (chemotype). There are 247 *P. methysticum* cultivars in 82 morphotypes overall (Russo 2001; Lebot, Merlin, Lindstrom 1992).

Historical and Cultural Perspective

Based on biochemical and linguistic evidence, *P. methysticum* may have been selectively cultivated beginning as long as 3,000 years ago. Ancient pottery intended for use in the Kava ritual provides archeological proof (Russo 2001; Lebot, Merlin, Lindstrom 1992).

Kava kava ("ava" or "awa" means "bitter drink") is the name of the herb as well as a ceremonial beverage. Origin myths often recount the observation of a rat or pig eating *P. methysticum* roots, leading to human discovery (Russo 2001). Early in its history, *P. methysticum* was an indulgence exclusive to higher-ranking members of society and the kahunas (priests). In some islands, use of *P. methysticum* was forbidden to premenopausal women unless they were of special social status. However, as it became abundant, its use became more democratic. *Piper methysticum* and the original *P. wichmannii* are the only members of the genus with recognized psychoactive kavalactones (Russo 2001).

Fresh *P. methysticum* root (there is some controversy as to whether it possesses a rhizome) was harvested between four and six years of growth. In the Tongan tradition, virgins chewed it; in the Fijian tradition, it was pounded or grated. In both methods, the pulp was mixed with water or coconut milk and then strained through palm fibers or coconut fronds. It is not fermented and contains no alcohol. It was served in coconut shells, and the individual was expected to drain the shell in one long drink. Typically, each individual drank one to three shells' worth (Mills, Bone 2000; Piscopo 1997; Lebot, Merlin, Lindstrom 1992).

P. methysticum's cultural role among Pacific Islanders has been compared to the social enjoyment of wine by Europeans, but without the hangover (Mills, Bone 2000). The first effect experienced by the Kava drinker is a numbing of the tongue and buccal mucosa due to the local anesthetic and astringent effect of *P. methysticum*. This is followed by a sense of euphoria and a heightened state of awareness, which apparently impacts the sense of hearing in particular. The overall enhancement of social interaction lasts for several hours and the sleep that follows is described as especially restful. Some varieties of *P. methysticum* are stronger than others. For instance, half a coconut shell of a very strong variety might induce sleep within thirty minutes (Piscopo 1997). In Vanuatu, a lichen of the genus Usnea may be added to Kava to boost its effects. This synergism may be due to lactonic acids in the lichen species (Lebot, Merlin, Lindstrom 1992).

Dutch explorers Jacob Le Mair and William Schouten were the first Europeans to document the ceremonial preparation of Kava (Schouten 1771). Parkinson, who accompanied Captain Cook to Tahiti on the ship *Endeavour*, gave the first scientific account (Parkinson 1773). Johann Georg Forster, botanist to Captain James Cook's second voyage aboard the *Resolution* to the Pacific Island region between 1772 and 1775, named the plant *Piper methysticum* ("intoxicating pepper") in reference to the plant's primary use as a social ceremonial drink. Captain Cook himself may have been the first European to partake of Kava. He also reported that the method of preparation was enough to discourage the rest of his crew from tasting it (Russo 2001).

Traditionally, *P. methysticum* also was used in the treatment of arthritis, asthma, tuberculosis, leprosy, skin infection, headache, migraine, insomnia, gonorrhea, syphilis, urinary tract infection, menstrual problems, and other complaints. It was also used to enhance lactation and fertility (Piscopo 1997). Plant ashes were rubbed on sick children, and ailing children chewed its buds to gain strength (Moerman 2002).

Use of *P. methysticum* by indigenous people was impacted by colonial rule. In particular, missionaries objected to its use and especially to the traditional method of preparation by chewing and spitting the macerated root into a communal bowl (Russo 2001). Missionary prohibition eradicated the use of *P. methysticum* in Tahiti and Hawaii (Russo 2001). *P. methysticum* was first listed in the British Pharmacopoeias in 1914. By 1950, it was marketed in the United State as "Gonosan" for the treatment of gonorrhea and as "Neurocardin" for the treatment of "nervous" disorders (Kilham 1996).

Today, *P. methysticum's* popularity persists and its cultivation is on the rise in Hawaii (Singh 1992). Renowned P. methysticum cultivars have been revived on Kauai (Ko'uko'u), Oahu (Hena), Maui (Lanakila) and the "big island" of Hawaii (Puna) (Singh 1992). On Vanuatu, men go to Kava bars (*nakamals*) before the evening meal. This local alternative to bars and pubs is growing in popularity (Russo 2001). In fact, *P. methysticum* farming has become increasingly important to island economies. French pharmaceutical companies alone purchase thirty tons of Vanuatu *P. methysticum* each year (Lebot, Merlin, Lindstrom 1992).

Ingredients

Resins are viscous plant secretions exuded on the surface or in response to injury. The sticky secretions soon harden, presumably to protect damage (see discussion of morphine and *Papaver somniferum*). Active components of *P. methysticum* are found in the lemon-yellow resin of the rootstock (Mills, Bone 2000). The major pharmacological effects of *P. methysticum* appear to be induced by compounds in the resin (lipid extract) rather than the aqueous extract (Jamieson, Duffield, Cheng et al. 1989).

Identified components include the kavalactones (also called kavapyrones) and flavonoids (or flavokavains). Also isolated from *P. methysticum* are three alkaloid components (two in the roots, one in the leaves: pipermethystin), flavokawains, an alcohol, a phytosterol, ketones, and organic acids (Russo 2001; Mills, Bone 2000; Piscopo 1997). The lateral roots, which may be as long as 3 m, usually contain the highest concentration of lactones (15%), followed by the rootstock (10%) and basal stems (5%) (Piscopo 1997).

The primary active components of *P. methysticum* are the kavalactones, which make up between 3 and 20% dry weight of the rootstock (depending upon the plant's age, variety, and geographical location). Of the fifteen kavalactones isolated, the six most prominent are methysticin, yangonin, dihydromethysticin, kawain (kavain), dihydrokavain, and demethoxyyangonin (Fig. 2-2). The first to be isolated (in 1860) was methysticin (kavakin, kavatin, kawakin, kanakin) (Russo 2001; Mills, Bone 2000; Singh 1992). Kavalactones are insoluble in water but are readily extracted in water from kava root because of saponins in the root that increase the solubility of lipophilic molecules via micelle formation (Mills, Bone 2000). Kavain and dihydrokavain cross the blood brain barrier most readily (Lebot, Merlin, Lindstrom 1992). Kavalactones contain no nitrogen and appear to be precursors of flavonoids with one less acetate unit (Russo 2001; Mills, Bone

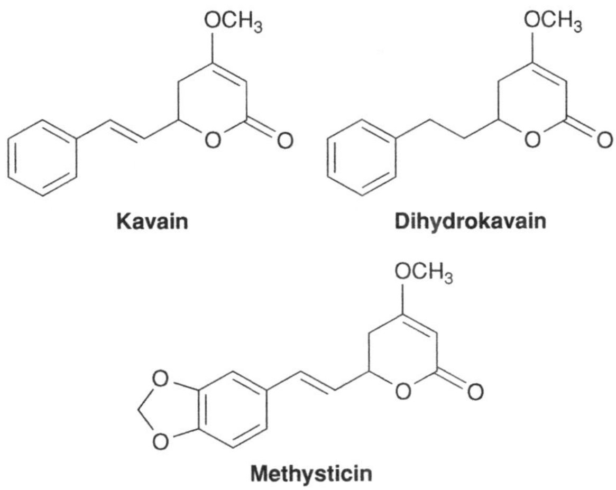

FIGURE 2-2. Active compounds of *Piper methysticum.* (Mills & Bone 2000)

2000). Kavalactones are chemically similar to myristicin, a component of nutmeg spice (Piscopo 1997).

Research has demonstrated that the chemical composition of specific cultivars of *P. methysticum* are characterized by distinct proportions of six major kavalactones: 1=desmethoxyyangonin, 2=dihydrokavain, 3=yangonin, 4=kavain, 5= dihydromethysticin, 6=methysticin (Lebot, Levesque 1989). Each cultivar was coded according to its proportional content of the six lactones, which were then listed in decreasing order. For example, the variety 256431 contained dihydrokavain in highest proportion and desmethoxyyangonin in lowest concentration. This variety was among the most potent varieties and was famous for inducing a "high" that lasted as long as two days, but was largely avoided because it often caused nausea. This cultivar is known in the pidgin of Vanuatu as tudei ("two day") (Russo 2001).

In rats, pharmacokinesis of an oral dose of kavalactones has been studied. Approximately half the dose of dihydrokavain can be found in urine, much in hydroxylated metabolites, within 48 hours. The other major *P. methysticum* compounds were revealed in lower concentration in urinary excretion. *P. methysticum* may be more bioactive and bioavailable in root extract preparations compared to isolated components of its resin. The bioavailability of kavalactones in extract is as much as three to five times higher compared to single components. In one study on mice, intraperitoneal injection of *P. methysticum* resin markedly increased the concentration of specific lactones compared to the injection of single compounds (Mills, Bone 2000).

In general, cultivars with high concentrations of kavain and low concentrations of dihydromethysticin (e.g., codes beginning with 426, 462, or 246) were the most popular among island cultures (Piscopo 1997). This important finding may not be used to advantage in current commercial preparations of *P. methysticum* available across the counter. Each component exerts a synergistic effect on the other, which may explain why the extract is more potent than isolated elements (Russo 2001). Synergistic mechanisms are recognized in *P. methysticum* and other herbal medicines (e.g., *Hypericum perforatum, Valeriana spp.*) (Spinella 2002). The synergistic or neutralizing effects of multiple compounds in any given plant must always be considered.

CNS Effects

It has been hypothesized that kavalactones potentiate GABA receptors, explaining their overlapping CNS effects with benzodiazepine. Although one study found no firm evidence to support this notion (Davies et al. 1992), it was subsequently found that kavalactones have a focal affinity for $GABA_A$ receptors in the amygdala, medulla oblongata, and hippocampus (Jussofie, Schmiz, Himke et al. 1994). Elsewhere, it was determined that kavalactones bind only slightly to $GABA_A$ receptors in the forebrain and not to $GABA_B$ receptors at all (Davies, Drew, Duffield et al. 1992).

Weak effects of kavalactones on GABA and benzodiazepine receptors in vitro were demonstrated (Davies, Drew, Duffield et al. 1992) and verified in another study, which showed a synergistic effect between kavalactones and other GABA-active sedatives (Jussofie, Schmiz, Himke 1994). An additive effect with benzodiazepines is possible in patients who use both physician-prescribed benzodiazepines and over-the-counter *P. methysticum* preparations because it acts on the same receptors and CNS areas as benzodiazepines (Almeida, Grimsley 1996).

Kavalactone extract and the isolated component dihydrokavain have been shown to inhibit $GABA_A$ receptors, supporting a role of these compounds in the regulation of GABAergic neurotransmission (Yuan, Dey, Wang, et al. 2002). However, another study suggests that *P. methysticum* extracts do not mediate their anxiolytic effects via the benzodiazepine binding sites on $GABA_A$ receptors (Garret, Basmadjian, Khan et al. 2003). No interaction with GABA (gamma-amino-butyric acid) or benzodiazepine binding sites has been demonstrated for either *P. methysticum* resin or kavalactones (Davies, Drew, Duffield et al. 1992).

Kawain and dihydromethysticin appear to exert an antiserotonin effect (Buckley et al. 1979). In one study, kawain and methysticin were virtually ineffective on monoamine and serotonin uptake (Seitz, Schule, Gleitz 1997). In a study of the guinea pig brain, kawain and dihydromethysticin were reported to have additive actions and may enhance the effects anxiolytic serotonin agonists. A serotonergic disturbance has been associated with anxiety and depression (Blier, de Montigny 1994). The basic mechanism of action of these kavalactones may be by activation of N-methyl-D-aspartate receptors and/or Ca^{++} channels in the hippocampus (Walden, von Wegerer, Winter et al. 1997).

Anticonvulsant and Neuroprotective Effects

Disturbance of intracellular Ca^{++} ion homeostasis has been described as part of the pathophysiology of affective disorders and epilepsy (Dubovsky 1993), and may provide a partial explanation of the mood stabilization and anti-epileptic effects of *P. methysticum*. Kavalactones possess anticonvulsant activity and were shown to be up to 10 times more effective than mephenesin in controlling strychnine-induced seizure (Kretzschmar, Meyer, Teschendorf 1970). The mechanism underlying Kava's anticonvulsant property has been demonstrated to be by both Na^{+} and Ca^{++} channel blockage, although the authors suggest that the Ca^{++} levels may be influenced indirectly by direct interaction with Na^{+} channels (Schirrmacher, Busselberg, Langosch et al. 1999; Gleitz et al. 1995, 1996a, 1996b). More recently, Na^{+} channel blockade has been implicated as the mechanism for the local anesthetic and neuroprotective effects of kavalactones (Hansel 1997-1998).

Kavalactones inhibit convulsions experimentally induced in animals by strychnine, electroshock, and pentylenetetrazole (Klohs, Keller, Williams et al. 1959; Kretzschmar, Meyer, Teschendork 1970; Meyer 1979).

A neuroprotective action against ischemic brain injury has also been described and may be mediated by the kavalactone methysticin (Backhauss, Krieglstein 1992).

The potency of a root extract of kavalactones was similar to the most potent lactone (dihydromethysticin) of the mixture, present at only 5% in controlling strychnine-induced seizures. However, despite promising experimental results, *P. methysticum* has not proven clinically useful for the treatment of epilepsy (Klohs, Keller, Williams et al. 1959), apparently because of the incidence of side effects such as Kava dermopathy associated with long-term use. Its mild anticonvulsant action makes it useful as an adjunct to conventional antiepileptics although this effect may not be potent enough to use without concomitant use of another anticonvulsant drug (Bone 1993/94).

Behavioral and Psychological Effects

Therapeutic indications for *P. methysticum* include the treatment of anxiety. It does not cause drowsiness and does not interact with mild consumption of alcohol, and there is no risk of tolerance or addiction. *P. methysticum* has a mild euphoric effect. Its mild antidepressant activity makes it particularly appropriate for the control of anxiety accompanied by mild depression (Bone 1993/94). It has been suggested that *P. methysticum* and *Valeriana spp.* should not be used for depression unless combined with other more stimulating herbs because of their sedative effects, although this is unfounded (Tillotson, Tillotson, Abel 2001).

P. methysticum produces apparently contradictory effects of increased relaxation and improved performance. In a double-blind crossover study, the effects of a standardized P. methysticum extract and the benzodiazepine oxazepam were compared. Oxazepam, but not *P. methysticum* extract, blunted cognitive performance in several psychometric tests (Munte, Heinze, Matzke et al. 1993). In another clinical trial, *P. methysticum* did not impair either reaction time or concentration, and at therapeutic doses, it improved cognitive performance (Heinz, Munthe, Steitz et al. 1994). Elsewhere, *P. methysticum* was well tolerated and as effective as buspirone and opipramol in the treatment of generalized anxiety disorder (Boerner, Sommer, Beger et al. 2003). Na^+ and Ca^{++} channel antagonism may underlie the anxiolytic effects of P. methysticum (Schirrmacher, Busselberg, Langosch et al. 1999).

In a recent study (Smith et al. 2003), newly hatched chicks were injected with chlordiazepoxide (5 mg/ml/kg), *P. methysticum* extract (30% kavalactones), or one of the six major *P. methysticum* components (kavain, dihydrokavain, methysticin, yangonin, dihydromethysticin, and desmethoxyyangonin at 30 mg/ml/kg). The change in response to social isolation compared to the presence of two other chicks was evaluated. Results indicated that chlordiazepoxide and kava extract reduced separation-related distress calls as well as stress-induced analgesia. Dihydrokavain reduced separation-related distress vocalizations only. The authors concluded that the anxiolytic effects of *P. methysticum* extract might be partially attributed to dihydrokavain.

In a randomized placebo-controlled double-blind clinical trial of 100 human patients conducted over a six-month period, *P. methysticum* extract (300 mg concentrated extract containing 210 mg of kavalactones, equivalent to 4 g of dried root) was tested in the control of non-psychotic anxiety disorders such as agoraphobia, specific phobia, and generalized anxiety disorder. Results support the use of *P. methysticum* extract as an alternative to tricyclic antidepressants and benzodiazepines in the treatment of anxiety. Adverse effects were infrequent in both groups but more common in the placebo group (Volz, Kieser 1997). Elsewhere, *P. methysticum* extract was effective in treating symptoms of nervousness, restlessness, sleep disturbance, muscle tension, anger, fear, and menopausal complaints (Mills, Bone 2002).

Hypnotic Effects

Although animal studies of psychotropic herbs are few, one study compared the neurophysiological effects of D,L-kavain extract (Neuronika®, Klinge Pharma, Munich Germany; 10–50 mg/kg IP), *P. methysticum* extract (50–100 mg pyrones/kg IP), placebo (0.9% NaCl, 3 ml IP), and pentobarbital (1 mg/kg IM) in laboratory cats. Only the *P. methysticum* extract exerted marked effects on the EEG, inducing high-amplitude delta waves and a continuous alpha or beta synchronization in the amygdalar complex. Muscle tone was diminished with both D,L-kavain and *P. methysticum* extract, but not consistently. Compared to placebo, both D,L-kavain and pentobarbital significantly shortened the duration of active wakefulness. Synchronized sleep was also significantly prolonged with these agents alone and in combination. This study suggests that limbic structures, and specifically the amygdalar complex, are the site of action for both D,L-kavain and *P. methysticum* extract. This may explain why *P. methysticum* extract and the isolated lactone kavain induce sleepiness without a sedative effect (Holm, Staedt, Heep et al). In rabbits, kavalactones produce EEG changes similar to sedative drugs (Kretzschmar, Teschendorf 1974).

Analgesic and Nociceptive Effects

Analgesic properties in animals were demonstrated with Kava resin, kavalactones, and lactone-free aqueous *P. methysticum* extract. The analgesic activity of *P. methysticum* is not reversed by the administration of naloxone, a morphine antagonist, indicating that opioid pathways are not involved. Naloxone, which inhibits morphine-induced analgesia, did not reverse the pain-controlling effect of *P. methysticum* extracts (Jamieson, Duffield 1990b).

Dihydrokavain (DHK) has a greater analgesic effect than aspirin but is less potent than morphine. Analgesic effects of 120 mg/kg of both dihydrokavain and dihydromethysticin were comparable to 2.5 mg/kg of morphine. A synergistic effect was found between dihydrokavain and aspirin. Caffeine did not affect the intensity of analgesia of dihydrokavain and dihydromethysticin, but did abbreviate their effects (Bruggenmann, Meyer 1963).

P. methysticum is useful for its analgesic effect on mucous membranes such as the oral cavity (e.g., toothache) and vagina (e.g., vaginal prolapse, child birth) (Bone 1993/1994). The local anesthetic effect of kavalactones is similar to cocaine and procaine (Meyer, Kretzschmar 1969). However, because of a narrow safety margin, one study concluded that kavain was unsuitable as a local anesthetic. In this study, subcutaneous injection of kavain in alcohol produced local anesthesia lasting as long as several days; at higher doses, paralysis of peripheral nerves was observed (Baldi 1980).

In one study, eight lipid soluble pyrones were investigated for their analgesic properties in mice. The most effective *P. methysticum* analgesic components included kavain, dihydrokavain, methysticin, and dihydromethysticin. Dihydrokavain was found to be the most potent but its effect was transient compared to dihydromethysticin, which was less potent but its effect was more prolonged. Methysticin was very similar in effect and duration to dihydromethysticin. Dihydrokavain had double the potency and a slightly longer duration of effect compared to kavain. The aqueous extract, but not the lipid-soluble fraction, was determined to be inactive if administered orally (Jamieson, Duffield, Cheng et al. 1989; Jamieson, Duffield 1990b).

Libidinal Effects

Commercial claims that *P. methysticum* possesses an aphrodisiac effect are not consistent with indigenous observation. In fact, Tongan users report that *P. methys-*

ticum can depress sexual urges (Lemert 1967). The participation of virgin members of the community in the preparation of the Kava beverage suggests recognition of its suppression of libido, or at least a separation of the use of *P. methysticum* and sexual behavior (Lebot, Merlin, Lindstrom 1992).

Cardiovascular Effects

Evidence suggests that *P. methysticum* exerts important cardiovascular benefits. Kavain has been shown to exert an antithrombotic effect on human platelets by means of a dose-dependent decrease in platelet aggregation, ATP release, and synthesis of both thromboxane A2 and prostaglandin E2 by virtue of primary inhibition of cyclooxygenase (Gleitz, Beile, Wilkens et al. 1997). *P. methysticum* reduced heart rate and blood pressure in a group of 54 healthy volunteers subjected to psychological stress in the laboratory (Cropley, Cave, Ellis 2002).

In a recent study inspired by evidence for cancer prevention by green tea in Japan, dihydrokavain showed strong inhibitory action in mice treated with tumor causing cells (Hashimoto, Suganuma, Fujiki et al. 2003). Another study examined the COX (cyclooxygenase)-I and COX-II inhibitory activities of P. methysticum compounds. Dihydrokavain and yangonin showed the highest inhibitory activities; yangonin and methysticin showed moderate antioxidant free radical scavenging activity (Wu, Yu, Nair et al. 2002). In another experiment, *P. methysticum* extract with hot water and methanol produced a number of novel compounds. All five compounds revealed significant COX-I and COX-II enzyme inhibition.

Myorelaxant Effects

In a study on rats and cats, a steam distillate of *P. methysticum* containing the water-soluble components kawain and dihydromethysticin produced a marked depression of spontaneous motor activity, skeletal muscle relaxation, ataxia, and moderate slowing of cortical, hypothalamic, and hippocampal activity (Buckley et al. 1979). *P. methysticum* is recommended for the treatment of muscle spasm and tension by virtue of its safe muscle relaxant effect (Bone 1993/94). Evidence for the myorelaxant effect of kavalactones suggests their superiority to common muscle relaxants such as benzodiazepines, benzazoles, and propanediol (Jossang, Molho 1970; Singh 1983). A similar effect has been demonstrated in smooth muscle, by means of K^+ channel blockade (Seitz, Ameri, Pelzer et al. 1997).

Antimicrobial Effects

P. methysticum is traditionally used for the treatment of sexually transmitted diseases such as gonorrhea; however, current data do not clearly support a bacteriostatic effect. In fact, one report describes the uninhibited growth of gram positive and gram negative, pathogenic and nonpathogenic bacteria in a growth medium containing kavalactones (Singh 1992). However, another report suggests that dihydrokavain was effective in inhibiting the growth of *Aspergillus niger* (Lebot,

Merlin, Lindstrom 1992); there is also some evidence for its antifungal activity (Locher, Burch, Mower 1995; Bone 1993/94). This aspect of *P. methysticum's* potential therapeutic use deserves further investigation.

Adverse Effects and Drug Interaction

In mice, the oral LD_{50} of dihydrokavain was 920 mg/kg and for dihydromethysticin was 1050 mg/kg. No evidence of chronic toxicity was found in mice given doses of 50 mg/kg of dihydrokavain three times a week over a three-month period (Meyer 1979). Other rodent studies of the LD_{50} of standardized *P. methysticum* extract (70% lactone content) record a wide range of values (370 mg/kg IP, 380 mg/kg IP, 1.8 g/kg PO, 16 g/kg PO) (Mills, Bone 2000).

Chronic and heavy consumption of high doses of *P. methysticum* is associated with a scaly skin eruption, which is characterized by hyperpigmentation and an ichthyosiform rash known as Kava dermopathy, or kani kani in Fijian (Singh 1992). Lesions typically appear in the face and descend to the feet; ocular photosensitivity may accompany skin lesions (Ruze 1990). The rash is followed by a desquamating keratosis, and palmar and plantar keratoderma. Skin lesions heal when *P. methysticum* consumption is withdrawn (Bone 1993/94).

An earlier study reported that daily doses of between 300 to 800 mg produced Kava dermopathy in many patients (Keller, Klohs 1963). Administration of 100 mg of nicotinamide per day did not relieve skin eruptions (Ruze 1990). Acute allergic reactions to *P. methysticum* have been reported, but these are distinct from Kava dermopathy (Suss, Lehmann 1996). Skin eruptions appear to be unrelated to vitamin B deficiency (Ruze 1990). The etiology of Kava dermopathy has not been determined. Suggested mechanisms have included niacin deficiency, skin accumulation of kavalactones, and chronic allergic dermatitis, but the cause remains unclear.

In recent reports, possible allergic dermatitis related to *P. methysticum* ingestion has been documented. In one case, significant lymphocytosis was triggered by *P. methysticum* extract. Based upon patient reports of poorer hair condition during *P. methysticum* treatment, it has been suggested that skin reactions may be related to cholesterol metabolism (Mills, Bone 2000).

Interestingly, the lesions leave no scars and the skin is smooth and clear following desquamation. Native cultures have used this effect to treat skin disease, much as tretinoin and other exfoliatives are used for the treatment of acne and other dermopathies (Russo 2001). *P. methysticum* may hold promise for this application as well and deserves further study.

Clinical reports of four patients with extrapyramidal signs following *P. methysticum* consumption may infer an underlying central dopaminergic antagonistic effect. A 22-year old woman exhibited involuntary oral and lingual dyskinesia, tonic head rotation, and painful twisting movements of the trunk within four hours of *P. methysticum* ingestion. A similar reaction was described in a 63-year-old woman after four days of *P. methysticum* consumption (Schelosky, Raffauf, Jendroska et al. 1995).

Aggravation of Parkinson's disease symptoms occurred in a 76-year-old woman. A 28-year-old man with a history of acute dystonia caused by anxiolytic drugs also developed involuntary neck extension and eye deviation within 90 minutes of taking *P. methysticum* for the first time (Schelosky, Raffauf, Jendroska et al. 1995). This evidence of a dopaminergic mechanism supports the possible benefit of *P. methysticum* to treat schizophrenia. Further, results suggest that *P. methysticum* should be used with caution in patients with Parkinson's disease and other conditions or medications that affect dopamine pathways. In fact, one case report describes *P. methysticum* -triggered Parkinsonian signs in a 45-year-old woman with a family history of Parkinson's disease (Meseguer, Taboada, Sanchez et al. 2002). *P. methysticum* can disrupt the effects of levodopa in Parkinson patients (Izzo, Ernst 2001).

Recent deaths and hepatic failure attributed to *P. methysticum* consumption are reported. In August 2002, Canadian authorities banned the sale and recall of all products containing *P. methysticum* or more than 30 different names of ingredients associated with *P. methysticum* components (Health Canada Online 2002). This action was prompted by findings of the Canadian health agency that *P. methysticum* use cause liver toxicity, muscle weakness, and incoordination. Four cases of suspected *P. methysticum*–induced hepatotoxicity were cited, none of which resulted in fatalities. However, the recall was also based on the reports of three deaths attributed to *P. methysticum* use in Europe. Between 1990 and 2002, 29 cases of hepatitis in Europe were recorded in association with *P. methysticum* intake; nine patients died, including two who succumbed after liver transplantation (Stickel, Baumuller, Seitz et al. 2003).

However, at least one report examines these cases more closely and proposes that an immune-mediated idiosyncratic mechanism is possible (Schulze, Raasch, Siegers 2003). Some suggest that the withdrawal of *P. methysticum* products may have been an "ill-founded over-reaction" (Schulze, Raasch, Siegers 2003). This is supported by another German study that examined the cases of *P. methysticum* hepatotoxicity and concluded that only one patient was consistent with *P. methysticum* toxicity. In 12 other patients, data was insufficient to confirm *P. methysticum* as the cause of disease. In five other cases, *P. methysticum* was excluded as a cause of liver disease. Nonetheless, caution was urged during the administration of *P. methysticum* (Teschke, Gaus, Loew 2003). A recent study suggests that electrophilic quinoid metabolites by hepatic microsomes may contribute to hepatotoxicity in people with preexisting genetic predisposition or drug interaction, but not under ordinary circumstances (Johnson, Qiu, Zhang et al. 2003).

Although *P. methysticum* products continue to be sold in the United States, a recent case of a 14-year-old girl who suffered acute hepatic failure and subsequently survived a liver transplant was reported. Liver biopsy showed hepatocellular necrosis consistent with chemical hepatitis. She had been taking a product containing *P. methysticum* for four months; however, the product itself was not subjected to chemical analysis (Humberston, Akhtar, Krenzelok 2003).

In a recent study on rats (Singh, Devkota 2003), a traditional aqueous infusion was administered in daily dosages of 200–500 mg/kg for two to four weeks. There was no elevation of enzymes known to be markers of liver toxicity (including alanine aminotransferase, aspartate aminotransferase, alkaline phosphatase, and lactate dehydrogenase); in some cases, in fact, these were significantly reduced. This supports the suggestions that commercial preparations differ in hepatotoxic potential compared to traditional *P. methysticum*. It has also been suggested that some *P. methysticum* products contain aerial portions of the plant that are not traditionally used. In a recent study of the major *P. methysticum* alkaloids, pipermethystine and not kavalactones appeared to induce cell apoptosis that may contribute to rare but worrisome hepatotoxicity associated with Kava consumption (Nerurkar, Dragull, Tang 2004).

The German Commission E monograph on the therapeutic use of *P. methysticum* advises that it is contraindicated for pregnant or nursing women and for the treatment of endogenous depression (Singh 1992). However, this is based on a lack of data rather than on evidence of adverse effects in these women (Mills, Bone 2000).

Drug interactions with kavalactones have been documented. These include a potentiation of barbiturate narcosis by dihydromethysticin in mice (Lebot, Merlin, Lindstrom 1992), and lethargy and disorientation (referred to as a "coma" by the authors in their title) in a 54-year-old man following use of *P. methysticum* and alprazolam (Xanax®) (Almeida, Grimsley 1996). *P. methysticum* may potentiate the effects of alprazolam (Izzo, Ernst 2001). However, the report of this solitary case of a patient who also used several other medications with the potential for CNS effects was poorly documented and conclusions were questionable.

In a recent study of 40 healthy human volunteers no negative effects of concomitant use of *P. methysticum* and alcohol were found (Herberg 1993); results suggested that *P. methysticum* could have counteracted the adverse effect of alcohol on cognitive performance. This is in contrast to another report of one individual who suffered transitory visual dysfunction approximately 30 minutes after drinking 500 ml of traditionally prepared *P. methysticum* (Garner, Klinger 1985). A study of *P. methysticum* and ethanol in mice determined that they both potentiate the other's toxicity in a dose-dependent manner (Jamieson, Duffield 1990a).

Given the current evidence for the potential of interaction with alcohol, barbiturates, benzodiazepines, sedatives, and antidepressants, their concomitant use with *P. methysticum* should be avoided (Bone 1993/94). This caution has serious implications for human and nonhuman surgical patients and underscores the importance of disclosing the use of all conventional and alternative medicines.

The potential abuse of substances with psychoactive effects should be a consideration. Reports of *P. methysticum* abuse have been described as a social epidemic among Australian Aborigines. Church workers who knew of the herb from contacts with Pacific Islanders introduced *P. methysticum* in the early 1980s to the Yolngu people in the Northern Territory of Australia. Their intent was to convince aboriginal alcohol abusers to use Kava instead of alcohol. However, by 1985, enormous quantities of *P. methysticum* were being consumed by as many as 80% of the adult male and 20% of the adult female aboriginal population (Lebot, Merlin, Linstrom 1992). Individuals consumed as much as 440 grams each week, which would be the equivalent of up to 100 times the quantity of normal consumption by Pacific indigenes, or more than one gallon of Kava every day (Lebot, Levesque 1989). One study (Mathews, Riley, Fejo et al. 1988), which arose from this unfortunate situation, concluded that *P. methysticum* was harmful. This was based on the poor health of the users (underweight 20%; serum biochemical changes that included decreased albumin, blood urea, and bilirubin, as well as elevated GGT (gamma-glutamyl-transferase). However, this study did not consider that many of the subjects heavily abused alcohol and tobacco, or the fact that aboriginal health is poor compared to other ethnic groups in Australia. Nonetheless, this phenomenon does indicate the potential for *P. methysticum* abuse, particularly when its use is not controlled by traditional or ritual checks.

Availability

P. methysticum is currently supplied in capsules of 100 mg, 125 mg, 128 mg, 150 mg, 250 mg, 390 mg, 400 mg, 425 mg, 455 mg, and 500 mg. It is available in liquid tinctures of 1:1 and 1:2, taken as 30 drops with water three times a day. It can also be taken as an infusion of one half cup twice a day. It should be taken with food or liquid to enhance absorption because of its lipid solubility (PDR 2000). Many polyherbal mixes are available for *P. methysticum.*

A bowl of Kava beverage contains approximately 250 mg of kavalactones. During traditional ceremonies, several bowls may be consumed (Bone 1993/94). The suggested dosages in people includes: standard preparations 100–200 mg of kavalactones divided/day; dried root/rhizome: 1.5–3 g/day; alcoholic 1:2 extract: 3 to 6 ml/day (20–40 ml/wk) (Bone 1993/94).

The American Herbal Products Association (AHPA) has suggested a total kavalactones intake of 300 mg/day and does not advocate its use for people younger than 18 years of age, when operating heavy equipment or automobiles, or in combination with alcohol (Anonymous 1999).

P. methysticum's hypnotic effect makes it an option for the treatment of mild insomnia (Bone 1993/94). A single bedtime dose of 150–210 mg of kavalactones is recommended to promote sleep in cases of insomnia and tension (Lebot, Levesque 1989).

The effects of Kavatrol®, a U.S.-marketed product, were reported to be safe and effective in an unpublished study at doses of up to 400 mg per day. However, this product is a cocktail of kavalactones, *Humulus lupulus* (Hops), *Passiflora incarnata* (Passionflower), *Matricaria chamomilla* (Chamomile), and *Schisandra chinensis* (Schisandra, Wu wei zi), and ingredient concentration is unclear on both the package and label (Russo 2001). It has been determined that modern pharmaceutical preparations of *P. methysticum* use dried rootstock or inferior-quality lateral roots. These are concentrated 12 to 2:1 in ethanol and water to produce 30% kavalactones, or a 70% yield in acetone and water (Schulz, Hansel, Tyler 1998). This complicates the calculation of required dosages, as well as the risk of side effects.

The recommended anxiolytic oral dose of *P. methysticum* varies according to the source. One recommendation is for 50–70 mg every eight hours (Lebot, Levesque 1989). However, a more current reference suggests the following dosages: 1.5–3 g/day of dried root or in decoction; 3–6 ml/day of 1:2 liquid extract; standardized preparation of 100–200 mg of kava lactones/day; standardized tablets of 60 mg, one tab 2–4 times/day.

The recommended hypnotic dose is the daily dose (undivided) one hour before bedtime. For other effects, similar or higher doses are needed to effect as required (Mills & Bone 2000). In mice, high doses of prolonged kava intake were associated with partial physiological tolerance. This effect was not observed at standard doses (Duffield, Jamieson 1991).

Clinical Application in Veterinary Behavior Medicine

P. methysticum is one of the better studied psychoactive herbs, but much remains to be clarified. Its proven effects make it an interesting option in the treatment of separation anxiety syndrome, generalized anxiety disorder, phobias, and agitated or hyperactive behaviors associated with anxiety. Feline house soiling due to psychosocial stress or feline interstitial cystitis would also be included in the list of anxiety-related disorders. This application would be consistent with its recommended uses in the nineteenth century, when *P. methysticum* preparations were advocated as treatment for inflammation of the neck of the bladder, painful micturition, nocturnal incontinence, and urethritis and dysuria, among many others (Felter, Lloyd 1898). In addition, its analgesic effect suggests its use in the treatment of self-mutilation and compulsive disorders such as tail chasing and psychogenic overgrooming. Preliminary evidence of its effectiveness in controlling mood disturbance associated with menopause suggests that it could be helpful in controlling irritable aggression. Its sedative effect and possible anticonvulsant effect suggest its use in cases of psychomotor seizure and feline hyperesthesia syndrome. Its hypnotic effects may also be helpful as an adjunct to treating geriatric pets with sleep disturbance associated with feline or canine cognitive dysfunction syndrome, or for young playful cats with crepuscular or nocturnal patterns of activity.

Notwithstanding its clinical potential, the risk of side effects associated with *P.*

methysticum must be considered. *P. methysticum* may be best used on an "as needed" basis (PRN) or for short periods of time. Excessive doses should be avoided and the patient carefully monitored. To minimize the risk of side effects and still take advantage of its beneficial effects, *P. methysticum* may be combined with other remedies to enhance the therapeutic response. Drug interactions must always be carefully considered between herbal and conventional drugs, and between herbal remedies.

References

Almeida JC, Grimsley EW. Coma from the health food store: interaction between kava and alprazolam. Ann Intern Med. 1996;125:940–941.

Anonymous. AHPA reissues kava label warning. HerbalGram. 1999;45:15.

Backhauss C, Krieglstein J. Extract of kava (*Piper methysticum*) and its methysticin constituents protect brain tissue against ischemic damage in rodents. Eur J Pharmacol. 1992;215:265–269.

Baldi D. Sulle proprieta farmacologische del *Piper methysticum*. Terapia Moderna. 1980;359–364.

Blier P, de Montigny C. Current advances and trends in the treatment of depression. Trends Pharmacol Sci. 1994;15:220–226.

Boerner RJ, Sommer H, Berger W et al. Kava-kava extract LI 150 is as effective as opipramol and buspirone in generalized Anxiety Disorder—an 8 week randomized, double-blind multi-centre clinical trial in 129 out-patients. Phytomedicine. 2003;10 Suppl 4:38–49.

Bone K. Kava: A safe herbal treatment for anxiety. Br J Phytother. 1993/94;3:147–152.

Bruggenmann F, Meyer HJ. Die analgetische Wirkung der Kawa-Inhaltsstoffe Dihydrokawain und Dihydromethysticin. Arzneim.-forsch. 1963;13:407–409.

Buckley JP, Furgiuele AR, O'Hara MJ. Pharmacology of kava. In: Efron DH (ed). Ethnopharmacologic search for psychoactive drugs. Raven Press, New York, NY. 1979;141–150.

Cropley M, Cave Z, Ellis J et al. Effect of kava and valerian on human physiological and psychological responses to mental stress assessed under laboratory conditions. Phytother Res. 2002:16:23–27.

Davies LP, Drew CA, Duffield P et al. Kava pyrones and resin: studies on $GABA_A$, $GABA_B$ and benzodiazepine binding sites in rodent brain. Pharmacol Toxicol. 1992;71:120–126.

Dubovsky SL. Calcium antagonists in manic-depressive illness. Neuropsychobiol. 1993;27:184–192.

Duffield PH, Jamieson DD. Development of tolerance to kava in mice. Clin Exper Pharmacol Physiol. 1991;18:571–578.

Felter HW, Lloyd JU. King's American Dispensatory. Ohio Valley Company, Cincinatti, OH. 1898. Available online at http://www.ibiblio.org/herbmed/eclectic/kings/

Garner LF, Klinger JD. Some visual effects caused by the beverage kava. J Ethnopharmacol. 1985;13: 307–311.

Garrett KM, Basmadjian G, Khan IA et al. Extracts of kava (*Piper methysticum*) induce acute anxiolytic-like behavioral changes in mice. Psychopharmacology. 2003;170:33–41.

Gleitz J, Beile A, Peters T. (+/-)-Kavain inhibits veratridine-activated voltage-dependent Na+ channels in synaptosomes prepared from rat cerebral cortex. Neuropharmacology. 1994;34:1133–1138.

Gleitz J, Friese J, Beile A, et al. Anticonvulsive action of (+/-)kkavain estimated from its properties on stimulated synaptosomes and Na+ channel receptor sites. Eur J Pharmacol. 1996;315:89–97.

Gleitz J, Beile A, Peters T. (+/-)-Kavain inhibits the veratridine- and KCl-induced increase in intracellular Ca2+ and glutamate-release of rat cerebrocortical synaptosomes. Neuropharmacology. 1996;35: 179–186.

Gleitz J, Beile A, Wildens P et al. Antithrombotic action of the kava pyrone (+/-) kavain prepared from *Piper methysticum* on human platelets. Planta Med. 1997;63:27–30.

Hansel R. Kava-kava (*Piper methysticum* G. Forster) in contemporary medical research: Portrait of a medicinal plant. European J Herb Med. 1997-1998;3:17–23.

Hashimoto T, Suganuma M, Fujiki H et al. Isolation and synthesis of TNF-alpha release inhibitors from Fijian Kawa (*Piper methysticum*). Phytomedicine. 2003;10:309–317.

Health Canada Online. Health Advisory: Health Canada Issues a stop-sale order for all products containing kava. August 21, 2002. http://www.hcsc.gc.ca/english/protection/warnings/2002/2002_56e.htm

Heinz HJ, Munthe TF, Steitz J et al. Pharmacopsychological effects of oxazepam and kava-extract in a visual search paradigm assessed with event-related potentials. Pharmacopsychiatry. 1994;27:224–230.

Holm E. Staedt U, Heep J, et al. Untersuchungen zum Wirkungsprofil von D,L-Kavain. Arzneim.-Forsch./Drug Res. 1991;41:673–683.

Herberg KW. Effect of Kava-Special Extract WS 1490 combined with ethyl alcohol on safety-relevant performance parameters. Blutalkohol. 1993;30:96–105.

Humberston CL, Akhtar J, Krenzelok EP. Acute hepatitis induced by kava kava. J Toxicol Clin Toxicol. 2003;41:109–113.

Izzo AA, Ernst E. Interactions between herbal medicines and prescribed drugs: a systematic review. Drugs 2001;61:2163–2175.

Jamieson DD, Duffield PH, Cheng D et al. Comparison of the CNS activity of the aqueous and lipid extract of kava (*Piper methysticum*). Arch Int Pharmacodyn. 1989;301:66–80.

Jamieson DD, Duffield PH. Positive interaction of ethanol and kava resin in mice. Clin Exp Pharmacol Physiol. 1990;17:509–514.

——. The antinociceptive actions of kava components in mice. Clin Exp Pharmacol Physiol. 1990;17: 495–508.

Johnson BM, Qiu SX, Zhang S et al. Identification of novel electrophilic metabolites of *Piper methysticum* Forst (kava). Chem Res Toxicol. 2003;16:733–740.

Jossang P, Molho D. Etude des constituents des feuilles de *Piper methysticum* Forst. Bulletin du Musee National D'Histoire Naturelle. 1970;440–447.

Jussofie A, Schmiz A, Himke C. Kavapyrone enriched extract from *Piper methysticum* as modulator of GABA binding site in different regions of rat brain. Psychopharmacology (Berlin). 1994;116: 469–474.

Keller F, Klohs MW. A review of the chemistry and pharmacology of the constituents of *Piper methysticum*. Lloydia. 1963;26:1–15.

Kilham C. Kava: Medicine Hunting in Paradise. Park Street Press, Rochester, VT. 1996;60–68.

Klohs MW, Keller F, Williams RE et al. A chemical and pharmacological investigation of *Piper methysticum* Forst. J Medication Pharm Chem. 1959;1:95–103.

Kretzschmar R, Meyer HJ, Teschendorf HJ. Strychnine antagonistic potency of pyrone compounds of the kava root (*Piper methysticum* Forst). Experientia. 1970;26:283–284.

Kretzschmar R, Teschendorf HJ. Pharmakologische Untersuchungen zur sedativ-tranquilisierenden Wirkung des Rauschpfeffers Piper methysticum Forst. Chemiker Zeitung. 1974;98:24.

Lebot V, Merlin M, Lindstrom L. Kava- the Pacific Elixir: the definitive guide to its ethnobotany, history and chemistry. Yale University Press, New Haven, CT. 1992:10–11.

Lebot V, Levesque J. The origin and distribution of kava: A phytochemical approach. Allertonia. 1989;5:223–280.

Lemert EM. Forms and pathology of drinking in three Polynesian societies. American Anthropologist. 1967;361–374.

Locher CP, Burch MT, Mower HF. Antimicrobial activity and anti-complement activity of extracts obtained from selected Hawaiian medicinal plants. J Ethnopharmacol. 1995;49:23–32.

Mathews JD, Riley MD, Fejo L et al. Effects of the heavy usage of kava on physical health: summary of a pilot survey in an aboriginal community. Med J Aust. 1988;148:548–555.

Meseguer E, Taboada R,Sanchez V, Mena MA, Campos V, Garcia De Yebenes J. Life-threatening parkinsonism induced by kava-kava. Mov Disord. 2002;17:195–196.

Meyer HJ. Pharmacology of kava. In: Efron DH, Holmsted B, Kline NA (eds). Ethnopharmacologic Search for Psychoative Drugs. Raven Press, New York, NY. 1979.

Meyer HJ, Kretzschmar R. Untersuchungen uber Beziehungen zwischen Molekularstruktur und pharmakologischer Wirkung C6-arylsubstituierter 4-Methoxy-alpha-pyrone vom Typ der Kawa-Pyrone. Arzneim-Forsch. 1969;19:617–623.

Mills S, Bone K. Principles and Practice of Phytotherapy. Churchill Livingstone, Philadelphia, PA. 2000;456–464.

Moerman DE. Native American Ethnobotany. Timber Press, Portland, OR. 2002;414–415.

Munte TF, Heinze HJ, Matzke M et al. Effects of oxazepam and an extract of kava roots (*Piper methysticum*) on event-related potentials in a word recognition task. Neuropsychobiology. 1993;27:46–53.

Nerurkar PV, Dragull K, Tang CS. In vitro toxicity of kava alkaloid, pipermethystine, in HepG2 cells as compared to kavalactones. Toxicol Sci. 2004;79:106–111.

Parkinson S. A journal of a voyage to the South Seas in His Majesty's ship the Endeavour (1768). S. Parkinson, London 1773.

PDR for Herbal Medicines (2nd ed) Medical Economics Company Inc., Montvale, NJ. 2000;443–446.

Piscopo G. Kava Kava: Gift of the Islands. Alternative Medicine Review. 1997;2:355–364.

Russo E. Handbook of Psychotropic Herbs: A Scientific Analysis of Herbal Remedies for Psychiatric Conditions. The Haworth Press, Binghamton, NY. 2001;160–179.

Ruze P. Kava-induced dermopathy: a niacin deficiency? Lancet. 1990;335:1442–1445.

Schelosky L, Raffauf C, Jendroska K et al. Kava and dopamine antagonism. J Neurol Neurosurg Psychiatry. 1995;58:639–640.

Schirrmacher K, Busselberg D, Langosch JM et al. Effects of (+/-)-kavain on voltage-activated inward currents of dorsal root ganglion cells from neonatal rats. European Neurophsychopharmacology. 1999;9:171–176.

Schouten W. The voyage of James Le Mair and William Schouten, 1616. In: Dalrymple A (ed). A historical collection of the several voyages and discoveries in the South Pacific Ocean: Dutch voyages. N. Israel, Amsterdam. 1771;2:1–64.

Schulz V, Hansel R, Tyler VE. Rational phytotherapy: A physicians' guide to herbal medicine. (3rd ed) Springer Verlag, New York, NY. 1998.

Schulze J, Raasch W, Siegers CP. Toxicity of kava pyrones, drug safety and precautions—a case study. Phytomedicine. 2003;10 Suppl 4:68–73.

Seitz U, Ameri A, Pelzer H et al. Relaxation of evoked contractile activity of isolated guinea-pig ileum by (+/-)-kavain. Planta Med. 1997;63:359–364.

Seitz U, Schule A, Gleitz J. [3H]-monoamine uptake inhibition properties of kava pyrones. Planta Med. 1997;63:548–549.

Singh YN. Effects of kava on neuromuscular transmission and muscle contractility. J Ethnopharmacol. 1983;7:267–276.

Singh YN. Kava: an overview. J Ethnopharmacol. 1992;37:13–45.

Singh YN, Devkota AK. Aqueous Kava extracts do not affect liver function tests in rats. Planta Med. 2003;69:496–499.

Spinella M. The importance of pharmacological synergy in psychoactive herbal medicines. Altern Med Rev. 2002;7:130–137.

Stickel F, Baumuller HM, Seitz K et al. Hepatitis induced by Kava. J Hepatol. 2003;39:62–67.

Suss R, Lehmann P. Hematogenous contact eczema caused by phytogenic drugs exemplified by kava root extract. Hautarzt. 1996;47:459–461.

Teschke R, Gaus W, Loew D. Kava extracts: safety and risks including rare hepatotoxicity. Phytomedicine. 2003;10:440–446.

Tillotson AK, Tillotson HS, Abel R. The One Earth Herbal Sourcebook. Kensington Publishing, New York, NY. 2001;338.

Volz HP, Kieser M. Kava-kava extract WS 1490 versus placebo in anxiety disorders: a randomized placebo-controlled 25 week outpatient trial. Pharmacopsychiat. 1997;30:1–5.

Walden J, Von Wegerer J, Winter U, et al. Effects of kawain and dihydromethysticin on field potential changes in the hippocampus. Prog Neuro-Psychopharmacol Biol Psychiat. 1997;21:697–706.

Wu D, Yu L, Nair MG et al. Cyclooxygenase enzyme inhibitory compounds with antioxidant activities from *Piper methysticum* (kava kava) roots. Phytomedicine. 2002;9:41–47.
Wu D, Nair MG, De Witt DL. Novel compounds from *Piper methysticum* Forst (Kava Kava) roots and their effect on cyclooxygenase enzyme. J Agric Food Chem. 2002;50:701–705.
Yuan CS, Dey L, Wang A et al. Kavalactones and dihydrokavain modulate GABAergic activity in a rat gastric-brainstem preparation. Planta Med. 2002;68:1092–1096.

Psilocybe spp.

Psilocybe mushroom species are found around the world (Hyde, Glancy, Omerod et al. 1978; Musha, Ishii, Tanaka et al. 1986; Allen, Merlin, Jansen 1991; Merlin, Allen 1993; Allen, Merlin 1992; Lehrer, Hughes, Altman et al. 1994; Marcano, Morales Mendez, Castellano et al. 1994; Borowiak, Ciechanowski, Waloszczyk 1998; Beck, Helander, Karlson-Stiber et al. 1998; Bogusz, Maier Schafer 1998; Lee, Cole, Linacre 2000; Pierrot, Josse, Raspiller et al. 2000; Moldavan, Grodzinskaya, Solomko et al. 2001; Carod Artal 2003) and have been used for medicinal and mystical practices (Carod Artal 2003). Recognized psychedelic fungi include *Panaelolus spp.* and the LSD-rich *Claviceps purpurea* (Carod Artal 2003). *Claviceps purpurea* was also the source of ergot, used medicinally to promote uterine contraction in cases of uterine inertia and hemorrhage, for example (Felter, Lloyd 1898). *L. williamsii* is discussed in detail elsewhere in this section.

In Thailand, some natives actively sell psychoactive fungi to tourists and foreign immigrants, as well as to restaurants for use in omelettes and soups. Marketing includes the sale of souvenir T-shirts, posters, and postcards celebrating the hallucinogenic fungi (Allen, Merlin 1992). Some Dutch coffee shops sell honey laced with psilocybe mushroom particles. Although this is legal in Holland, these illicit honey preparations have become increasingly popular elsewhere (Bogusz, Maier, Schafer et al. 1998).

Ingredients

Psilocybin and psilocin are the primary psychoactive compounds; these are not necessarily found in psychoactive fungal species other than *Psilocybe spp.* (Merlin, Allen 1993). Psychoactive fungi containing these alkaloids are often called "magic mushrooms" (Musshoff, Madea, Beike 2000). These compounds are derived from tryptamine and are characterized by an indole nucleus (Pierrot, Jose, Raspiller et al. 2000).

CNS Effects

In vitro Psilocybin extract was recently shown to reduce spike activity of hippocampal pyramidal neurons and to suppress glutamate transmission (Moldavan, Grodzinskaya, Solomko et al. 2001). Recreational ingestion of hallucinogenic fungi is an increasing problem around the world, prompting many forensic laboratories to conduct further research (Gross 2000; Lee, Cole, Linacre 2000; Musshoff, Madea, Beike 2000).

Behavioral and Psychological Effects

Psilocybe mushrooms have been suggested as a possible treatment for obsessive-compulsive disorders in people. In one report, compulsive counting, showering, and ritualistic washing of the hands, body, and clothes were controlled in one patient who self-medicated with daily Psilocibe ingestion over a four-year period. His compulsive symptoms disappeared but returned two years after he had discontinued the mushroom preparation. During Psilocibe ingestion, he did not suffer hallucinogenic effects because of an acquired tolerance. It is thought that a down-regulation of 5-HT_{2A} receptors by psychedelic drugs such as LSD, psilocybin (in Psilocybe mushrooms), and mescaline (in *L. williamsii*, the Peyote cactus) may explain a beneficial effect on OCD, and that this may alleviate other diseases such as anorexia nervosa (Perrine 1999).

Adverse Effects

Phenylethylamine has been implicated as playing a role in adverse reactions to Psilocybe mushroom consumption (Beck, Helander, Karlson-Stiber et al. 1998). Toxic effects include: sympathomimetic signs, transient psychotic states, schizoid reactions (Hyde, Glancy, Omerod et al. 1978); psychedelic states with dream consciousness, complete amnesia (Musha, Ishii, Tanaka et al. 1986); cardiac toxicity including Wolff-Parkinson-White syndrome, arrhythmia, myocardial infarction (Borowiak, Ciechanowski, Waloszczyk 1998), tachycardia (Beck, Helander, Karlson-Stiber 1998). Complications may be fatal and diagnosis can be difficult (Pierrot, Jose, Raspiller et al. 2000).

Wild *Psilocybe cubensis* is so widespread in the United States and in Europe that it constitutes the most potent allergen source in its category. Basidiospore reactivity is most often associated with symptoms of atopy, asthma, and rhinitis (Lehrer, Hughes, Altman et al. 1994).

Clinical Application in Veterinary Behavior Medicine

Illegal substances have no place in clinical veterinary practice.

References

Allen JW, Merlin MD. Psychoactive mushroom use in Koh samui and Koh Pha-Ngan, Thailand. J Ethnopharmacol 1992;35:205–228.

Allen JW, Merlin MD, Jansen KL. An ethnomycological review of psychoactive agarics in Australia and New Zealand. J Psychoativ Drugs. 1991;23:39–69.

Beck O, Helander A, Karlson-Stiber C et al. Presence of phenylethylamine in hallucinogenic Psilocybe mushroom: possible role in adverse reactions. J Anal Toxicol. 1998;22:45–49.

Bogusz MJ, Maier RD, Schafer AT et al. Honey with Psilocybe mushrooms: a revival of a very old preparation on the drug market? Int J Legal Med. 1998;111:147–150.

Carod Artal FJ. Neurological syndromes associated with the ingestion of plants and fungi with a toxic component (II). Hallucinogenic fungi and plants, mycotoxins and medicinal herbs. Rev Neurol. 2003;36:951–960.
Felter HW, Lloyd JU. King's American Dispensatory. Ohio Valley Company, Cincinatti, OH. 1898. Available online at http://www.ibiblio.org/herbmed/eclectic/kings/
Gross ST. Detecting psychoactive drugs in the developmental stage of mushrooms. J forensic Sce. 2000; 45:527–537.
Hyde C, Glancy G, Omerod P et al. Abuse of indigenous psilocybin mushrooms: a new fashion and some psychiatric complications. Br J Psychiatry. 1978:132:602–604.
Lee JC, Cole M, Linacre A. Identification of members of the genera Panaeolus and Psilocybe by a DNA test. A preliminary test for hallucinogenic fungi. Forensic Sci Int. 2000;112:123–133.
Lehrer SB, Hughes JM, Altman LC et al. Prevalence of basidiomycete allergy in the USA and Europe and its relationship to allergic respiratory symptoms. Allergy. 1994;49:460–465.
Marcano V, Morales Mendez A, Castellano F et al. Occurrence of psilocybin and psilocin in *Psilocybe pseudobullacea* (Petch) Pegler from the Venezuelan Andes. J Ethnopharmacol. 1994;43:157–159.
Merlin MD, Allen JW. Species identification and chemical analysis of psychoactive fungi in the Hawaiian islands. J Ethnopharmacol. 1993;40:21–40.
Moldavan MG, Grodzinskaya AA, Solomko EF et al. The effect of *Psilocybe cubensis* extract on hippocampal neurons in vitro. Fiziol Zh. 2001;47:14–23.
Musha M, Ishii A, Tanaka F et al. Tohoku J Exp Med. 1986;148:73–78.
Musshoff F, Madea B, Beike J. Hallucinogenic mushrooms on the German market: simple instructions for examination and identification. Forensic Sci Int. 2000;113:389–395.
Perrine DM. Hallucinogens and obsessive-compulsive disorder. Am J Psychiatry 1999;156:1123.
Pierrot M, Josse P, Raspiller MF et al. Intoxications by hallucinogenic mushrooms. Ann Med Interne (Paris) 2000;151 (Suppl B):B16–19.

Salvia spp.

Salvia officinalis (Common Sage, Garden Sage, Kitchen Sage, Dalmatian Sage), a small shrub up to 60 cm high, is a native to the Mediterranean, where it is still harvested today (Fig. 2-3; color plate 2-2). *S. officinalis* is a member of the family *Labiatae (Lamiacaea)*; the subfamily *Nepetoideae* includes *Lavandula, Nepeta, Prunella, Melissa, Monarda,* and *Salvia* clades, all of which include psychoactive members that are described elsewhere in this book (Kaufmann, Wink 1994). Many varieties of Salvia species, such as *S. syriaca*, exist around the world. *Salvia miltiorrhiza* (Dan shen) is an Asian species that is described in detail in the Oriental herb section.

Salvia officinalis has naturalized everywhere in Europe (and in parts of the United States) where it is a favorite for culinary and medicinal use. Its traditional uses include gargles and infusions for infections of the mouth, throat, and digestive tract, and inhibition of perspiration and libido (Felter, Lloyd 1898; PDR 2000). *S. officinalis* has proven antibacterial antifungal, antiviral, antihypertensive, antiperspirant, and antispasmodic properties; an antidiabetic effect is also suggested (PDR 2000).

Because significant variation in the major compounds of the essential oil occurs during the year, *S. officinalis* is best harvested in the autumn or winter when thujone levels (see below) are highest (Santos-Gomes, Fernandes-Ferreira 2001; PDR

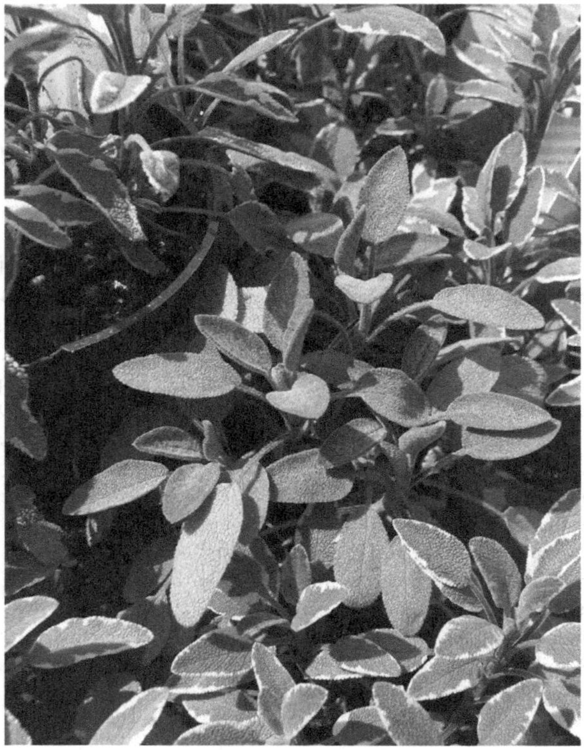

FIGURE 2-3. Varieties of *Salvia officinalis.* (Photo courtesy of Dr. Stefanie Schwartz)

2000d; Perry, Anderson, Brennan et al. 1999). *S. officinalis* is best prepared by drying in well-ventilated drying chambers with no humidity to preserve the maximum amount of volatile oil. Recent interest has focused on the use of ultrasound to more efficiently extract the major bioactive compounds from cultivated plants (PDR 2000; Salisova, Toma, Mason 1997).

Historical Perspective

It is likely that the *S. officinalis* was brought by English settlers and eventually introduced to the Native Americans. The Cherokee drank infusions of *S. officinalis* and *S. lyrata* (Lyreleaf Sage) to remedy "nervous debility." The Chinese, too, enjoyed tea made from *S. officinalis* to improve digestion and other complaints (Moerman 2002; Hamel, Chiltoskey 1975).

S. divinorum has hallucinogenic properties that were used ritually and medicinally by the Mazatec Indians of Mexico. Its psychoactive effects are comparable to psilocybin mushrooms, discussed elsewhere in this text (Valdes, Diaz, Paul 1983). It is used as a marijuana substitute today in many countries around the world

(Giroud, Felber, Augsburger et al. 2000). Recreational use of the "magic mint" is of increasing concern because it is not yet specifically banned in many places. Its popularity is on the rise in Europe and in the United States (Roth, Baner, Westkaemper et al. 2002; Giroud, Felber, Augsburger et al. 2000).

Ingredients

Bioactive compounds include: the volatile oil (e.g., humuline; linalool; alpha-, beta-thujone); caffeic acid derivatives (e.g., rosmarinic acid); diterpenes; flavonoids (e.g., apigenin glucoside, genkwanin); and triterpenes (Ulubelen 2003; PDR 2000d). New diterpenoid compounds (divinatorins and salvinorins) have recently been identified (Bigham, Munro, Rizzacasa et al. 2003; Munro, Rizzacasa 2003).

CNS and Neuroprotective Effects

Thujone, the primary active compound of *S. officinalis* and other varieties of *Salvia spp.*, is also the active compound in oil of *Artemisia absinthium* (Wormwood), a plant that was exploited for its hallucinogenic properties ("absinthism") in the nineteenth and early twentieth centuries. Small quantities administered to rabbits and dogs were observed to cause tremors, intoxication, and loss of sensibility; larger doses could be fatal (Felter, Lloyd 1898).

At one time, it was speculated that thujones bound to cannabinoid receptors, but this has been disproved (Meschler, Howlett 1999). The alpha- and beta-thujones are now recognized as noncompetitive blockers of the GABA Cl^- channel. They also act as seizure triggers (PDR 2000d; Burkhard, Burkhardt, Haenggeli et al. 1999; Millet, Jouglard, Steinmetz et al. 1981). Flavone constituents of *S. officinalis* (apigenin, hispidulin, and cirsimaritin) have shown competitive affinity for benzodiazepine receptors (Kavvadias, Monschein, Sand et al. 2003).

The dried root of *S. miltiorrhiza* Bunge, known as Dan shen in Chinese and Tan-shen in Japanese, is an important traditional Chinese medicine often used for the treatment of stroke and other cerebrovascular disease (Lam, Lo, Sun et al. 2003). The primary active compounds have been identified as the lipid soluble tanshinones. Tanshinones IIA and IIB showed easy penetration of the blood brain barrier of mice and possessed significant neuroprotective properties (Lam, Lo, Sun et al. 2003). Tanshinone VI had a positive impact on cardiac contractility and myocardial energy production following hypoxia (Takeo, Tanonaka, Hirai et al. 1990). *S. miltiorrhiza* produced significant improvement on cirrhosis and portal hypertension in rats by inhibiting nitric oxide, adding more proof of its antioxidant properties (Wang, Chen, Qiu 2003). *S. miltiorrhiza* is discussed in detail in Chapter 4 (Oriental Psychoactive Herbs).

Behavioral and Psychological Effects

Salvia species have drawn interest as treatments for Alzheimer's disease. In a four-month, double-blind, and placebo-controlled Iranian study of patients with mild to moderate Alzheimer's disease, *S. officinalis* extract produced significant improvement in cognitive function and less agitation in the treatment group compared to placebo (Akhondzadeh, Noroozian, Mohammadi et al. 2003). Side effects were consistent with cholinergic stimulation (or cholinesterase inhibition) and data indicating the role of cholinergic mechanisms in Alzheimer's disease. In other research, *S. lavandulaefolia* (Spanish Sage) has inhibited AChE *in vitro* and *in vivo*. This anticholinesterase property, along with antioxidant, estrogenic, and anti-inflammatory effects, led British researchers to suggest its clinical study in Alzheimer's patients (Perry, Houghton, Sampson et al. 2001).

The active component of *S. divinorum* is salvinorin A, which has high affinity for kappa-opioid receptors in rhesus monkeys (Butelman, Harris, Kreek 2003) and in cloned human kappa-opioid receptors (Chavkin, Sud, Jin et al. 2004). Kappa opioid receptors are important in the modulation of human perception. Salvinorin A's selectivity for these receptors suggest its therapeutic potential in the treatment of diseases such as schizophrenia, dementia, and bipolar disorders that are characterized by perceptual distortion (Roth, Baner, Westkaemper et al. 2002).

Fresh leaves of the herb are traditionally chewed or consumed as a beverage. Salvinorin A is deactivated by digestion, and absorption depends on absorption through the oral mucosa (Siebert 1994). In an isolated case report, an Australian patient with chronic depression self-medicated with *S. divinorum* leaves, which she chewed and held for fifteen minutes in her mouth. A therapeutic course on sertraline had previously failed to provide relief from her depression. She reported a resolution of her depressive symptoms with long-term use of the herb despite the clinician's warning against the use of a clinically uncertain remedy (Hanes 2001).

Miscellaneous Effects

In rodents, *S. leriifolia* has recently been shown to exert significant and dose-dependent anti-inflammatory properties, and may also have supraspinal antinociceptive effects via opioid receptors (Hosseinzadeh, Haddadkhodaparast, Arash 2003). Components obtained from the aerial parts of *S. officinalis* induced an immunomodulatory response (Capek, Hribalova, Svandova et al. 2003). In a Greek study of aqueous infusions of *S. officinalis*, a number of compounds showed antioxidant activity (Matsingou, Petrakis, Kapsokefalou et al. 2003).

The essential oil of *S. officinalis*, among other culinary spices and herbs tested, possessed significant antimicrobial properties that support some of its traditional uses (Kalemba, Kunicka 2003).

Adverse Effects

Although *S. officinalis* is not thought to be addictive, further research is needed to elucidate its effects and potential as a legitimate pharmaceutical compound (Halpern 2003).

Effects on cytochrome P450 oxidation further emphasize the need for more study into the toxicity and drug interaction potential of medicinal *Salvia spp.* (Hold, Sirisoma, Casida 2001; Sirisoma, Hold, Casida 2001). For example, *S. miltiorrhiza* extract stimulated cytochrome P450 activity and resulted in reduced plasma concentration of diazepam treated rats (Jinping, Peiling, Yawei et al. 2003). Evidence of interaction between herbal and conventional medicines is of growing concern, particularly since many do not reveal the use of alternative remedies for themselves or their pets to their physicians or veterinarians.

Clinical Application in Veterinary Behavior Medicine

S. officinalis is the most clinically interesting among *Salvia spp.*, in particular for its potential in the treatment of cognitive dysfunction. If clinical evidence of its efficacy in the treatment of Alzheimer's disease continues to accumulate, for example, it will become of real interest for pets suffering from cognitive dysfunction syndrome.

References

Akhondzadeh S, Noroozian M, Mohammadi M et al. *Salvia officinalis* extract in the treatment of patients with mild to moderate Alzheimer's disease: a double blind, randomized and placebo-controlled trial. J Clin Pharm Ther. 2003;28:53–59.

Bigham AK, Munro TA, Rizzacasa MA et al. Divinatorins A-C, new neoclerodane diterpenoids from the controlled sage *Salvia divinorum.* J Nat Prod. 2003;66:1242–1244.

Burkhard PR, Burkhardt K, Haenggeli CA et al. Plant-induced seizures: reappearance of an old problem. J Neurol. 1999;246:667–670.

Butelman ER, Harris TJ, Kreek MJ. The plant-derived hallucinogen, salvinorin A, produces kappa-opioid agonist-like discriminative effects in rhesus monkeys. Psychopharmacology (Berl). 2003;172: 220–224.

Capek P, Hribalova V, Svandova E et al. Characterization of immunomodulatory polysaccharides from *Salvia officinalis* L. Int J Biol Macromol. 2003;33:113–119.

Chavkin C, Sud S, Jin W et al. Salvinorin A, an active component of the hallucinogenic sage *Salvia divinorum,* is a highly efficacious kappa opioid receptor agonist: structural and functional considerations. J Pharmacol Exp Ther. 2004;308:1197–1203.

Felter HW, Lloyd JU. King's American Dispensatory. Ohio Valley Company, Cincinatti, OH. 1898. Available online at http://www.ibiblio.org/herbmed/eclectic/kings/

Giroud C, Felber F, Augsburger M et al. *Salvia divinorum*: an hallucinogenic mint which might become a new recreational drug in Switzerland. Forensic Sci Int. 2000;112:143–150.

Halpern JH. Hallucinogens: an update. Curr Psychiatry Rep. 2003;5:347–354.

Hamel PB, Chiltoskey MU. Cherokee Plants and Their Uses: A 400-Year History. Herald Publishing Co., Sylva, NC. 1975.

Hanes KR. Antidepressant effects of the herb *Salvia divinorum*: a case report. J Clin Psychopharmacol. 2001;21:634–635.

Hold KM, Sirisoma NS, Casida JE. Detoxification of alpha- and beta-Thujones (the active ingredients of absinthe): site specificity and species differences in cytochrome P450 oxidation in vitro and in vivo. Chem Res Toxicol. 2001;14:589–595.

Hosseinzadeh H, Haddadkhodaparast MH, Arash AR. Antinociceptive, antiinflammatory and acute toxicity effects of *Salvia leriifolia* Benth seed extract in mice and rats. Phytother Res. 2003;17: 422–425.

Jinping Q, Peiling H, Yawei L et al. Effects of the aqueous extract from *Salvia miltiorrhiza* Bg on the pharmacokinetics of diazepam and on liver microsomal cytochrome P450 enzyme activity in rats. J Pharm Pharmacol. 2003;55:1163–1167.

Kalemba D, Kunicka A. Antibacterial and antifungal properties of essential oils. Curr Med Chem. 2003;10:13–829.

Kaufmann M, Wink M. Molecular systematics of the nepetoideae (family *Labiatae*) phylogenetic implications form rbcL gene sequences. Z Naturforsch. 1994;49:635–645.

Kavvadias D, Monschein V, Sand P et al. Constituents of sage (*Salvia officinalis*) with in vitro affinity to human brain benzodiazepine receptors. Planta Med. 2003;69:113–117.

Lam BY, Lo AC, Sun X et al. Neuroprotective effects of tanshinones in transient focal cerebral ischemia in mice. Phytomedicine. 2003;10:286–291.

Matsingou TC, Petrakis N, Kapsokefalou M et al. Antioxidant activity of organic extracts from aqueous infusions of sage. J Agric Food Chem. 2003;51:6696–6701.

Millet Y, Jouglard J, Steinmetz MD et al. Toxicity of some essential plant oils. Clinical and experimental study. Clin Toxicol. 1981;18:1485–1498.

Moerman DE. Native American Ethnobotany. Timber Press, Portland, OR. 2002; 509–511.

Munro TA, Rizzacasa MA. Salvinorins D-F, new neoclerodane diterpenoids from *Salvia divinorum*, and an improved method for the isolation of salvinorin A. J Nat Prod. 2003;66:703–705.

PDR for Herbal Medicines. (2nd ed) Medical Economics Company Inc., Montvale, NJ. 2000;655–657.

Perry NB, Anderson RE, Brennan NJ et al. Essential oils from Dalmatian sage (*Salvia officinalis* l.): variations among individuals, plant parts, seasons, and sites. J Agric Food Chem. 1999;47:2048–2054.

Perry NS, Houghton PJ, Sampson J et al. In vitro activity of *S. lavandulaefolia* (Spanish sage) relvant to treatment of Alzeimer's disease. J Pharm Pharmacol. 2001;53:1347–1356.

Roth BL, Baner K, Westkaemper R et al. Salvinorin A: a potent naturally occurring nonnitrogenous kappa opioid selective agonist. Proc Natl Acad Sci USA. 2002;99:11934–11939.

Salisova M, Toma S, Mason TJ. Comparison of conventional and ultrasonically assisted extractions of pharmaceutically active compounds from *Salvia officinalis*. Ultrason Sonochem. 1997;4:131–134.

Santos-Gomes PC, Fernandes-Ferreira M. Organ- and season-dependent variation in the essential oil composition of *Salvia officinalis* L. cultivated at two different sites. J Agric Food Chem. 2001;49: 2908–2916.

Seibert DJ. *Salvia divinorum* and salvinorin A: new pharmacologic findings. J Ethnopharmacol. 1994; 43:53–56.

Sirisoma NS, Hold KM, Casida JE. Alpha- and beta-Thujones (herbal medicines and food additives): synthesis and analysis of hydroxy and dehydroxy metabolites. J Agric Food Chem. 2001;49:1915–1921.

Takeo S, Tanonaka K, Hirai K et al. Beneficial effect of tan-shen, an extract from the root of Salvia, on post-hypoxic recovery of cardiac contractile force. Biochem Pharmacol. 1990;40:1137–1143.

Ulubelen A. Cardioactive and antibacterial terpenoids from some Salvia species. Phytochemistry 2003; 64:395–399.

Valdes LJ, Diaz JL, Paul AG. Ethnopharmacology of ska Maria Pastora (*Salvia divinorum* Eplig & Jativa-M.). J Ethnopharmacol. 1983;7:287–312.

Wang H, Chen XP, Qiu FZ. *Salvia miltiorrhizae* ameliorates cirrhosis and portal hypertension by inhibiting nitric oxide in cirrhotic rats. Hepatobiliary Pancreat Dis Int. 2003;2:391–396.

Sanguinaria canadensis

Sanguinaria canadensis (Bloodroot, family *Papaveraceae*) is a perennial plant that is native to the northeastern United States. It is also referred to as Canadian Bloodroot, Indian Paint, Red Root, Coon Root, Snakebite, Sweet Slumber, Indian Plant, Paucon, Pauson, and Tetterwort. The whole plant and the thick, round rhizome are the medicinal parts. The rhizome grows between 2.5 and 10 cm in length and has orange-red rootlets. The plant itself is small, reaching only 15 cm high; a single gray-green and palmate leaf appears following bloom time (PDR 2000). Its name derives from a blood-like secretion from the injured root (Felter, Lloyd 1898).

Bloodroot bears mention because it was used as a love medicine by a number of Native American tribes. The Micmac used it as an aphrodisiac (Moerman 2003; Rousseau 1948). Ponca bachelors rubbed the root into the palms of their hands as a love charm (Moerman 2003; Gilmore 1919). The Algonquin also used *S. canadensis* as a love charm. However, as its alternative name "Indian Paint" implies, they also used it as a red dye for clothing, weapons, and skin decoration. During the nineteenth century, it was considered effective in treating respiratory, gynecological, dermatological (e.g., syphilis-related dermatopathy, eczema), and gastrointestinal (e.g., jaundice, dysentery) complaints. It was also used to treat impotence and other male sexual dysfunction (Felter, Lloyd 1898). An aphrodisiac effect has not been documented in modern research to date (Moerman 2003; Bradley 1936).

Ingredients

Active compounds include isoquinoline alkaloids, which include sanguinarine, chelerythrine, berberine, and others (PDR 2000).

CNS Effects

Although one study concluded that the alkaloids sanguinarine, chelerythrine, and others could be responsible for the inhibition of $GABA_A$ receptors (Haberlein, Tschiersch, Boonen et al. 1996), another determined that sanguinarine had an inhibitory effect on rat brain glutamate decarboxylase, which catalyzes GABA synthesis, implying an indirect inhibition of GABA receptors (Netopilova, Drsata, Ylrichova 1996). More recently, sanguinarine showed noncompetitive inhibition of MAO activity in mouse brain, suggesting that it contributes to catecholamine regulation (Lee, Kai, Lee 2001).

Sanguinarine is also of particular interest because of its similarity to morphine, the alkaloid of another member of the *Papaveraceae* (*Papaver somniferum*)(Bird, Franceschi, Facchini 2003). Its effect on opioid systems remains to be investigated, although a recent study of berberine bridge enzyme and other key enzymes of the *P. somniferum* that are also involved in the biosynthesis of sanguinarine determined that their impact occurs at the level of cellular DNA (Bird, Franceschi, Facchini 2003).

Miscellaneous Effects

Sanguinarine has antimicrobial and anti-inflammatory properties (Vrba, Hrbac, Ulrichova et al. 2004; Agarwal, Piesco, Peterson et al. 1997; Godowski 1989). It has documented ability to combat plaque and gingivitis and is still used as a component of some toothpastes and mouthwashes despite recent reports of the development of oral leukoplakia with one product line (Allen, Loudon, Mascarenhas 2001; PDR 2000; Godowski 1989).

Traditional application of Sanguinaria preparations for digestive complaints is supported by recent findings of *S. canadensis* extract activity against Helicobacter pylori, which has been identified as the microbe responsible for gastric or peptic ulcers (Mahady, Pendland, Stoia et al. 2003). Its potent nematocidal activity (e.g., *Toxocara canis*) is also consistent with Native American applications of this herb; however, Japanese researchers were concerned with its cytotoxicity and did not recommend sanguinarine for future antihelminthic application (Satou, Akao, Matsuhashi et al. 2002, Moerman 2002).

Sanguinarine may also have anticancer properties (Adhami, Aziz, Mukhtar et al. 2003; Ahmad, Gupta, Husain et al. 2000; Godowski 1989), although one study determined that its apparent effect was due to potent cytotoxicity without any specificity for cancer cells (Debiton, Madelmont, Legault et al. 2003).

Adverse Effects

S. canadensis induces vomiting at higher dosages and can also cause diarrhea and severe cramping (PDR 2000). It has been identified as one of two alkaloids responsible for Epidemic Dropsy, which results from consumption of food contaminated with another sanguinarine-containing, plant-derived argemone oil. Symptoms include vomiting, diarrhea, hepatotoxicity, edema, erythema, respiratory distress, glaucoma, and cardiac arrest; sporadic epidemics have been reported in India, South Africa and Fiji (Das, Khanna 1997).

Sanguinarine is a dose-dependent positive inotrope by inhibition of myocardial Na+, K+-ATPase, which must also be considered as a potential adverse effect, particularly in patients with concomitant heart disease (Seifen, Adams, Riemer 1979).

The acute oral LD50 in rats of sanguinarine was 1658 mg/kg (the rat LD 50 IV was 29 mg/kg); however, other alkaloid extracts had lower LD50 calculations (Becci, Schwartz, Barnes et al. 1987). In a recent study of the safety of sanguinarine and chelerythrine as feed additives in pigs, a daily dose of up to 5 mg/kg proved to be safe (Kosina, Walterova, Ulrichova et al. 2004).

Clinical Application in Veterinary Behavior Medicine

Further research will clarify the psychoactive effects of Sanguinaria species and their components. The risk of toxicity associated with *Sanguinaria canadensis* prohibits its use at this time, pending the establishment of appropriate dosages for each species. More important, this vulnerable plant is protected by the U.S. Department of Agriculture; its survival precludes its use for any purpose (USDA 2004).

References

Aarwal S, Piesco NP, Peterson DE et al. Effects of sanguinarium, chlorhexidine and tetracycline on neutrophil viability and functions in vitro. J Periodontal Res. 1997;32:335–344.

Adhami VM, Aziz MH, Mukhtar et al. Activation of prodeath Bcl-2 family proteins and mitochondrial apoptosis pathway by sanguinarine in immortalized human HaCaT keratinocytes. Clin Cancer Res. 2003;9:3176–3182.

Ahmad N, Gupta S, Husain MM et al. Differential antiproliferative and apoptotic response of sanguinarine for cancer cells versus normal cells. Clin Cancer Res. 2000;6:1524–1528.

Allen CL, Loudon J, Mascarenhas AK. Sanguinaria-related leukoplakia: epidemiologic and clinicopathologic features of a recently described entity. Gen Dent. 2001;49:608–614.

Becci PJ, Schwartz H, Barnes HH et al. Short-term toxicity studies of sanguinarine and of two alkaloid extracts of *Sanguinaria canadensis* L. J Toxicol Environ Health. 1987;20:199–208.

Bird DA, Franceschi VR, Facchini PJ. A tale of three cell types: alkaloid biosynthesis is localized to sieve elements in opium poppy. Plant Cell. 2003;15:2626–2635.

Bradley WT. Medical Practices of the New England Aborigines. J Am Pharm Assoc 1936;25:138–147.

Das M, Khanna SK. Clinicoepidemiological, toxicological, and safety evaluation studies on argemone oil. Crit Rev Toxicol. 1997;27:273–297.

Debiton E, Madelmont JC, Legault J et al. Sanguinarine-induced apoptosis is associated with an early and severe cellular glutathione depletion. Cancer Chemother Pharmacol. 2003;51:474–482.

Felter HW, Lloyd JU. King's American Dispensatory.Ohio Valley Company, Cincinatti, OH. 1898. Available online at http://www.ibiblio.org/herbmed/eclectic/kings/

Gilmore R. Uses of Plants by the Indians of the Missouri River Region. SI-BAE Annual Report, 1919.

Godowski KC. Antimicrobial action of sanguinarine. J Clin Dent. 1989;1:96–101.

Haberlein H, Tschiersch KP, Boonen G et al. *Chelidonium majus* L.: components with in vitro affinity for the GABAA receptor. Positive cooperation of alkaloids. Planta Med. 1996;62:227–231.

Kosina P, Walterova D, Ulrichova J et al. Sanguinarine and chelerythrine: assessment of safety on pigs in ninety days feeding experiment. Food Chem Toxicol. 2004;42:85–91.

Lee SS, Kai M, Lee MK. Inhibitory effects of sanguinarine on monoamine oxidase activity in mouse brain. Phytother Res. 2001;15:167–69.

Mahady GB, Pendland SL, Stoia A et al. In vitro susceptibility of Helicobacter pylori to isoquinoline alkaloids from *Sanguinaria canadensis* and *Hydrastis canadensis*. Phytother Res. 2003;17:217–221.

Moerman DE. University of Michigan—Dearborn. Native American Ethnobotany Database, 2003. http://herb.umd.umich.edu/

Moerman DE. Native American Ethnobotany. Timber Press, Portland, OR. 2002;108–109.

Netopilova M, Drsata J, Ulrichova J. Influence of sanguinarine on the GABA synthesizing enzyme glutamate decarboxylase in vitro. Pharmazie. 1996;51:589–591.

PDR for Herbal Medicines. (2nd ed) Medical Economics Company Inc., Montvale, NJ. 2000;108–109.

Rousseau J. Ethnobotanique et ethnozoologie gaspesiennes. Archives de Folklore. 1948;3:51–64.

Satou T, Akao N, Matsuhashi R et al. Inhibitory effect of isoquinoline alkaloids on movement of second-stage larvae of *Toxocara canis*. Biol Pharm Bull. 2002;25:1651–1654.

Seifen E, Adams RJ, Riemer RK. Sanguinarine: a positive inotropic alkaloid which inhibits cardiac Na+,K+-ATPase. Eur J Pharmacol. 1979;60:373–377.

United States Department of Agriculture, 2004; http://plants.usda.gov/cgi_bin/

Vrba J, Hrbac J, Ulrichova J et al. Sanguinarine is a potent inhibitor of oxidative burst in DMSO-differentiated HL-60 cells by a non-redox mechanism. Chem Biol Interact. 2004;147:35–47.

Scutellaria spp.

Scutellaria lateriflora (Scullcap, Skullcap, American Scullcap, Blue Skullcap, Quaker Bonnet, Blue Pimpernel, Madweed, Mad-Dog Weed, Helmet Flower, Hoodwort; family *Lamiaceae*) is a perennial native to North America and is also cultivated in Europe. *S. lateriflora* grows as high as 60 cm. It has pink or blue flowers and heavily branched, hairy stems. Foliage is oval to lanceolate and may be crenate. The medicinal part of the plant is the aerial portion of mature plants, which are not harvested before the third bloom during the month of June (PDR 2000; Russo 2001). Traditionally, *S. lateriflora* has been used for the treatment of seizures, delirium tremens, irritable digestive disorders, insomnia, tension headache, hysteria, irritability, and nervousness (Mills, Bone 2000; PDR 2000; Felter, Lloyd 18981). Scullcap species have been shown to possess antispasmodic, anti-inflammatory, and sedative effects (PDR 2000) (color plate 2-3).

The most active research is currently focused on the Chinese medicinal herb *Scutellaria baicalensis* (*Huang qin*, Chinese Scullcap), an Asian species that is used in Traditional Chinese Medicine (TCM) for the treatment of bronchitis and digestive conditions, among other applications; it has also shown sedative effects and impressive antioxidant properties. According to TCM principles, *S. baicalensis* affects the liver, lung, heart, gallbladder, and large intestine meridians (channels). It is used for excessive liver yang characterized by irritability, red eyes, flushed face associated with hypertension, and other ailments. Traditionally, it is applied as a calming agent because it dispels heat (it is "cold" in energy) and toxins (Tierra 1998).

Historical Perspective

The Cherokee used a decoction of *Scutellaria incana* (Hoary Skullcap), *S. elliptica* (Hairy Skullcap), or *S. lateriflora* for nerves and breast pain (Moerman 2003; Moerman 2002; Hamel, Chiltoskey 1975). *S. lateriflora's* name of "mad-dog" alludes to its traditional use to treat human exposure to rabies (Russo 2001). The plant enjoyed popularity as a nervine tea for headache, sedation, and a variety of ailments associated with nervousness and anxiety well through the nineteenth century (Felter, Lloyd 1898).

Ingredients

Active compounds of skullcap species include iridoids, volatile oil, tannins, and flavonoids (e.g., scutellarin, wogonin, baicalein, baicalin) (Lee, Yang, Wang et al. 2003; PDR 2000). The root of *S. baicalensis*, for example, contains a concentration of more than 35% in flavonoids, which are very important to its antioxidant, antimicrobial, anticancer, and anxiolytic activity (Wolfson, Hoffmann 2003).

CNS and Neuroprotective Effects

A Korean research team has shown that wogonin, a flavonoid isolated from the root of *S. baicalensis*, inhibits the pathogenic inflammatory response and exerts a significant neuroprotective effect (Lee, Kim, Kim et al. 2003). In China, researchers found that the flavonoid baicalein is the most potent neuroprotector compared to baicalin and wogonin (Lee, Yang, Wang et al. 2003). In addition to having antioxidant effects, baicalein and baicalin appeared to antagonize acetylcholine (Huang, Wong, Lau et al. 2004).

Behavioral and Psychological Effects

Recent study has begun to shed light on the psychoactive effects of Scutellaria species. For example, 5,7,2′-trihydroxy-6,8-dimethoxyflavone, a newly identified flavonoid isolated from *S. baicalensis*, has shown significant anxiolytic properties comparable to diazepam but without any sedative, myorelaxant, or ataxic effects. It showed an affinity for benzodiazepine receptors and potentiated $GABA_A$ receptors (Huen, Hui, Leung et al. 2003). In an earlier report (Wang, Hui, Xu et al. 2002;), this flavonoid along with another new flavone 6,2′-dihydroxy-5,7,86′-tetramethoxyflavone showed affinity for the benzodiazepine site of the $GABA_A$ receptor complex. At least two-dozen new flavonoids isolated from *S. baicalensis* exhibit binding affinity for the benzodiazepine receptor (Wang, Hui, Chen et al. 2002).

Wogonin, an important monoflavonoid of this herb, showed significant affinity for the benzodiazepine site on the $GABA_A$ receptor complex, with low toxicity and without sedation or myorelaxation in mice (Hui, Huen, Wang et al. 2002). Current research is focused on novel compounds that do not have the adverse effects attributed to benzodiazepine anxiolytics. However, preliminary evidence suggests that *S. baicalensis* may improve cognitive deficits as well as neuropathological and immune system changes in mice (Shang, Gong, Zhou et al. 2001), which could become of great clinical importance in the future.

Scutellaria flavones baicalin and baicalein, common to *S. baicalensis* as well as *S. lateriflora*, are also known to bind to the benzodiazepine site of the $GABA_A$ receptor. In fact, a Canadian study suggests that *S. lateriflora* also possesses significant anxiolytic properties (Awad, Arnason, Trudeau et al. 2003). Recently, *S. lateriflora* extract bound to the 5-HT(7) receptor and inhibited binding of [3H]-LSD to the receptor. They also identified a new bioactive flavone compound, lateriflorin (Gafner, Bergeron, Batcha et al. 2003). Finally, in a double blind, placebo-controlled study of healthy volunteers, *S. lateriflora* was associated with significant anxiolytic effects (Wolfson, Hoffman 2003). Much more clinical study is warranted.

Miscellaneous Effects

The clinical potential of Scutellaria flavones appears to be in its infancy as additional biological activities and compounds are identified. For example, baicalein was compared to the soy isoflavone genistein and was determined to be a more potent antagonist of estrogen receptors (Po, Chen, Tsang et al. 2002). This property has a number of clinical uses including the treatment of estrogen-sensitive cancers.

S. baicalensis has recognized antiviral activity against the respiratory syncytial virus (Ma, Du, But et al. 2002), hepatitis B virus (Huang, Chen, Huang et al. 2000), and the human immunodeficiency virus (HIV) (Wu, Attele, Zhang et al. 2001).

Scutellaria species are drawing interest in the treatment of cancer. *S. baicalensis* possesses antinausea activity that may be of therapeutic benefit to cancer patients undergoing chemotherapy (Aung, Dey, Mehendale et al. 2003). *S. barbatae*, another Chinese variety, showed important cytotoxicity against ovarian and breast cancer cells (Powell, Fung, Jackson et al. 2003). In another study, baicalein and baicalin possessed an anti-angiogenesis potential that could be of additional importance in cancer research (Liu, Huang, Cheng et al. 2003). Researchers at the Mount Sinai School of Medicine in New York City demonstrated that *S. baicalensis* inhibited the proliferation of squamous cell carcinoma, breast cancer, prostate carcinoma, hepatocellular carcinoma, and colon cancer *in vitro* (Zhang, Wu, Ye et al. 2003; Ye, Xui, Yi et al. 2002).

Adverse Effects

Adverse effects have not been reported with therapeutic dosages (PDR 2000), although cases of possible hepatotoxicity have been described (Foster, Tyler 1999).

Availability

Many commercial preparations of Scutellaria species are available and include powder and liquid extract; capsules contain 425 mg. A 200 mg dosage of *S. lateriflora* was most effective as an anxiolytic in a study of healthy human volunteers, but benefits were also reported at 100 mg (Wolfson, Hoffmann 2003).

Clinical Application in Veterinary Behavior Medicine

Although traditional uses of Scutellaria preparations for psychoactive application have been unsubstantiated to date, recent preliminary evidence of their affinity for benzodiazepine, GABA, and serotonin (5-HT) receptors suggest that Scutellaria species hold much clinical promise in veterinary behavior medicine. Additional research will clarify their use.

References

Aung HH, Dey L, Mehendale S et al. *Scutellaria baicalensis* extract decreases cisplatin-induced pica in rats. Cancer Chemother Pharmacol. 2003;52:453–458.

Awad R, Arnason JT, Trudeau V et al. Phytochemical and biological analysis of skullcap (*Scutellaria lateriflora* L.): a medicinal plant with anxiolytic properties. Phytomedicine. 2003;10:640–649.

Felter HW, Lloyd JU. King's American Dispensatory. Ohio Valley Company, Cincinatti OH. 1898. Available online at http://www.ibiblio.org/herbmed/eclectic/kings/

Foster S, Tyler VE. Tyler's honest herbal: A sensible guide to the use of herbs and related remedies (4th ed). The Haworth Herbal Press, Binghamton, NY. 1999; 350–351.

Gafner S, Bergeron C, Batcha LL et al. Inhibition of [3H]-LSD binding to 5-HT7 receptors by flavonoids from *Scutellaria lateriflora*. J Nat Prod. 2003;66:535–537.
Hamel PB, Chiltoskey MU. Cherokee Plants and Their Uses: A 400-Year History. Herald Publishing Co., Sylva, NC. 1975.
Huang RL, Chen CC, Huang HL et al. Anti-hepatitis B virus effects of wogonin isolated from *Scutellaria baicalensis*. Planta Med. 2000;66:694–698.
Huang Y, Wong CM, Lau CW et al. Inhibition of nitric oxide/cyclic GMP-mediated relaxation by purified flavonoids, baicalin and baicalein, in rat aortic rings. Biochem Pharmacol. 2004;67:787–794.
Huen MS, Hui KM, Leung JW et al. Naturally occurring 2'-hydroxyl-substituted flavonoids as high-affinity benzodiazepine site ligands. Biochem Pharmacol. 2003;66:2397–2407.
Hui KM, Huen MS, Wang HY et al. Anxiolytic effect of wogonin, a benzodiazepine receptor ligand isolated from *Scutellaria baicalensis* Georgi. Biochem Pharmacol. 2002;64:1415–1424.
Lee H, Kim YO, Kim H et al. Flavonoid wogonin from medicinal herb is neuroprotective by inhibiting inflammatory activation of microglia. FASEB J. 2003;17:1943–1944.
Lee HH, Yang LL, Wang CC et al. Differential effects of natural polyphenols on neuronal survival in primary cultured central neurons against glutamate- and glucose-deprivation-induced neuronal death. Brain Res. 2003;986:103–113.
Liu JJ, Huang TS, Cheng WF et al. Baicalein and baicalin are potent inhibitors of angiogenesis: Inhibition of endothelial cell proliferation, migration and differentiation. Int J Cancer. 2003;106: 559–565.
Ma SC, Du J, But PP, Deng XL et al. Antiviral Chinese medicinal herbs against respiratory syncytial virus. J Ethnopharmacol. 2002;79:205–211.
Mills S, Bone K. Principles and Practice of Phytotherapy. Churchill Livingstone, Philadelphia, PA. 2000;232–234.
Moerman DE. Native American Ethnobotany. Timber Press, Portland, OR. 2002;524.
Moerman DE. University of Michigan—Dearborn. Native American Ethnobotany Database, 2003. http://herb.umd.umich.edu/
PDR for Herbal Medicines. (2nd ed) Medical Economics Company Inc., Montvale, NJ. 2000;678–679.
Po LS, Chen ZY, Tsang DS et al. Baicalein and genistein display differential actions on estrogen receptor (ER) transactivation and apoptosis in MCF-7 cells. Cancer Lett. 2002;187:33–40.
Powell CB, Fung P, Jackson J et al. Aqueous extract of herba *Scutellaria barbatae*, a Chinese herb used for ovarian cancer, induces apoptosis of ovarian cancer cell lines. Gynecol Oncol. 2003;91:332–340.
Russo E. Handbook of Psychotropic Herbs: A Scientific Analysis of Herbal Remedies for Psychiatric Conditions. The Haworth Press, Binghamton, NY. 2001;132–134.
Shang YZ, Gong MY, Zhou XX et al. Improving effects of SSF on memory deficits and pathological changes of neural and immunological systems in sensescent mice. Acta Pharmacol Sin. 2001;22:1078–1083.
Tierra M. The Way of Chinese Herbs. Pocket Books, New York, NY. 1998;174–175.
Wang H, Hui KM, Xu S et al. Two flavones from *Scutellaria baicalensis* Georgi and the binding affinities to the benzodiazepine site of the GABAA receptor complex. Pharmazie. 2002;57:857–858.
Wang H, Hui KM, Chen Y et al. Structure-activity relationships of flavonoids, isolated from *Scutellaria baicalensis*, binding to benzodiazepine site of GABA(A) receptor complex. Planta Med. 2002;68: 1059–1062.
Wolfson P, Hoffmann DL. An investigation into the efficacy of *Scutellaria lateriflora* in healthy volunteers. Altern Ther Health Med. 2003;9:74–78.
Wu JA, Attele AS, Zhang L et al. Anti-HIV activity of medicinal herbs: usage and potential development. Am J Chin Med. 2001;29:69–81.
Ye F, Xui L, Yi J et al. Anticancer activity of *Scutellaria baicalensis* and its potential mechanism. J Altern Complement Med. 2002;8:567–572.
Zhang DY Wu J, Ye F et al. Inhibition of cancer cell proliferation and prostaglandin E(2) synthesis by *Scutellaria baicalensis*. Cancer Res. 2003;63:4037–3043.

Miscellaneous Native American Psychotropic Herbs

Anemone spp.

Anemone species (*Asteraceae*) were used as psychological aids by the Meskwaki and Iroquois. *Anemone cylindrica*, for example, was used by the Meskwaki to cure "crazy people" (Moerman 2002a; Smith 1928). *Anemone virginiana* was used by the Iroquois to prepare a love medicine to attract either sex; it was also used to counteract the effects of a love potion (Moerman 2002a; Herrick 1977).

During the 1800s, *Anemone patens* (referred to as American Paulsatilla) was used to treat genital complaints in both men and women, as well as skin eruptions, gastric pain, and chronic irritation of the nerves (Felter, Lloyd 1898). The medicinal use of *Anemone spp.* appears to be unsupported by scientific data at this time.

Aquilegia spp.

Aquilegia spp. (Columbine, *Ranunculaceae*) are flowering plants native to Europe, the eastern United States and Asia. Flowers may be blue, violet, pink, or white and have five spreading sepals that resemble petals; however, different species can have marked variation in flower morphology. Stems are erect with several branches. The leaf shape varies slightly depending on their location on the plant and may be simple or lobed, crenate to serrate, and generally ovate. The medicinal parts of the plant are the aerial elements, which are harvested during bloom and dried. Some parts of the plant contain trace amounts of cyanide; however, these are not considered to be in toxic concentrations (PDR 2000f; Hodges, Arnold 1994).

Columbine preparations have been traditionally used to cure scurvy, jaundice, and menopausal discomfort. Columbine has also been used as a sedative to treat agitation and anxiety (PDR 2000f). The Meskwaki, Omaha, Pawnee, and Ponca tribes valued the seeds of *Aquilegia canadensis* (Red Columbine) as love charms. The Meskwaki also smoked Columbine (Moerman 2003; Moerman 2000h; Smith 1928; Gilmore 1919). Women of the Thompson tribe used *A. formosa* as a love medicine to attract men (Moerman 2003; Moerman 2000h; Steedman 1928).

The flavonoid compound isocytisoside has a hepatoprotective effect (Adamska, Mlynarczyk, Jodynis-Liebert et al. 2003). Newly isolated glycosides called quilegiosides appear to have an immunosuppressive property (Nishida, Yoshimitsu, Okawa et al. 2003). A recently identified alkaloid has a potential anticancer effect (Chen, Gao, Li et al. 2002; Bylka, Matlawska 1997). The flavonoid apigenin, found in other psychoactive plants such as Chamomile and Passion Flower (Zanoli, Avallone, Baraldi 2000), has been isolated from Columbine (Chen, Gao, Leung et al. 2001). This compound has been shown to exert an antidepressant (Nakazawa, Yasuda, Ueda et al. 2003) and anxiolytic effect (Zanoli, Avallone, Baraldi 2000). A dopaminergic mechanism was suspected based on apigenin's

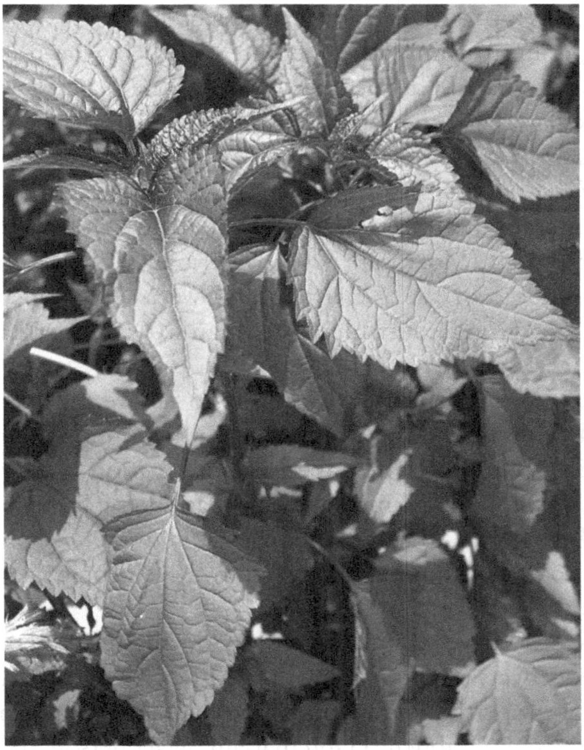

FIGURE 2-4. *Eupatorium rugosum* (Chocolate Joepyeweed shown) is a toxic medicinal plant native to the United States. (Photo courtesy of Dr. Stefanie Schwartz)

ability to decrease dopamine turnover in the amygdala and increase hypothalamic dopamine turnover. Although new compounds of Aquilegia species continue to be identified, there are no data to support their aphrodisiac effects to date.

Eupatorium spp.

Eupatorium spp. are members of the *Asteraceae* family; varieties are found around the world. The three most prominent native varieties of the eastern United States are *E. perfoliatum*, *E. maculatum*, and *E. purpurum*. The Cherokee, Micmac, Mohegan, Penobscot, Chippewa, Delaware, Iroquois, and Menominee were among the tribes that used Eupatorium species to control fever, flu, gynecological complaints, urinary tract problems, analgesia, and many other symptoms (Fig. 2-4).

E. perfoliatum (Boneset, Indian Sage, Thoroughwort, Crosswort, Feverwort, Agueweed, Sweating Plant, Teasel, Vegetable Antimony) is a tall, flowering perennial herb of North America that prefers to grow along streams and swampy ground. Stems have bristly hairs and can reach up to 1.5 m. Leaves are long (10–15 cm), tapering to shiny yellow points caused by the resin excreted from glands at the undersurface. The medicinal parts of the plant include the horizontal hairy rootstock as well as the aerial portions after bloom. The Iroquois used the root of *E. perfoliatum* to help overcome addiction to alcohol. They also prepared a decoction of *E. maculatum* (Spotted Joepyeweed) that was used as a wash by the Iroquois to counteract the effects of a love medicine, and by the Chippewa to calm babies or children (Moerman 2003; Moerman 2000i; Herrick 1977). The Meskwaki kept a piece of the *E. purpurum* (Sweetscented Joepyeweed, Gravel Root) to nibble on during courtship (Moerman 2003; Moerman 2000i; Smith 1928).

During the nineteenth century, it was used to relieve the muscular aches and pains associated with influenza (from which its common name of "boneset" stems) and similar complaints described in conjunction with rheumatism and syphilis. The plant was used as an emetic and diaphoretic in cases of fever and inflammation (Felter, Lloyd 1898). Nonetheless, *Eupatorium spp.* are toxic plants that can be fatal to grazing animals and even to those people who ingest the milk of exposed cattle.

Eupatorium species have stimulating effects on the immune system as well as anti-inflammatory effects (Habtemariam 2001; PDR 2000g). Some species possess weak antibacterial properties and cytotoxic properties that are similar to those of the anticancer drug chlorambucil (Habtemariam, Macpherson 2000). A strong antifungal effect was found in *E. aschenbornianum*, which is used traditionally by native Mexican herbalists (Navarro Garcia, Gonzalez, Fuentes et al. 2003; Fernandez, Cerda Zolezzi, Risco et al. 2002). So far, there have been no psychoactive properties confirmed. Concerns regarding adverse effects further reduce the clinical interest of Eupatorium species in veterinary behavior medicine and beyond.

Geum spp.

The Iroquois decocted *Geum canadense* (White Avens; *Rosaceae*) as a love medicine. They also used *Geum aleppicum* (Yellow Avens) to trigger emesis as a cure for a love medicine (Moerman 2003; Moerman 2002j; Herrick 1977). Men of the Thompson tribe used a variety of *Geum spp.* as love charms to gain female affection (Moerman 2003; Moerman 2002j; Steedman 1928). The roots of *Geum triflorum* (Prairiesmoke) were made into an infusion by women of the Okanagan-Colville to win back the affections of a man (Moerman 2003; Moerman 2002j; Turner, Bouchard, Kennedy 1980).

A number of Geum species were used medicinally in North America, Europe, and Asia. *Geum rivale* (Water Avens) and *Geum urbane*, for example, have both used for inflammations and infection of the skin and digestive system (PDR 2000e; Mills, Bone 2000). During the 1800s, *Geum spp.* were used as remedies for gastrointestinal ailments and hemorrhage (Felter, Lloyd 1898).

The primary compounds are tannins and eugenol, found in the volatile oil fraction (PDR 2000e). Their use is not as popular as other herbal remedies today; however, such use may be underreported.

A recent report of a possible drug interaction in a kidney transplant patient in Chile is worth mention. Apparently, use of a Geum remedy was not disclosed to the surgeons, and the patient's cyclosporin level was increased despite having taken the dosage as directed. This was eventually attributed to the patient's consumption of *Geum chiloense*; cyclosporin levels returned to normal when the herb was discontinued (Duclos, Goecke 2001).

There is documented evidence that Geum species possess antimicrobial properties (Panizzi, Catalano, Miarelli et al. 2000; McCutcheon, Ellis, Hancock et al. 1994). Geumonoid, a new triterpene isolated from *Geum japonicum*, showed inhibitory activity against the human immunodeficiency virus (HIV) (Xu, Ming, Dong et al. 2000). Eugeniin, another component of *G. japonicum* that targets viral DNA synthesis, showed a potent inhibition of the herpes virus (Kurokawa, Hozumi, Basnet et al. 1998). Components of *G. japonicum* also showed potent anticoagulant activity (Dong, Chen, Kini et al. 1998). At this time, there does not appear to be evidence for an aphrodisiac effect, or any other cognitive and behavioral effect, for Geum species.

Juniperus spp.

Juniper species were popular with several tribes. The Pawnee used smoke from *Juniperus virginiana* (Eastern Red Cedar; Cupressaceae) to combat nervousness and nightmares (Moerman 2002d, 2003; Gilmore 1919); the Seminole relied upon smoke of the southern variety of Red Cedar to cure insanity (Moerman 2003; Sturtevant 1954). The Cheyenne used *J. communis* (Common Juniper), *J. horizontalis* (Creeping Juniper) and *J. scopulorum* (Rocky Mountain Juniper) to make flutes used for courtship (Fig. 2-5). The Kiowa created their love flutes from the red, aromatic wood of *J. virginiana* (Moerman 2003; Vestal, Shultes1939).

During the 1800s, Juniper preparations were considered to be effective diuretics and were applied to treat ascites in children, as well as venereal disease and urinary tract infections or inflammations (Felter, Lloyd 1898).

A recent study in Japan compared a number of essential oils, including juniper oil, to the effect of benzodiazepine on stressed mice. Juniper oil was ineffective in this study (Umezu 2000). The effect of inhaled Juniper oil on the human brain would be interesting to determine what impact, if any, its aroma might produce on human arousal and behavior. There is no current evidence to support a psychological benefit for using Juniper.

Lactuca canadensis

Lactuca canadensis (Canada Lettuce) was known to the Cherokee and prepared as a tea to calm "nerves" and induce sleep. Interestingly, they also used it as a stim-

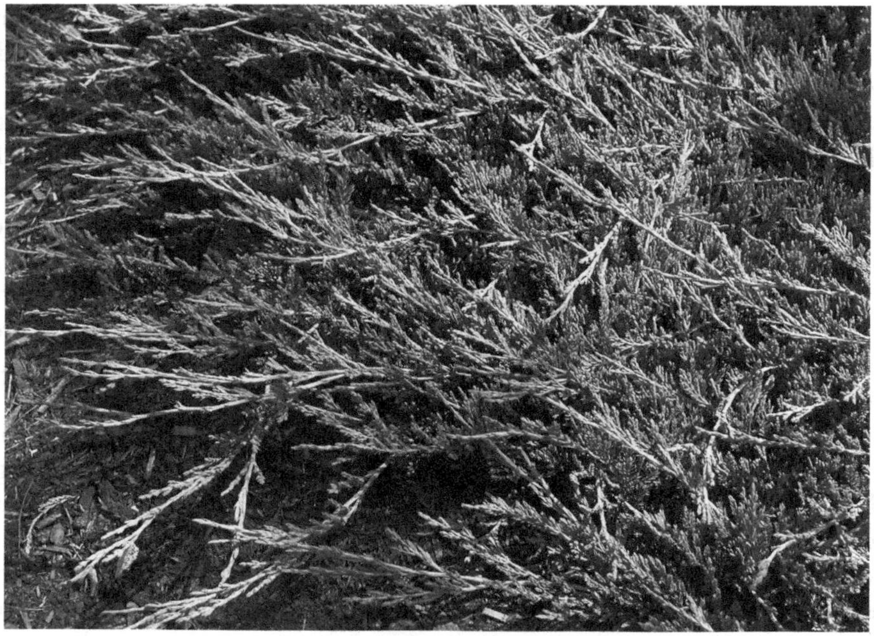

FIGURE 2-5. Creeping juniper, *Juniperus horizontalis.* (Photo courtesy of Dr. Stefanie Schwartz)

ulant (Moerman 2003, 2002c). The European native *Lactuca virosa* was used for similar purpose (discussed elsewhere in this book); however, the application for either Lactuca species as a psychological aid remains unsubstantiated on either continent.

Lonicera spp.

Lonicera spp. (Honeysuckle species) were well known to many tribes and used for a wide range of symptoms including psychological applications (Moerman 2002f). Lonicera is a group of deciduous, flowering vines and shrubs classified as *Caprifoliaceae,* indicating their preference by browsing goats, that grow in mainly temperate climates around the world (PDR 2000). The Iroquois prepared an infusion of the bark *L. canadensis* (American Fly Honeysuckle) as a sedative for "children who cry all night" and valued *L. dioica* (Limber Honeysuckle) as an antilove and love medicine. They also used an infusion of the bark of *L. oblongifolia* (Swamp Fly Honeysuckle) as a sedative for restlessness and to alleviate loneliness. Thompson Indians used *L. ciliosa* (Orange Honeysuckle vine) in medicinal baths for the treatment of seizures and as a sedative and soporific tucked under the pillow. People of the Nitinaht tribe ate the springtime buds of *L. involucrata* (Twinberry Honeysuckle) or rubbed its bark on the body to cure nervous breakdowns. The Nootka and Manhousat also used it during long whaling expeditions to relieve sexual urges (Moerman 2003; Moerman 2002f).

L. japonica (*Jin yin hua*) is considered a heat-clearing and toxin-resolving herb and is commonly used in Traditional Chinese formulas (Zhong, Wiseman, Ellis 1996). This species may be less toxic and is the only Lonicera species in common use (Dr. Susan Wynn, personal communication 2004), although it does not appear to have psychological or behavioral activity.

Lonicera spp. have shown anti-inflammatory effects in recent studies (Tae, Han, Yoo et al. 2003; Kwak, Han, Chang et al. 2003).

Active compounds include saponins (PDR 2000a), and new compounds continue to be discovered (Machida, Sasaki, Iijima et al. 2002; Peng, Mei, Jiang et al. 2002; Kita, Kigoshi, Uemura 2001; Kumar, Sati, Semwal et al. 2000; Peng, Mei, Jiang et al. 2000). Although new therapeutic applications for Lonicera species are emerging, including protection against hepatotoxicity (Xiang, Xiong, Ketut et al. 2001; Liu, Liu, Jia et al. 1991), risks of side effects such as nausea, vomiting, renal injury, and clotting disorders suggest that it should be used with extreme caution at this time (PDR 2000a; Chang, Hsu 1992).

Monarda spp.

Monarda didyma (Scarlet Beebalm, Oswego Tea Beebalm) is a perennial member of the *Lamiaceae* family. Its active compounds include cyclitols, polyynes, and flavonoids (PDR 2000b). The essential oil has 26 compounds, including thymol, d-limonene, linalool, and hydrothymoquinone. In addition, flavonoids in leaves and flowers include rutin, hyperoside, quercitrin, luteolin, and quercetin, which are common to other psychoactive plants discussed elsewhere in this text (PDR 2000b; Savickiene, Dagilyte, Barsteigiene et al. 2002). It continues to be used today most often as an infusion known as Oswego tea (Savickiene, Dagilyte, Barsteigiene et al. 2002; PDR 2000b).

The Blackfoot and Creek Indians administered a decoction of *Monarda punctata* (American Horsemint, Wild Bergamot) as a sedative for delirium (Moerman 2002g, 2003; PDR 2000c; Taylor 1940; Swanton 1928). The Cherokee gave *Monarda didyma* and *Monarda fistulosa* (Wild Bergamot Beebalm) as sedatives for the treatment of "hysterics and restful sleep" (Moerman 2002g, 2003; Hamel, Chiltoskey 1975) (Fig. 2-6).

Physicians of the nineteenth century applied *Monarda spp.* to calm dyspepsia characterized by vomiting and nausea, and as a diuretic for ailments of the urinary tract (Felter, Lloyd 1898).

Although other relatives of *Monarda spp.* (e.g., lavender, lemon balm, catnip) possess interesting psychoactive and medicinal properties (Kaufmann, Wink 1994), there is, regrettably, no evidence to report in support of a psychoactive application of Monarda species at this time.

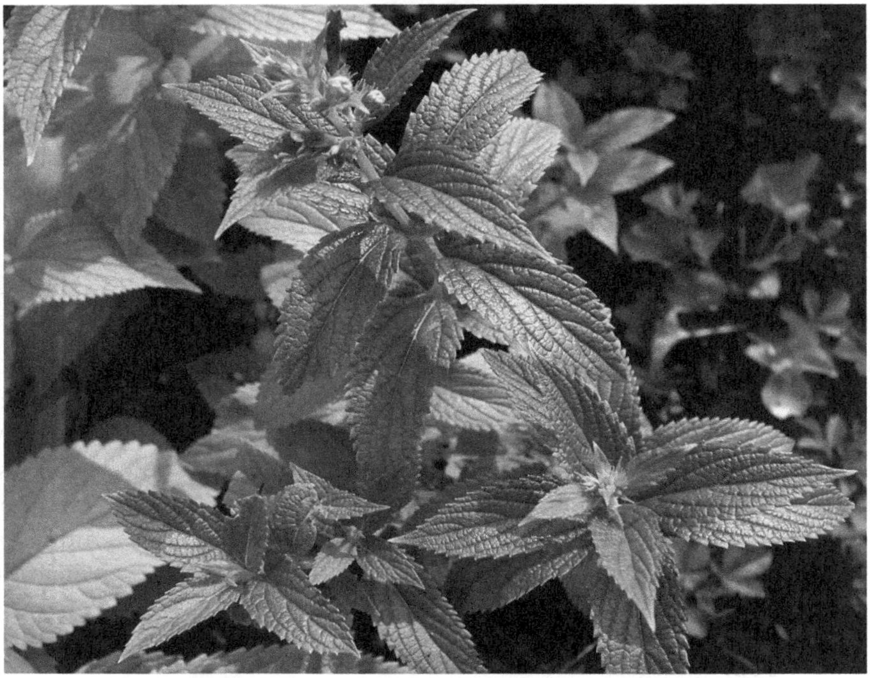

FIGURE 2-6. *Monarda didyma* hybrid budding in the author's garden and showing leaves and characteristic square stem. (Photo courtesy of Dr. Stefanie Schwartz)

Nepeta cataria

Nepeta cataria (Catnip; family *Lamiaceae*) was used by the Iroquois as a hypnotic for children and to calm restless babies (Moerman 2002e; Herrick 1977). The Cherokee used it as a stimulant as well as in the treatment of hysteria (Moerman 2002e). *N. cataria* is discussed separately in this book (Chapter 1, Western Psychoactive Herbs).

Penstemon spp.

Native Americans used *Penstemon spp.* (*Scrophulariaceae*) as psychological aids. The Iroquois, for example, used *Penstemon fruticosus* (Bush Penstemon) as an antilove medicine. They prepared a decoction that produced vomiting to combat the effects of a love medicine (Moerman 2003; Herrick 1977).

To cure grief, people of the Karok tribe drank an infusion of *P. laetus* (Mountain Blue Penstemon) or used it in a steam bath (Schenck, Gifford 1952).

Phenylethanoid, phenylpropanoid and iridoid glycosides, including verbascoside derivatives, have been isolated from Penstemon species; some of these glycosides appear to have anticancer activity (Skrzypek, Wysokinska, Swiatek et al.

1999; Krull, Stermitz, Franzyk et al. 1998; Zhou, Bahler, Hofmann et al. 1998; Ismail, el-Azizi, Khalifa et al. 1995). No significant medicinal, cognitive, or behavioral effects have been found to date.

Prunus species

Prunus emarginata (Bitter Cherry, *Rosaceae*), *Ribes divaricatum* (Spreading Gooseberry, *Grossulariaceae*), *Ribus lobii* (Gummy Gooseberry, *Grossulariaceae*) and *Ribes lacustre* (Prickly Currant, *Grossulariaceae*) were used by the Saanich people of Vancouver Island to enhance the intelligence and obedience of children, among other applications (Moerman 2002b; Turner, Hebda 1990; Turner 1971). Aside from an apparent spermicidal activity by *Prunus emarginata* (Farnsworth, Waller 1982), there is no evidence to support its medicinal use.

However, *Prunus virginiana* (Wild Cherry) was considered by nineteenth-century physicians to be beneficial in treating a variety of digestive (e.g., hepatitis) and respiratory (e.g., whooping cough, pneumonia, bronchitis) ailments; it was thought to have a sedative action that was applied to control "nervous disease" (Felter, Lloyd 1898). These uses appear to be unsubstantiated by current data.

Verbascum thapsus

Verbascum thapsus (Common Mulein, *Scrophulariaceae*) is a biennial plant that grows between 1 and almost 3 m tall. The Hopi smoked it as a treatment for people who were psychologically disturbed, and the Navajo smoked its dried leaves wrapped in cornhusk to "clear the mind if lost" (Moerman 2002i). The plant and related species have been used to treat respiratory symptoms (e.g., asthma, cough), skin disorders (e.g., itching, eczema, insect bites), intestinal complaints (e.g., diarrhea, hemorrhoids), urinary complaints, ear infection and other problems (Felter, Lloyd 1898).

Although one contemporary study confirms its antibacterial property and potential of antitumor activity (Turker, Camper 2002), there is little evidence to support its use for medicinal purposes and no current evidence to support the use of Verbascum species as psychological aids.

References

Adamska T, Mlynarczyk W, Jodynis-Liebert J et al. Hepatoprotective effect of the extract and isocytisoside from *Aquilegia vulgaris*. Phytother Res. 2003;17:691–696.

Bylka W, Matlawska I. Flavonoids from *Aquilegia vulgaris* L. Part II. Derivatives of apigenin and luteolin. Acta Pol Pharm. 1997;54:335–337.

Chang WC, Hsu FL. Inhibition of platelet activation and endothelial cell injury by polyphenolic compounds isolated from *Lonicera japonica*. Prostaglandins Leukot Essent Fatty Acids. 1992;45:307–312.

Chen SB, Gao GY, Leung HW et al. Aquiledine and isoaquiledine, novel flavonoid alkaloids from *Aquilegia ecalcarata*. J Nat Prod. 2001;64:85–87.

Chen SB, Gao GY, Li YS et al. Cytotoxic constituents from *Aquilegia ecalcarata*. Planta Med. 2002;68: 554–556.

Dong H, Chen SX, Kini RM et al. Effects of tannins from *Geum japonicum* on the catalytic activity of thrombin and factor Xa of blood coagulation cascade. J Nat Prod. 1998;61:1356–1360.

Duclos J, Goecke H. Hierba del clavo (*Geum chiloense*) modifying cyclosporine levels: potential risk for transplanted people. Rev Med Chil. 2001;129:789–790.

Farnsworth NR, Waller DP. Current status of plant products reported to inhibit sperm. Res Front Fertil Regul. 1982;2:1–16.

Felter HW, Lloyd JU. King's American Dispensatory. Ohio Valley Company, Cincinatti, OH. 1898. Available online at http://www.ibiblio.org/herbmed/eclectic/kings/

Fernandez T, Cerda Zolezzi P, Risco E et al. Immunomodulating properties of Argentine plants with ethnomedicinal use. Phytomedicine. 2002;9:546–552.

Gilmore R. Uses of Plants by the Indians of the Missouri River Region. SI-BAE Annual Report, 1919.

Habtemariam S. Antiinflammatory activity of the antirheumatic herbal drug, gravel root (*Eupatorium purpureum*): further biological activities and constituents. Phytother Res. 2001;15:687–690.

Habtemariam S, Macpherson AM.Cytotoxicity and antibacterial activity of ethanol extract from leaves of a herbal drug, boneset (*Eupatorium perfoliatum*). Phytother Res. 2000;14:575–577.

Hamel PB, Chiltoskey MU. Cherokee Plants and Their Uses: A 400-Year History. Herald Publishing Co., Sylva, NC. 1975.

Hart JA. The Ethnobotany of the Northern Cheyenne Indians of Montana. J Ethnopharm. 1981;4:1–55.

Herrick JW. Iroquois Medical Botany. State University of New York, Albany, NY. PhD Thesis. 1977.

Hodges SA, Arnold ML. Columbines: a geographically widespread species flock. Proc Natl Acad Sci USA. 1994;91:5129–5132.

Ismail LD, el-Azizi MM, Khalifa TI et al. Verbascoside derivatives and iridoid glycosides from *Penstemon crandallii*. Phytochemistry. 1995;39:1391–1393.

Kaufmann M, Wink M. Molecular systematics of the nepetoideae (family *Labiatae*) phylogenetic implications from rbcL gene sequences. Z Naturforsch. 1994;49:635–45.

Kita M, Kigoshi H, Uemura D. Isolation and structure of korolkoside, a bis-iridoid glucoside from *Lonicera korolkovii*. J Nat Prod. 2001;64:1090–1092.

Krull RE, Stermitz FR, Franzyk H et al. Iridoid glycoside biosynthesis in *Penstemon secundiflorus*. Another H-5, H-9 trans-iridoid glycoside. Phytochemistry. 1998;49:1605–1608.

Kumar S, Sati OP, Semwal VD et al. Iridoid glycosides from *Lonicera quinquelocularis*. Phytochemistry. 2000;53:499–501.

Kurokawa M, Hozumi T, Basnet P et al. Purification and characterization of eugeniin as an antiherpesvirus compound from *Geum japonicum* and *Syzygium aromaticum*. J Pharmacol Exp Ther. 1998;284:728–735.

Kwak WJ, Han CK, Chang HW et al. Loniceroside C, an antiinflammatory saponin from *Lonicera japonica*. Chem Pharm Bull (Tokyo). 2003;51:333–335.

Liu YP, Liu J, Jia XS et al. Protective effects of fulvotomentosides on acetaminophen-induced hepatotoxicity. Zhongguo Yao Li Xue Bao. 1992;13:209–212.

Machida K, Sasaki H, Iijima T et al. Studies on the constituents of Lonicera species. XVII. New iridoid glycosides of the stems and leaves of *Lonicera japonica* THUNB. Chem Pharm Bull (Tokyo). 2002;50:1041–1044.

McCutcheon AR, Ellis SM, Hancock RE et al. Antifungal screening of medicinal plants of British Columbian native peoples. J Ethnopharmacol. 1994;44:157–169.

Meschler JP, Howlett AC. Thujone exhibits low affinity for cannabinoid receptors but fails to evoke cannabimimetic responses. Pharmacol Biochem Behav. 1999;62:473–480.

Mills S, Bone K. Principles and Practice of Phytotherapy. Churchill Livingstone, Philadelphia, PA. 2000;170.

Moerman DE. Native American Ethnobotany. Timber Press, Portland, OR. 2002;72–7a; 439–448b; 294c; 282–293d; 353–354e; 317–319f; 346–348g; 509–511h; 532–533i; 247–248j;80h;229–230i.

Moerman DE. University of Michigan—Dearborn. Native American Ethnobotany Database, 2003. http://herb.umd.umich.edu/

Nakazawa T, Yasuda T, Ueda J et al. Antidepressant-like effects of apigenin and 2,4,5-trimethoxycinnamic acid from *Perilla frutescens* in the forced swimming test. Biol Pharm Bull. 2003;26:474–480.

Navarro Garcia VM, Gonzalez A, Fuentes M et al. Antifungal activities of nine traditional Mexican medicinal plants. J Ethnopharmacol. 2003;87:85–88.

Nishida M, Yoshimitsu H, Okawa M et al. Four new cycloartane glycosides from *Aquilegia vulgaris* and their immunosuppressive activities in mouse allogeneic mixed lymphocyte reaction. Chem Pharm Bull (Tokyo). 2003;51:683–687.

Panizzi L, Catalano S, Miarelli C et al. In vitro antimicrobial activity of extracts and isolated constituents of *Geum rivale*. Phytother Res. 2000;14:561–563.

PDR for Herbal Medicines. (2nd ed) Medical Economics Company Inc., Montvale, NJ. 2000;399–401a; 562–563b; 407–408c; 655–657d; 796–797e; 211–212f; 113–114g.

Peng LY, Mei SX, Jiang B et al. Constituents from *Lonicera japonica*. Fitoterapia. 2000;71:713–715.

Savickiene N, Dagilyte A, Barsteigiene Z et al. Analysis of flavonoids in the flowers and leaves of *Monarda didyma* L. Medicina (Kaunas). 2002;38:1119–1122.

Schenck SM, Gifford EW. Karok Ethnobotany. Anthropol Rec. 1952;13:377–392.

Skrzypek Z, Wysokinska H, Swiatek L et al. Phenylpropanoid glycosides from *Penstemon serrulatus*. J Nat Prod. 1999;62:127–129.

Smith HH. Ethnobotany of the Menomini Indians. Bulletin of the Public Museum of the City of Milwaukee. 1923;4:1–174.

Smith HH. Ethnobotany of the Meskwaki Indians. Bulletin of the Public Museum of the City of Milwaukee. 1928;4:175–326.

Steedman EV. The Ethnobotany of the Thompson Indians of British Columbia. SI-BAE Annual Report. 1928;45:441–522.

Sturtevant W. The Mikasuki Seminole: Medical Beliefs and Practices. Yale University, PhD Thesis. 1954.

Sumner J. The natural history of medicinal plants. Timber Press, Portland, OR. 2000;75.

Swanton JR. Religious Beliefs and Medical Practices of the Creek Indians. SI-BAE Annual Report. 1928;42:473–672.

Tae J, Han SW, Yoo JY et al. Anti-inflammatory effect of *Lonicera japonica* in proteinase-activated receptor 2-mediated paw edema. Clin Chim Acta. 2003;330:165–171.

Taylor LA. Plants Used As Curatives by Certain Southeastern Tribes. Botanical Museum of Harvard University, Cambridge, MA. 1940.

Turner NC, Bell MA. The Ethnobotany of the Coast Salish Indians of Vancouver Island, I and II. Economic Botany. 1971;25:63–104; 335–339.

Turner NJ, Bouchard R, Kennedy DI. Ethnobotany of the Okanagan-Colville Indians of British Columbia and Washington. British Columbia Provincial Museum, Victoria, British Columbia. 1980;126.

Turner NJ, Hebda RJ. Contemporary use of bark for medicine by two Salishan native elders of southeast Vancouver Island, Canada. J Ethnopharmacol. 1990;29:59–72.

Umezu T. Behavioral effects of plant-derived essential oils in the geller type conflict test in mice. Jpn J Pharmacol. 2000;83:150–153.

Vestal PA, Schultes RE. The Economic Botany of the Kiowa Indians. Botanical Museum of Harvard University, Cambridge, MA. 1939.

Xiang T, Xiong QB, Ketut AI et al. Studies on the hepatocyte protective activity and the structure-activity relationships of quinic acid and caffeic acid derivatives from the flower buds of *Lonicera bournei*. Planta Med. 2001;67:322–325.

Xu HX, Ming DS, Dong H et al. A new anti-HIV triterpene from *Geum japonicum*. Chem Pharm Bull (Tokyo). 2000;48:1367–1369.

Zanoli P, Avallone R, Baraldi M. Behavioral characterisation of the flavonoids apigenin and chrysin. Fitoterapia. 2000;71(Suppl 1):S117–S123.

Zhong YX, Wiseman N, Ellis A. Fundamentals of Chinese medicine. Paradigm Publications; Brookline, MA. 1996;301.

Zhou BN, Bahler BD, Hofmann GA et al. Phenylethanoid glycosides from *Digitalis purpurea* and *Penstemon linarioides* with PKCalpha-inhibitory activity. J Nat Prod. 1998;61:1410–1412.

Table 2-1a. List of Herbs Used by Native Americans for the Treatment of Psychological Symptoms or to Inspire and Stimulate Specific Emotions

TRIBE	ADDICTION to TOBACCO/ ALCOHOL	CONTROL of ANGER / TEMPER	CONTROL of SEXUAL AROUSAL or PERVERSION	COURAGE	DEPRESSION, LONELINESS & GRIEF
ABNAKI	...	...	***Nuphar sp.***; *Nymphaeaceae*	...	...
ALGONQUIN	...	...	...	...	***Fraxinus pennsylvanica*** Green Ash; *Oleaceae*
	...	...	...	...	***Sorbus americana*** American Mountain Ash; *Rosaceae*
CHEROKEE	...	...	...	...	***Solanum nigrum*** Black Nightshade; *Solanaceae*
	...	...	...	...	***Solanum tu***berosum Irish Potato; *Solanaceae*
CHEYENNE	...	...	***Madia glomerata*** Mountain Tarweed; *Asteraceae*	...	...
CREE	...	...	...	***Acorus calamus*** Calamus; *Acoraceae*	...
CREEK	...	...	...		...
DAKOTA	...	...	...	***Acorus calamus*** Calamus; *Acoraceae*	...
HOPI	...	***Datura wrightii*** Sacred Thornapple; *Solanaceae*	...	...	...
	...	***Plantago patagonica*** Woolly Plantain; *Plantaginaceae*	...	...	...
IROQUOIS	***Eupatorium perfoliatum*** Common Boneset; *Asteraceae*	...	***Nicotiana rustica*** Aztec Tobacco; *Solanaceae*	...	***Corylus cornuta*** Beaked Hazelnut; *Betulaceae*
	Lobelia inflata Indian Tobacco; *Campanulaceae*	...	...	...	***Gentiana andrewsii*** Closed Bottle Gentian; *Gentianaceae*
	...	...	...	...	***Laportea canadensis*** Canadian Woodnettle; *Urticaceae*
	...	...	...	...	***Lobelia cardinalis*** Cardinalflower; *Campanulaceae*
	...	...	...	...	***Lonicera canadensis*** American Fly Honeysuckle; *Caprifoliaceae*
	...	...	...	...	***Pinus strobus*** Eastern White Pine; *Pinaceae*
	...	...	...	...	***Prunella vulgaris*** Common Selfheal; *Lamiaceae*

Table 2-1a. List of Herbs Used by Native Americans for the Treatment of Psychological Symptoms or to Inspire and Stimulate Specific Emotions (*continued*)

TRIBE	ADDICTION to TOBACCO/ ALCOHOL	CONTROL of ANGER / TEMPER	CONTROL of SEXUAL AROUSAL or PERVERSION	COURAGE	DEPRESSION, LONELINESS & GRIEF
	...	...	...	...	***Quercus alba*** White Oak; *Fagaceae*
	...	...	...	...	***Salix discolor*** Pussy Willow; *Salicaceae*
KAROK	...	...	...		***Osmorhiza berteroi*** Sweetcicely; *Apiaceae*
	...	...	...	...	***Penstemon laetus*** Mountain Blue Penstemon; *Scrophulariaceae*
KERES	...	...	...	***Berlandiera lyrata*** Lyreleaf Greeneyes; *Asteraceae*	***Crepis runcinata*** Fiddleleaf Hawksbeard; *Asteraceae*
	...	...	...	...	***Eriogonum jamesii*** James' Buckwheat; *Polygonaceae*
	...	...	...	...	***Packera fendleri*** Fendler's Ragwort; *Asteraceae*
NITINAHT	...	...	***Conocephalum conicum***; *Conocephalaceae*	...	***Sambucus racemosa*** Pacific Red Elder; *Caprifoliaceae*
	...	...	***Tellima grandiflora*** Bigflower Tellima; *Saxifragaceae*	...	...
OMAHA	***Echinocactus williamsii*** Mescal; *Cactaceae*	...	...	...	...
RAPPAHANNOCK	...	...	***Liriodendron tulipifera*** Tuliptree; *Magnoliaceae*	...	...
SEMINOLE	...	...	...	...	***Persea borbonia*** Redbay; *Lauraceae*

Table 2-1b. List of Herbs Used by Native Americans for the Treatment of Psychological Symptoms or to Inspire and Stimulate Specific Emotions

TRIBE	IMPROVEMENT of MEMORY or COGNITIVE FUNCTION	INSOMNIA	INSANITY or DELIRIUM	LOVE & SEX	SEDATIVE for Nervousness/ Anxiety
ABNAKI	...	...	...	***Nuphar sp.*** Yellow Pond Lily; *Nymphaeaceae*	...
ALABAMA	...	***Pseudognaphalium obtusifolium*** Rabbit Tobacco; *Asteraceae*	...	...	***Pseudognaphalium obtusifolium*** Rabbit Tobacco; *Asteraceae*
ALGONQUIN	...	...	...	***Sanguinaria canadensis*** Bloodroot; *Papaveraceae*	...
CHEHALIS	...	...	...	***Eriophyllum lanatum*** Woolly Eriophyllum; *Asteraceae*	...
CHEROKEE	***Cynoglossum virginianum*** Wild Comfrey; *Boraginaceae*	...	...	***Fragaria virginiana*** Virginia Strawberry; *Rosaceae*	***Angelica atropurpurea*** Purplestem Angelica; *Apiaceae*
	Hackelia virginiana Beggarslice; *Boraginaceae*	***Lactuca canadensis*** Canada Lettuce; *Asteraceae*	...	***Hackelia virginiana*** Beggarslice; *Boraginaceae*	***Asarum canadense*** Canadian Wildginger; *Aristolochiaceae*
	...	...	...	**Phoradendron leucarpum*** Oak Mistletoe; *Viscaceae*	***Caulophyllum thalictroides***; Blue Cohosh; *Berberidaceae*
	...	...	...	...	***Cichorium intybus*** Chicory; *Asteraceae*
	...	...	...	...	***Clematis virginiana*** Devil's Darning Needles; *Ranunculaceae*
	...	...	...	...	***Fragaria virginiana*** Virginia Strawberry; *Rosaceae*
	...	...	...	...	***Galax urceolata*** Beetleweed; *Diapensiaceae*
	...	...	...	...	***Lactuca canadensis*** Canada Lettuce; *Asteraceae*
	...	...	...	...	***Leonurus cardiaca*** Common Motherwort; *Lamiaceae*
	...	...	...	...	***Liquidambar styraciflua*** Sweetgum; *Hamamelidaceae*

Table 2-1b. List of Herbs Used by Native Americans for the Treatment of Psychological Symptoms or to Inspire and Stimulate Specific Emotions (*continued*)

TRIBE	IMPROVEMENT of MEMORY or COGNITIVE FUNCTION	INSOMNIA	INSANITY or DELIRIUM	LOVE & SEX	SEDATIVE for Nervousness/ Anxiety
	...	...	...	...	***Mentha piperita*** *(pro sp.) [aquatica × spicata]* Water Mint; *Lamiaceae*
	...	...	...	...	***Mentha spicata*** Spearmint; *Lamiaceae*
	...	...	...	...	***Oxydendrum arboreum*** Sourwood; *Ericaceae*
	...	...	...	...	***Panax quinquefolius*** American Ginseng; *Araliaceae*
	...	...	...	...	***Panax trifolius*** Dwarf Ginseng; *Araliaceae*
	...	...	...	...	***Phytolacca americana*** American Pokeweed; *Phytolaccaceae*
	...	...	...	...	***Ribes rotundifolium*** Appalachian Gooseberry; *Grossulariaceae*
	...	...	...	...	***Salvia lyrata*** Lyreleaf Sage; *Lamiaceae*
	...	...	...	...	***Salvia officinalis*** Kitchen Sage; *Lamiaceae*
	...	...	...	...	***Scutellaria elliptica*** Hairy Skullcap; Lamiaceae
	...	...	...	...	***Scutellaria incana*** Hoary Skullcap; *Lamiaceae*
	...	...	...	...	***Scutellaria lateriflora*** Blue Skullcap; *Lamiaceae*
	...	...	...	...	***Solidago odora*** Anise-scented Goldenrod; *Asteraceae*
	...	...	...	...	***Sonchus arvensis*** Field Sowthistle; *Asteraceae*
	...	...	...	...	***Taraxacum officinale*** Common Dandelion; *Asteraceae*
	...	...	...	...	***Xanthorhiza simplicissima*** Yellowroot; *Ranunculaceae*

(continued)

Table 2-1b. List of Herbs Used by Native Americans for the Treatment of Psychological Symptoms or to Inspire and Stimulate Specific Emotions (*continued*)

TRIBE	IMPROVEMENT of MEMORY or COGNITIVE FUNCTION	INSOMNIA	INSANITY or DELIRIUM	LOVE & SEX	SEDATIVE for Nervousness/ Anxiety
CHEYENNE	...	***Artemisia ludoviciana*** Foothill Sagewort; *Asteraceae*	***Arctostaphylos uva-ursi*** Kinnikinnick; *Ericaceae*	***Juniperus communis*** Common Juniper; *Cupressaceae*	***Juniperus communis*** Common Juniper; *Cupressaceae*
	...	***Ericameria nauseosa*** Rubber Rabbitbrush; *Asteraceae*	***Lithospermum incisum*** Narrowleaf Gromwell; *Boraginaceae*	***Juniperus horizontalis*** Creeping Juniper; *Cupressaceae*	...
	...	...	...	***Juniperus scopulorum*** Rocky Mountain Juniper; *Cupressaceae*	...
	...	...	...	***Madia glomerata*** Mountain Tarweed; *Asteraceae*	...
	...	...	...	***Mentha arvensis*** Wild Mint; *Lamiaceae*	...
CHICKASAW	...	...	***Gaylussacia sp.*** Huckleberry; *Ericaceae*	...	***Gaylussacia sp.*** Huckleberry; *Ericaceae*
CHIPPEWA	...	...	***Apocynum androsaemifolium*** Spreading Dogbane; *Apocynaceae*	***Onosmodium molle*** Softhair Marbleseed; *Boraginaceae*	***Eupatorium maculatum*** Spotted Joeypyeweed *Asteraceae*
	...	...	***Vaccinium angustifolium*** Lowbush Blueberry; *Ericaceae*	...	...
COSTANOAN	...	...	...	***Datura wrightii*** Sacred Thornapple; *Solanaceae*	...
COWLITZ	...	...	...	***Galium aparine*** Stickywilly; *Rubiaceae*	...
CREE	...	...	...	***Valeriana dioica*** Woods Valerian; *Valerianaceae*	...
CREEK	...	...	***Monarda sp.*** Horsemint; *Lamiaceae*		...
DAKOTA	...	...	...	***Lomatium foeniculaceum*** Desert Biscuitroot; *Apiaceae*	...
DELAWARE	...	...	...	***Podophyllum peltatum*** Mayapple; *Berberidaceae*	***Humulus lupulus*** Common Hop; *Cannabaceae*
HAWAIIAN	...	...	***Cucurbita maxima*** Winter Squash; *Cucurbitaceae*	***Alocasia macrorrhizos*** Giant Taro; *Araceae*	***Cibotium chamissoi*** Chamisso's Manfern; *Cyatheaceae*

Table 2-1b. List of Herbs Used by Native Americans for the Treatment of Psychological Symptoms or to Inspire and Stimulate Specific Emotions (*continued*)

TRIBE	IMPROVEMENT of MEMORY or COGNITIVE FUNCTION	INSOMNIA	INSANITY or DELIRIUM	LOVE & SEX	SEDATIVE for Nervousness/ Anxiety
	...	...	***Microlepia strigosa*** Palapalai; *Dennstaedtiaceae*	...	***Cordyline fruticosa*** Tiplant; *Agavaceae*
HOPI	...	...	***Macromeria viridiflora*** Gianttrumpets; *Boraginaceae*	...	...
	...	...	***Verbascum thapsus*** Common Mullein; *Scrophulariaceae*	...	...
HOUMA	...	...	...	...	***Scirpus sp.*** Rat Grass; *Cyperaceae*
IROQUOIS	***Cannabis sativa*** Marijuana; *Cannabaceae*	***Asarum canadense*** Canadian Wildginger; *Aristolochiaceae*	***Cornus sericea*** Redosier Dogwood; *Cornaceae*	****Adiantum pedatum*** Northern Maidenhair; *Pteridaceae*	***Cardamine diphylla*** Crinkleroot; *Brassicaceae*
	...	***Lonicera oblongifolia*** Swamp Fly Honeysuckle; *Caprifoliaceae*	***Gentiana andrewsii*** Closed Bottle Gentian; Gentianaceae	****Anemone virginiana*** Tall Thimbleweed; *Ranunculaceae*	***Cypripedium parviflorum*** Lesser Yellow Lady's Slipper; *Orchidaceae*
	...	...	***Ilex verticillata*** Common Winterberry; *Aquifoliaceae*	***Anemone virginiana*** Tall Thimbleweed; *Ranunculaceae*	***Leonurus cardiaca*** Common Motherwort; *Lamiaceae*
	...	...	***Juglans nigra*** Black Walnut; *Juglandaceae*	***Aster sp.;*** Asteraceae	***Lonicera oblongifolia*** Swamp Fly Honeysuckle; *Caprifoliaceae*
	...	...	***Mitchella repens*** Partridgeberry; Rubiaceae	****Caltha palustris*** Yellow Marsh-marigold; *Ranunculaceae*	***Nepeta cataria*** Catnip; *Lamiaceae*
	...	...	...	***Cardamine concatenata*** Cutleaf Toothwort; *Brassicaceae*	***Plantago sp.*** Plantain; *Plantaginaceae*
	...	...	...	****Cardamine diphylla*** Crinkleroot; *Brassicaceae*	***Toxicodendron pubescens*** Atlantic Poison Oak; *Anacardiaceae*
	...	...	...	***Corallorrhiza maculata*** Summer Coralroot; *Orchidaceae*	...
	...	...	...	***Dirca palustris*** Eastern Leatherwood; *Thymelaeaceae*	...
	...	...	...	****Eupatorium maculatum*** Spotted Joepyeweed; *Asteraceae*	...

(*continued*)

Table 2-1b. List of Herbs Used by Native Americans for the Treatment of Psychological Symptoms or to Inspire and Stimulate Specific Emotions (*continued*)

TRIBE	IMPROVEMENT of MEMORY or COGNITIVE FUNCTION	INSOMNIA	INSANITY or DELIRIUM	LOVE & SEX	SEDATIVE for Nervousness/ Anxiety
	...	...	...	***Galium triflorum*** Fragrant Bedstraw; ***Rubiaceae***	...
	...	...	...	***Geranium maculatum*** Spotted Geranium; *Geraniaceae*	...
	...	...	...	*****Geum aleppicum*** Yellow Avens; ***Rosaceae***	...
	...	...	...	***Geum canadense*** White Avens; *Rosaceae*	...
	...	...	...	*****Laportea canadensis*** Canadian Woodnettle; ***Urticaceae***	...
	...	...	...	***Lilium philadelphicum*** Wood Lily; *Liliaceae*	...
	...	...	...	*****Linaria vulgaris*** Butter And Eggs; *Scrophulariaceae*	...
	...	...	...	***Lobelia cardinalis*** Cardinalflower; *Campanulaceae*	...
	...	...	...	°***Lobelia inflata*** Indian Tobacco; *Campanulaceae*	...
	...	...	...	*****Lobelia kalmii*** Ontario Lobelia; *Campanulaceae*	...
	...	...	...	***Lobelia spicata*** Palespike Lobelia; *Campanulaceae*	...
	...	...	...	°***Lonicera dioica*** Limber Honeysuckle; *Caprifoliaceae*	...
	...	...	...	***Malva neglecta*** Common Mallow; *Malvaceae*	...
	...	...	...	***Mitchella repens*** Partridgeberry; *Rubiaceae*	...
	...	...	...	*****Osmorhiza sp.*** Sweet Cicely; *Apiaceae*	...
	...	...	...	*****Penstemon fruticosus*** Bush Penstemon; *Scrophulariaceae*	...

Table 2-1b. List of Herbs Used by Native Americans for the Treatment of Psychological Symptoms or to Inspire and Stimulate Specific Emotions (*continued*)

TRIBE	IMPROVEMENT of MEMORY or COGNITIVE FUNCTION	INSOMNIA	INSANITY or DELIRIUM	LOVE & SEX	SEDATIVE for Nervousness/ Anxiety
	...	...	...	***Phytolacca americana*** American Pokeweed; *Phytolaccaceae*	...
	...	...	...	***Polygonum arenastrum*** Ovalleaf Knotweed; *Polygonaceae*	...
	...	...	...	****Populus alba*** White Poplar; *Salicaceae*	...
	...	...	...	***Prenanthes trifoliolata*** Gall Of The Earth; *Asteraceae*	...
	...	...	...	***Rumex crispus*** Curly Dock; *Polygonaceae*	...
	...	...	...	***Sarracenia purpurea*** Purple Pitcherplant; *Sarraceniaceae*	...
	...	...	...	****Solidago canadensis*** Canada Goldenrod; *Asteraceae*	...
	...	...	...	****Spiraea sp.;*** Rosaceae	...
	...	...	...	***Symphyotrichum novae-angliae*** New England Aster; *Asteraceae*	...
	...	...	...	***Taraxacum officinale*** Common Dandelion; *Asteraceae*	...
	...	...	...	***Viburnum lantanoides*** Hobblebush; *Caprifoliaceae*	...
	...	...	...	***Vicia americana*** American Vetch; *Fabaceae*	...
	...	...	...	***Vicia sativa*** Common Vetch; *Fabaceae*	...
KAROK	...	...	...	***Acer circinatum*** Vine Maple; *Aceraceae*	...
	...	...	...	***Calystegia occidentalis*** Chaparral False Bindweed; *Convolvulaceae*	...
	...	...	...	***Clinopodium douglasii*** Yerba Buena;	...
			...	*Lamiaceae*	

(*continued*)

Table 2-1b. List of Herbs Used by Native Americans for the Treatment of Psychological Symptoms or to Inspire and Stimulate Specific Emotions (*continued*)

TRIBE	IMPROVEMENT of MEMORY or COGNITIVE FUNCTION	INSOMNIA	INSANITY or DELIRIUM	LOVE & SEX	SEDATIVE for Nervousness/ Anxiety
	...	...	...	***Galium triflorum*** Fragrant Bedstraw; *Rubiaceae*	...
	...	...	...	***Monardella odoratissima*** Pacific Monardella; *Lamiaceae*	...
	...	...	...	***Populus balsamifera*** Black Cottonwood; *Salicaceae*	...
KASHAYA POMO	...	...	...	***Arbutus menziesii*** Pacific Madrone; *Ericaceae*	...
KERES	***Zinnia acerosa*** Desert Zinnia; *Asteraceae*	***Gaura mollis*** Velvetweed; *Onagraceae*	...	...	***Chrysothamnus sp.*** Rabbit Brush; *Asteraceae*
	...	...	...	...	***Pectis angustifolia*** Narrowleaf Pectis; *Asteraceae*
KIOWA	...	...	...	***Juniperus virginiana*** Eastern Redcedar; *Cupressaceae*	...
KLALLAM	...	...	...	***Conium maculatum*** Poison Hemlock; *Apiaceae*	...
KWAKIUTL	...	...	...	***Aruncus dioicus*** Bride's Feathers; *Rosaceae*	...
	...	...	...	***Drosera rotundifolia*** Roundleaf Sundew; *Droseraceae*	...
	...	...	...	***Monotropa hypopithys*** Pinesap; *Ericaceae*	...
	...	...	...	***Platanthera stricta*** Modoc Bog Orchid; *Orchidaceae*	...
LOLAHNKOK	...	...	...	***Angelica sp.*** *Apiaceae*	...
MAHUNA	...	***Clinopodium douglasii*** Yerba Buena; *Lamiaceae*	...	...	...
MAKAH	...	...	...	***Prosartes hookeri*** Oregon Drops Of Gold; *Liliaceae*	...
	...	...	...	***Prosartes smithii*** Largeflower Fairybells; *Liliaceae*	...
	...	...	...	***Trillium ovatum*** Pacific Trillium; *Liliaceae*	...

Table 2-1b. List of Herbs Used by Native Americans for the Treatment of Psychological Symptoms or to Inspire and Stimulate Specific Emotions (*continued*)

TRIBE	IMPROVEMENT of MEMORY or COGNITIVE FUNCTION	INSOMNIA	INSANITY or DELIRIUM	LOVE & SEX	SEDATIVE for Nervousness/ Anxiety
	...	...	...	***Vicia nigricans*** Giant Vetch; *Fabaceae*	...
MENDOCINO	...	***Angelica sp.*** Angelica Root; *Apiaceae*	***Frangula californica*** California Buckthorn; *Rhamnaceae*	...	***Prunus virginiana*** Western Chokecherry; *Rosaceae*
MENOMINEE	***Diervilla lonicera*** Northern Bush Honeysuckle; *Caprifoliaceae*	***Mitchella repens*** Partridgeberry; *Rubiaceae*	...	***Castilleja coccinea*** Scarlet Indian Paintbrush; *Scrophulariaceae*	***Valeriana uliginosa*** Mountain Valerian; *Valerianaceae*
	Panax quinquefolius American Ginseng; *Araliaceae*	...	...	***Dicentra cucullaria*** Dutchman's Breeches; *Papaveraceae*	...
	...	...	...	***Echinocystis lobata*** Wild Cucumber; *Cucurbitaceae*	...
	...	...	...	***Pedicularis canadensis*** Canadian Lousewort; *Scrophulariaceae*	...
MESKWAKI	***Solidago canadensis*** Canada Goldenrod; *Asteraceae*	***Arisaema triphyllum*** Jack In The Pulpit; *Araceae*	***Anemone cylindrica*** Candle Anemone; *Ranunculaceae*	***Aquilegia canadensis*** Red Columbine; Ranunculaceae	***Ambrosia trifida*** Great Ragweed; *Asteraceae*
		Humulus lupulus Common Hop; *Cannabaceae*	***Gymnocladus dioicus*** Kentucky Coffeetree; *Fabaceae*	***Cypripedium acaule*** Pink Lady's Slipper; *Orchidaceae*	...
	...	...	***Maianthemum racemosum*** Feather Solomon's Seal; *Liliaceae*	***Filipendula rubra*** Queen Of The Prairie; *Rosaceae*	...
	...	...	***Pseudognaphalium obtusifolium*** Rabbit Tobacco; *Asteraceae*	***Iodanthus pinnatifidus*** Purplerocket; *Brassicaceae*	...
	...	...	***Symphyotrichum lateriflorum*** Calico Aster; *Asteraceae*	***Lobelia cardinalis*** Cardinalflower; *Campanulaceae*	...
	...	...	***Tradescantia occidentalis*** Prairie Spiderwort; *Commelinaceae*	***Lobelia siphilitica*** Great Blue Lobelia; *Campanulaceae*	...
	...	...	***Vitis vulpina*** Frost Grape; *Vitaceae*	***Panax quinquefolius*** American Ginseng; *Araliaceae*	...
	...	...	...	***Pedicularis canadensis*** Canadian Lousewort; *Scrophulariaceae*	...
	...	...	...	***Phlox pilosa*** Downy Phlox; *Polemoniaceae*	...

(*continued*)

Table 2-1b. List of Herbs Used by Native Americans for the Treatment of Psychological Symptoms or to Inspire and Stimulate Specific Emotions (*continued*)

TRIBE	IMPROVEMENT of MEMORY or COGNITIVE FUNCTION	INSOMNIA	INSANITY or DELIRIUM	LOVE & SEX	SEDATIVE for Nervousness/ Anxiety
	...	...	...	***Thalictrum dasycarpum*** Purple Meadowrue; *Ranunculaceae*	...
MICMAC	...	...	...	***Sanguinaria canadensis*** Bloodroot; *Papaveraceae*	***Cypripedium acaule*** Pink Lady's Slipper; *Orchidaceae*
MOHEGAN	...	...	...	...	***Humulus lupulus*** Common Hop; *Cannabaceae*
NAVAJO	...	***Arabis perennans*** Perennial Rockcress; *Brassicaceae*	***Adiantum capillus-veneris*** Common Maidenhair; *Pteridaceae*	***Tradescantia occidentalis*** Prairie Spiderwort; *Commelinaceae*	***Ceanothus fendleri*** Fendler's Ceanothus; *Rhamnaceae*
	...	***Eriogonum jamesii*** James' Buckwheat; *Polygonaceae*	***Frasera speciosa*** Showy Frasera; *Gentianaceae*	***Vitis arizonica*** Canyon Grape; *Vitaceae*	***Frasera speciosa*** Showy Frasera; *Gentianaceae*
	...	***Thymophylla pentachaeta*** Five-needle Pricklyleaf; *Asteraceae*	***Verbascum thapsus*** Common Mullein; *Scrophulariaceae*	...	***Gutierrezia sarothrae*** Broom Snakeweed; *Asteraceae*
	...	...	...	...	***Quercus ×pauciloba Rydb. (pro sp.)*** *[gambelii × turbinella]* Wavyleaf Oak; *Fagaceae*
	...	...	...	...	***Thelesperma megapotamicum*** Hopi Tea, Greenthread; *Asteraceae*
NEVADA	...	...	...	***Castilleja sp.*** Indian Paint Brush; *Scrophulariaceae*	...
NITINAHT	...	***Conocephalum conicum***; *Conocephalaceae*	***Lonicera involucrata*** Twinberry Honeysuckle; *Caprifoliaceae*	...	***Lonicera involucrata*** Twinberry Honeysuckle; *Caprifoliaceae*
	...	...	***Postelsia palmaeformis*** Sea Palm; *Lessioniaceae*	...	***Sambucus racemosa*** Pacific Red Elder; *Caprifoliaceae*
NOOTKA	...	...	...	***Lonicera involucrata*** Twinberry Honeysuckle; *Caprifoliaceae*	...
OJIBWA	...	...	...	***Coeloglossum viride*** Longbract Frog Orchid; *Orchidaceae*	...
	...	...	...	***Pedicularis canadensis*** Canadian Lousewort; *Scrophulariaceae*	...

Table 2-1b. List of Herbs Used by Native Americans for the Treatment of Psychological Symptoms or to Inspire and Stimulate Specific Emotions (*continued*)

TRIBE	IMPROVEMENT of MEMORY or COGNITIVE FUNCTION	INSOMNIA	INSANITY or DELIRIUM	LOVE & SEX	SEDATIVE for Nervousness/ Anxiety
OKANAGAN	...	...	...	***Apocynum androsaemifolium*** Spreading Dogbane; *Apocynaceae*	***Sedum spathulifolium*** Broadleaf Stonecrop; *Crassulaceae*
	...	...	...	***Arnica cordifolia*** Heartleaf Arnica; *Asteraceae*	...
	...	...	...	***Arnica latifolia*** Broadleaf Arnica; *Asteraceae*	...
	...	...	...	***Geum triflorum*** Prairiesmoke; *Rosaceae*	...
	...	...	...	***Matricaria discoidea*** Disc Mayweed; *Asteraceae*	...
OKLAHOMA	...	...	...	***Aquilegia canadensis*** Red Columbine; *Ranunculaceae*	***Humulus lupulus*** Common Hop; *Cannabaceae*
OMAHA	...	...	...	***Artemisia dracunculus*** Wormwood; *Asteraceae*	...
	...	...	...	***Lomatium foeniculaceum*** Desert Biscuitroot; *Apiaceae*	...
	...	...	...	***Lomatium sp.*** Biscuit Root; *Apiaceae*	...
OREGON	...	...	...	***Aquilegia canadensis*** Red Columbine; *Ranunculaceae*	...
PAIUTE	...	...	***Mirabilis alipes*** Winged Four O'clock; *Nyctaginaceae*	***Cuscuta compacta*** Compact Dodder; *Cuscutaceae*	...
PAWNEE	...	...	...	***Lobelia cardinalis*** Cardinalflower; *Campanulaceae*	***Ipomoea leptophylla*** Bush Morningglory; *Convolvulaceae*
	...	...	...	***Lomatium foeniculaceum*** Desert Biscuitroot; *Apiaceae*	***Juniperus virginiana*** Eastern Redcedar; *Cupressaceae*
	...	...	...	***Panax quinquefolius*** American Ginseng; *Araliaceae*	...
PENOBSCOT	...	...	...	...	***Cypripedium acaule*** Pink Lady's Slipper; *Orchidaceae*

(*continued*)

Table 2-1b. List of Herbs Used by Native Americans for the Treatment of Psychological Symptoms or to Inspire and Stimulate Specific Emotions (*continued*)

TRIBE	IMPROVEMENT of MEMORY or COGNITIVE FUNCTION	INSOMNIA	INSANITY or DELIRIUM	LOVE & SEX	SEDATIVE for Nervousness/ Anxiety
PIMA	...	...	...	...	***Pluchea sericea*** Arrowweed; *Asteraceae*
PONCA	...	...	...	***Aquilegia canadensis*** Red Columbine; *Ranunculaceae*	...
	...	...	...	***Lomatium foeniculaceum*** Desert Biscuitroot; *Apiaceae*	...
	...	...	...	***Sanguinaria canadensis*** Bloodroot; *Papaveraceae*	...
	...	...	...	***Thalictrum dasycarpum*** Purple Meadowrue; *Ranunculaceae*	...
POTAWATOMI	...	...	...	***Menziesia ferruginea*** Rusty Menziesia; *Ericaceae*	...
	...	...	...	***Platanthera ×media (Rydb.) Luer (pro sp.) [dilatata × hyperborea]*** Bog Orchid; *Orchidaceae*	...
	...	...	...	***Schoenoplectus tabernaemontani*** Softstem Bulrush; *Cyperaceae*	...
	...	...	...	***Thalictrum dasycarpum*** Purple Meadowrue; *Ranunculaceae*	...
QUILEUTE	...	...	...	***Galium triflorum*** Fragrant Bedstraw; *Rubiaceae*	...
QUINAULT	...	...	...	***Vicia nigricans*** Giant Vetch; *Fabaceae*	...
RAPPAHANNOCK	...	...	...	***Liriodendron tulipifera*** Tuliptree; *Magnoliaceae*	...
SEMINOLE	***Ilex vomitoria*** Yaupon; *Aquifoliaceae*	***Ilex vomitoria*** Yaupon; *Aquifoliaceae*	***Hyptis pectinata*** Comb Bushmint; *Lamiaceae*	***Chrysobalanus icaco*** Icaco Coco Plum; *Chrysobalanaceae*	***Chenopodium ambrosioides*** Mexican Tea; *Chenopodiaceae*
	...	...	***Juniperus virginiana*** Southern Redcedar; *Cupressaceae*	***Chrysophyllum oliviforme*** Satinleaf; *Sapotaceae*	...

Table 2-1b. List of Herbs Used by Native Americans for the Treatment of Psychological Symptoms or to Inspire and Stimulate Specific Emotions (*continued*)

TRIBE	IMPROVEMENT of MEMORY or COGNITIVE FUNCTION	INSOMNIA	INSANITY or DELIRIUM	LOVE & SEX	SEDATIVE for Nervousness/ Anxiety
	...	...	***Lagenaria siceraria*** Bottle Gourd; *Cucurbitaceae*	*****Conyza canadensis*** Canadian Horseweed; *Asteraceae*	...
	...	...	***Licania michauxii*** Gopher Apple; *Chrysobalanaceae*	***Morella cerifera*** Southern Bayberry; *Myricaceae*	...
	...	...	***Osmunda regalis*** Royal Fern; *Osmundaceae*	***Panax quinquefolius*** American Ginseng; *Araliaceae*	...
	...	...	***Persea borbonia*** Redbay; *Lauraceae*	***Persea borbonia*** Redbay; *Lauraceae*	...
	...	...	***Phlebodium aureum*** Golden Polypody; *Polypodiaceae*	***Quercus phellos*** Willow Oak; *Fagaceae*	...
	...	...	***Polypodium incanum*** Resurrection Fern; *Polypodiaceae*	***Quercus virginiana*** Live Oak; *Fagaceae*	...
	...	...	***Vittaria lineata*** Appalachian Shoestring Fern; *Vittariaceae*	***Salix caroliniana*** Coastal Plain Willow; *Salicaceae*	...
	...	...	***Thelypteris kunthii*** Kunth's Maiden Fern; *Thelypteridaceae*	***Sideroxylon foetidissimum*** False Mastic; *Sapotaceae*	...
SONGISH	...	...	...	***Osmorhiza purpurea*** Purple Sweetroot; *Apiaceae*	...
SWINOMISH	...	...	...	***Osmorhiza berteroi*** Sweetcicely; *Apiaceae*	...
THOMPSON	...	...	***Populus tremuloides*** Quaking Aspen; *Salicaceae*	***Aquilegia formosa*** Western Columbine; *Ranunculaceae*	***Sedum spathulifolium*** Broadleaf Stonecrop; *Crassulaceae*
	...	...	...	***Cornus nuttallii*** Pacific Dogwood; *Cornaceae*	...
	...	...	...	***Delphinium menziesii*** Menzies' Larkspur; *Ranunculaceae*	...
	...	...	...	***Dodecatheon jeffreyi*** Tall Mountain Shootingstar; *Primulaceae*	...
	...	...	...	***Geranium viscosissimum*** Sticky Geranium; *Geraniaceae*	...

(continued)

Table 2-1b. List of Herbs Used by Native Americans for the Treatment of Psychological Symptoms or to Inspire and Stimulate Specific Emotions (*continued*)

TRIBE	IMPROVEMENT of MEMORY or COGNITIVE FUNCTION	INSOMNIA	INSANITY or DELIRIUM	LOVE & SEX	SEDATIVE for Nervousness/ Anxiety
	...	...	...	***Geum sp.*** Avens; *Rosaceae*	...
	...	...	...	***Platanthera dilatata var. leucostachys (Lindl.) Luer*** Bog Orchid; *Orchidaceae*	...
	...	...	...	***Sagittaria latifolia*** Broadleaf Arrowhead; *Alismataceae*	...
WINNABEGO	...	...	...	***Aquilegia canadensis*** Red Columbine; *Ranunculaceae*	...
	...		...	***Lomatium foeniculaceum*** Desert Biscuitroot; *Apiaceae*	
ZUNI	...	...	***Dimorphocarpa wislizeni*** Touristplant; *Brassicaceae*	...	

* Counteracts effects of a love medicine.

° Used to inspire and discourage feelings of love.

References

Akana A. Hawaiian Herbs of Medicinal Value. Pacific Book House, Honolulu, HI. 1922.

Baker MA. The Ethnobotany of the Yurok, Tolowa and Karok Indians of Northwest California. Humboldt State University, MA Thesis. 1981.

Bocek BR. Ethnobotany of Costanoan Indians, California. Based on Collections by John P. Harrington. Economic Botany. 1984;38:240–255.

Chandler FR, Freeman L, Hooper SN. Herbal Remedies of the Maritime Indians. J Ethnopharm. 1979;1:49–68.

Chestnut VK. Plants Used by the Indians of Mendocino County, California. Contributions from the U.S. National Herbarium. 1902;7:295–408.

Colton HS. Hopi History And Ethnobotany. In: Horr DA (ed), Hopi Indians. Garland: New York, NY. 1974.

Curtin LS. By the Prophet of the Earth. San Vicente Foundation, Sante Fe, NM. 1949.

Densmore F. Uses of Plants by the Chippewa Indians. SI-BAE Annual Report. 1928;44:273–379.

Elmore FH. Ethnobotany of the Navajo. School of American Research, Sante Fe, NM. 1944.

Gilmore MR. Uses of Plants by the Indians of the Missouri River Region. SI-BAE Annual Report. 1919.

Grinnell GB. The Cheyenne Indians—Their History and Ways of Life Vol.2. University of Nebraska Press, Lincoln, NE. 1972.

Goodrich J, Lawson C. Kashaya Pomo Plants. Los Angeles. American Indian Studies Center, University of California, Los Angeles, CA. 1980.

Gunther E. Ethnobotany of Western Washington. University of Washington Press, Seattle, WA. 1973.
Hamel PB, Chiltoskey MU. Cherokee Plants and Their Uses: A 400-Year History. Herald Publishing Co., Sylva, NC. 1975.
Hart JA. The Ethnobotany of the Northern Cheyenne Indians of Montana. J Ethnopharm. 1981;4:1–55.
Herrick JW. Iroquois Medical Botany. State University of New York, Albany, NY. PhD Thesis. 1977.
Hocking GM. Some Plant Materials Used Medicinally and Otherwise by the Navajo Indians in the Chaco Canyon, New Mexico. El Palacio 1956;56:146–165.
Merriam HC. Ethnographic Notes on California Indian Tribes. University of California Archaeological Research Facility, Berkeley, CA. 1966.
Murphey E. Indian Uses of Native Plants. Meyerbooks, Glenwood, Illinois. 1990.
Moerman DE. Native American Ethnobotany. Timber Press, Portland, OR. 2002.
Moerman DE. University of Michigan—Dearborn. Native American Ethnobotany Database, 2003. http://herb.umd.umich.edu/
Perry F. Ethno-Botany of the Indians in the Interior of British Columbia. Museum and Art Notes. 1952; 2:36–43.
Raymond M. Notes Ethnobotaniques Sur Les Tete-de-Boule de Manouan. Contributions de l'Institut Botanique de l'Universite de Montreal. 1945;55:113–134.
Romero JB. The Botanical Lore of the California Indians. Vantage Press, Inc., New York, NY. 1954.
Rousseau J. Ethnobotanique Abenakise. Archives de Folklore. 1947;11:145–182.
Rousseau J. Le Folklore Botanique De L'Ile Aux Coudres. Contributions de l'Institut Botanique de l'Universite de Montreal 1945;55:75–111.
Schenck SM, Gifford EW. Karok Ethnobotany. Anthropol Rec. 1952;13:377–392.
Smith HH. Ethnobotany of the Menomini Indians. Bulletin of the Public Museum of the City of Milwaukee. 1923;4:1–174.
Smith HH. Ethnobotany of the Meskwaki Indians. Bulletin of the Public Museum of the City of Milwaukee. 1928;4:175–326.
Smith HH. Ethnobotany of the Ojibwe Indians. Bulletin of the Public Museum of Milwaukee. 1932;4: 327–525.
Smith HH. Ethnobotany of the Forest Potawatomi Indians. Bulletin of the Public Museum of the City of Milwaukee. 1933;7:1–230.
Speck FG. Medicine Practices of the Northeastern Algonquians. Proceedings of the 19th International Congress of Americanists. 1917;303–321.
Speck FG. A List of Plant Curatives Obtained From the Houma Indians of Louisiana. Primitive Man. 1941;14:49–75.
Speck FG, Hassrick RB, Carpenter ES. Rappahannock Herbals, Folk-Lore and Science of Cures. Proceedings of the Delaware County Institute of Science. 1942;10:7–55.
Steedman EV. The Ethnobotany of the Thompson Indians of British Columbia. SI-BAE Annual Report. 1928;45:441–522.
Stevenson MC. Ethnobotany of the Zuni Indians. SI-BAE Annual Report. 1915.
Sturtevant W. The Mikasuki Seminole: Medical Beliefs and Practices. Yale University, PhD Thesis. 1954.
Swank GR. The Ethnobotany of the Acoma and Laguna Indians. University of New Mexico, MA Thesis. 1932.
Swanton JR. Religious Beliefs and Medical Practices of the Creek Indians. SI-BAE Annual Report. 1928;42:473–672.
Tantaquidgeon G. Mohegan Medicinal Practices, Weather-Lore and Superstitions. SI-BAE Annual Report. 1928;43:264–270.
Tantaquidgeon G. A Study of Delaware Indian Medicine Practice and Folk Beliefs. Pennsylvania Historical Commission, Harrisburg, PA. 1942.
Tantaquidgeon G. Folk Medicine of the Delaware and Related Algonkian Indians. Historical Commission Anthropological Papers, Harrisburg, PA. 1972.

Taylor LA. Plants Used As Curatives by Certain Southeastern Tribes. Botanical Museum of Harvard University, Cambridge, MA.1940.

Train P, Henrichs JR, Archer WA. Medicinal Uses of Plants by Indian Tribes of Nevada. U.S. Department of Agriculture, Washington DC. 1941.

Turner NC, Bell MA. The Ethnobotany of the Coast Salish Indians of Vancouver Island, I and II. Economic Botany 1971; 25:63–104, 335–339.

Turner NC, Bell MA. The Ethnobotany of the Southern Kwakiutl Indians of British Columbia. Economic Botany 1973;27:257–310.

Turner NC, Bouchard R, Kennedy DI. Ethnobotany of the Okanagan-Colville Indians of British Columbia and Washington. British Columbia Provincial Museum, Victoria, BC. 1980.

Turner NC, Thomas J, Barry F et al. Ethnobotany of the Nitinaht Indians of Vancouver Island. British Columbia Provincial Museum, Victoria, BC. 1983.

Turner NC, Thompson LC, Thompson MT et al. Thompson Ethnobotany: Knowledge and Usage of Plants by the Thompson Indians of British Columbia. Royal British Columbia Museum, Victoria, BC. 1990.

Vestal PA, Schultes RE. The Economic Botany of the Kiowa Indians. Botanical Museum of Harvard University, Cambridge, MA. 1939.

Whiting AF. Ethnobotany of the Hopi. Museum of Northern Arizona Bulletin. 1939.

Wyman LC, Harris SK. The Ethnobotany of the Kayenta Navaho. The University of New Mexico Press, Albuquerque, NM. 1951.

Chapter 3

Ayurvedic Psychoactive Herbs

"The plants that are brown, and those that are white; the red ones and the speckled ones; the sable and the black plants, all these do we invoke.

May they protect this man from the disease sent by the gods, the herbs whose father is the sky, whose mother is the earth, whose root is the ocean. The waters and the heavenly plants are foremost; they have driven out from every limb thy disease, consequent upon sin.

The plants that spread forth, those that are bushy, those that have a single sheath, those that creep along, do I address; I call in thy behalf the plants that have shoots, those that have stalks, those that divide their branches, those that are derived from all the gods, the strong plants that furnish life to man.

With the might that is yours, ye mighty ones, with the power and strength that is yours, with that do ye, O plants, rescue this man from this disease!

I now prepare a remedy."

—*Hymn of Universal Remedy to All Magic and Medicinal Plants, Atharvaveda*

Historical Perspective of Ayurveda

Ayurveda is the classical Indian system of holistic healing. It has its origins in the Hindu scriptures, some of which date back at least 10,000 years and represent the first recorded knowledge of the human race. By 3147 BC, physician-priests had recorded much of the empirical wisdom of the oral tradition in four Sanskrit scriptures (*Rugveda*, *Yajurveda*, *Atharvaveda*, and *Samaveda*) collectively called the *Vedas* (Anjaria, Parabia, Dwivedi 2002; Lad 2002; Vivekananda 2003). These *Sutras* (Sanskrit origin of "to suture") in the form of poetry and verse represent the condensed thread of knowledge with emphasis on deriving medicine from plants and living in balance with nature. Ayurveda stems from the Atharvaveda. The *Rasayanas* are the traditional medicines used to promote mental and physical health, boost the immune system, and prolong life.

The *Maharshi Shalihotra* wrote the first text of veterinary Ayurveda (*Ashva Ayurveda*) around 2350 BC. On view at Gujarat Ayurveda University in India, it details the care of horses and also mentions elephants, the great vehicles of war of ancient times. *Palakapya* composed the great text of elephant healing (*Gaja Ayurveda*) around 1500 BC. Bovine medicine is described in a number of ancient texts (e.g., *Agni Purana*) but its practice originates with the philosophies of *Lord Krishna* around 1000 BC. *King Ashoka* ordered the construction of the first veterinary hospital in 300 BC and is responsible for the formalized use of Ayurvedic remedies for animals (Dr. Jayvir Anjaria, personal communication 2004; Anjaria, Parabia, Dwivedi 2002).

The second Ayurvedic period occurred during the Buddhist era (1873 to 1793 BC) when teachings of the Buddha (Sanskrit for "enlightened one") were integrated into Ayurvedic wisdom. Buddha was the Indian prince Siddhartha Gautama, who was well known for his compassion for nonhuman animals and preached against their abuse. Ayurvedic principles of spirituality, the importance of mental balance and moderation, and the practice of meditation and yoga for therapeutic purpose are to a large degree due to his expanded consciousness. Ayurvedic knowledge of the *marmani* (singular *marma*), energy points on the body, is used as a diagnostic tool and treatment of disease. It is a method of therapeutic massage and is similar to Chinese acupuncture (Anjaria, Parabia, Dwivedi 2002; Lad 2002).

The oldest surviving Sanskrit text of Ayurveda (*Charaka Samhita*) has been dated to 1220 BC. It is attributed to the physician Charakcharya, who first presented the doshic classification of vata, pitta, and kapha. It also contains a famous section of veterinary Ayurveda known as the *Mrig Ayurveda*. The second great treatise of Ayurveda (*Sushruta Samhita*), written by Nagarjuna, contains the first descriptions of surgery and the subdoshas of pitta. Many great works followed (Anjaria, Parabia, Dwivedi 2002; Lad 2002).

Although this book is not meant to be a text of philosophy, it would be impossible to understand or appreciate the clinical application of Ayurvedic herbs without providing the basis of how and why to use them. Delving into Ayurvedic principles requires the novice to abandon much of his or her Western nomenclature and bias, although Ayurveda has integrated modern medical knowledge as well. An introduction to Ayurvedic philosophy follows, with the hope that it will improve the reader's appreciation of a healing art that will likely become of increasing importance to Western healers.

Introduction to *Ayur Vidya*

Ayurveda's fundamental doctrine is that health is a state of physical, mental, social, and spiritual well being (*Niramaya*) and can be considered the original method of holistic medicine. Ayurveda teaches that the body is merely an objective experience whereas the mind is a subjective experience. The spirit (soul or *atman*) is pure consciousness and is as important to treating disease as is curing the body and mind. Ayurveda comes from the Sanskrit *Ayur Vidya*, "Knowledge of Life," which underscores just how much the healing power of Nature is to be revered. Physicians and veterinarians are, therefore, vehicles for this healing power, whether or not they are aware of it. Ayurveda requires the individual to take responsibility for his or her own health and teaches that every individual is a microcosm of the great forces of the cosmos. Each individual should strive to express the divinity within, embracing all of Creation, to attain the highest level of health and spiritual purity and balance. The body is a vehicle for the spirit or soul. Heaven is not a geographical place but rather a quality of consciousness or a state of "mind."

Much of herbal medicine has its roots in Ayurveda, as does Traditional Chinese Medicine. Extending from India, Ayurvedic principles have influenced all Eastern healing practices including Arab medicine, which had such great impact on the origins of Western medicine as well. The influences of regional philosophies such as Buddhism were also absorbed into Ayurveda. Although the British required the suppression of Ayurveda during colonial occupation of India, it has enjoyed great resurgence and revitalization. There is no concept of specialization in Ayurveda as there is in Western medicine; the whole person must be balanced to heal a focal point of disease. Furthermore, just as a person should be treated as a whole, so should the herbal remedy that treats the person be used as a whole. Just as Ayurveda does not focus on any one aspect of an individual's well-being, Ayurveda has incorporated new scientific knowledge and remains a vital and important practice in Indian medicine and, increasingly, in the West.

The *Shad Darsham* (*Shad* = six; *Darsham* = perceptions) are the six Ayurvedic philosophies of life (Anjaria, Parabia, Dwivedi 2002; Lad 2002; Vivekananda 2003). These lead the individual toward self-actualization and the alleviation of pain and suffering. One's actions (*karmas*) toward self-fulfillment and toward others will impact one's spiritual evolution and well-being. To act out of love and compassion will not only benefit everyone you come in contact with but also elevate your inner self and benefit the quality of your own life, now and into the next life. The six perceptions are as follows:

- *Sankhya*—"to know the truth": There are 24 manifestations of the universe, which include the five senses, the five actions (speech, grasping, walking, procreation, elimination), and the five elements (Ether, Water, Air, Fire, Earth). The five elements and their significance in Ayurveda are discussed in more detail below. Consciousness is derived from the senses that provide energy channels from the world around us toward the world within us. *Mahad*, the corporal intelligence at the cellular level, is energized not only by the nourishment we take but also by the flow of *Prana,* the life force that governs intercellular communication, neuromotor function, and sensory perception. Prana is the equivalent of *Qi* (*Chi*) in Traditional Chinese Medicine and philosophy.

- *Vaisheshika*: The nine consecutive substances of the Universe are ether, air, fire, water, earth, soul (*atman*), mind (*manas*), time (*kala*), and direction (*dig*). Cognitive awareness of the mind is made possible by subconscious or conscious sensory input. Psychological time is the movement of thought, compared to chronological time, which is the movement of past into the present and the future.
- *Nyaya*: Teaches how to deal with the nine substances of the universe and presents the four sources of valid knowledge: perception, inference, comparison, and testimony, which are based on the five ordinary senses and extraordinary perception, if the individual is open to this level of awareness. Intuition can be a diagnostic tool for use in addition to the findings of a physical examination.
- *Mimamsa*—"to analyze/understand the truth": The meaning of life can be attained through religious awareness but also by performing duties (*dharmas*). Meditation and ritual can help us to attain a higher level of self. Rituals are part of the healing sciences as well.
- *Yoga*: The practice of yoga allows the *yogi* to maintain a healthy and flexible body. Breathing is controlled and slowed, thereby regulating the flow of Prana and extending one's longevity. The practice of yoga is also a form of meditation in that it helps to clear the mind and go beyond its boundaries. Yoga promotes the union of lower and higher self to expand the individual consciousness into cosmic consciousness.
- *Vedanta*—"the ending of knowledge": Ultimately, one cannot learn about life or truth by reading a book. Our physical reality is artificial because *Brahman* (God) is in all of Creation.

The Five Elements

Because humankind is viewed as a microcosm of the universal Cosmos, the five basic elements are also considered to exist in balance within each individual. The five elements (*Maha Bhutas*), summarized in Table 3-1, are the basic building blocks of Ayurvedic medical principles and are key to understanding the medical perspective of Ayurveda.

Ether represents the omnipresent spiritual energy that permeates everything and fills all spaces and cavities. It corresponds to the sense of hearing and therefore to the production of sound by the vocal chords. Air represents movement such as the beating heart, breathing, and neurotransmission. It corresponds to the skin and in particular the hands, which are highly sensitive to the sense of touch. Fire symbolizes the heat of metabolism such as that generated by the digestive system, or the energy of the brain. Because the eyes direct our locomotion, the eyes

Table 3-1: Summary of the Five Elements Of Ayurveda and Their Respective Spiritual and Physical Roles According to Ayurvedic Philosophy

ELEMENT	ENERGY	CHARACTERISTICS & FUNCTION	BODY PART	SENSE & KEY BODY PART	MANIFESTATION
ETHER	NUCLEAR	Space; Pure substrate of spiritual energy	Nose, GI tract, buccal cavity, abdomen, chest respiratory tract, vasculature, intercellular space	HEARING/Ears	Speech, Vocal cords
AIR	ELECTRICAL	Movement; Keeps the body in motion	Heartbeat, respiration, nerve impulses	TOUCH/Hands	Skin
FIRE	RADIANT	Metabolism; Carries heat to the cells in blood & plasma	Digestive system, brain, eyes, body T°	VISION/Eyes	Walking, Legs
WATER (Liquids)	CHEMICAL	Hydration; Permeates every cell with energy	Blood, plasma, Lymph, cerebrospinal fluid, digestive secretions	TASTE/Tongue	Procreation, Genitals
EARTH (Solids)	MECHANICAL	Solid structures	Bone, muscle, teeth, cartilage skin, hair	SMELL/Nose	Defecation, Anus

(Anjaria, Parabia, Dwivedi 2002; Lad 2002)

and legs are associated with the element of Fire. Water (alternatively referred to as Liquid) corresponds to Taste, so the tongue and digestive secretions are all part of this element. It is manifested by sex and the genitalia because these were viewed as the "lower tongue" by Ayurvedic physician/priests. Finally, Earth (also known as Solids) encompasses all solid structures of the body and corresponds to the sense of smell because of its association to solid waste produced as excrement.

In Ayurvedic medicine, the fire element (*Agni*) is of primary concern. Agni is the Sanskrit root of "ignite," from the Latin "ignis." Agni is the heat of living tissue, and there are no fewer than forty different subtypes of agni. Agni brings laughter, joy, and a light spirit. An allusion to a "healthy glow" is a direct reflection of the fire element in balance. It is by virtue of healthy agni that food energy is metabolized to become Prana. Agni governs perception, sensation, and neurotransmitters. Without the heat and light of agni, the individual becomes a shadow, plagued with the gloom of depression, sadness, grief, and disease. Depression is attributed to the suppression of agni. If agni is decreased or suppressed, the metabolism is reduced and kapha ailments and qualities predominate. If agni is excessive, the metabolism is increased and results in aggressive behavior, inflammatory disease, hypoglycemia, and compulsivity. If agni is irregular, the individual becomes anxious, insecure, fearful, and prone to neurological problems or emotional disturbance.

The importance of the five elements is recognized in TCM as well. They are also central to the practice of *Fung Shui*, the Chinese tradition of appropriate placement, orientation, and color of the homes we build, the furniture we fill them with, and even the clothing we wear, all based on a healthy flow of Qi to promote health and well-being. Although it is not as well known, the Ayurvedic practice of *Vastu Shilpa Shastra* preceded the art of Fung Shui and incorporates the five elements and other criteria to bring balance within a home and beyond as well.

The five elements reemerge in the Ayurvedic philosophy of nutrition. The body may be merely a container for the spirit, but it must be lovingly nurtured nonetheless. Western science instructs us about the four basic food groups. Ayurveda teaches a system of nutrition based on the five elements and six tastes or *Rasas* (sweet, sour, salty, pungent, bitter, and astringent). Consuming an excess of astringent-tasting foods, for example, will result in anxiety and depression. Not only should eating be a spiritual experience, but every step of its preparation should be performed in total awareness. In addition, any food or medicine that is placed in the mouth will first be experienced through the sense of taste. What a particular taste "feels like," not only in the mouth but also throughout the body, is the potent energy of that substance, known as *Virya*. Virya translates as "active principle" or "potency" and is another system of Ayurveda called the *Ashthavidha Virya* (eight types of Virya), derived from the list of twenty gunas explained in the next section. Ultimately, the Heating (*Ushna*) and Cooling (*Sheeta*) Viryas are the two predominant qualities acting on agni (digestive fire)

Table 3-2: Summary of the Six Tastes and Their Typical Corresponding Viryas in Descending Order of Their Cooling (*Sheeta Virya*) or Heating (*Ushna Virya*) Properties, and the Effects of Taste on the Doshas Vata (V), Pitta (P), and Kapha (K)

Rasa (Taste)	Virya (Active Principle)	Effect of Rasa on the Doshas
Astringent (*kashaya*)	Cooling ***Sheeta Virya***	V ↑ P ↓ K ↓
Bitter (*tikta*)	Cooling ***Sheeta Virya***	V ↑ P ↓ K ↓
Sweet (*madhura*)	Cooling ***Sheeta Virya***	V ↓ P ↓ K ↑
Sour (*amla*)	Heating ***Ushna Virya***	V ↓ P ↑ K ↑
Salty (*lavana*)	Heating ***Ushna Virya***	V ↓ P ↑ K ↑
Pungent (*katu*)	Heating ***Ushna Virya***	V ↑ P ↑ K ↓

(Anjaria, Parabia, Dwivedi 2002; Lad 2002)

and metabolism. With some exceptions, the six tastes generally correspond to either ushna or sheeta (Table 3-2).

The Three Doshas (Tridoshas) and Twenty Gunas

Ayurveda categorizes three distinct body types according to psychophysiological and functional criteria determined by the individual's constitution at the time of conception. These three categories, called the *Doshas*, are also derived from the five elements. Dosha means "impurity." When the balance of any of the dosha is disrupted, the energy of the Dosha is transformed and becomes the toxic element underlying disease. The three doshas are *Vata*, *Pitta*, and *Kapha*. These also correspond to three major personality types (*Prakriti*). Vata is comprised of Ether and Air and also corresponds to a melancholic personality profile; Pitta comes from Fire and Water (bilious profile); Kapha is the combination of Water and Earth (phlegmatic profile) (Table 3-3).

The doshas move through the body along physical and energetic channels known as the *Srotamsi* or *Patha*. It is interesting to note that the word "path" and its derivatives originate from the Sanskrit *patha*. The relative balance of the Doshas is also normally influenced by the season. Pitta is elevated in summer. Vatta increases in the fall. Kapha is increased during winter months. Food will also modify the balance of the doshas.

Vata is the energy of movement and is associated with the elements of ether and air. Prana is the essence of vata dosha. By visualizing the body parts that move as a vital function, one can easily understand that vata governs respiration, eye blink, heartbeat, muscle contraction, and cellular movement. Think of the word "inspiration." It connotes being filled with divine breath. Balanced vata brings creative inspiration and other benefits. In keeping with the theme of air and space, vata imbalance will be associated with volatility, including fearfulness and other anxiety-related conditions.

Table 3-3: Summary of the Three Doshas and Their Function in Health and Disease

DOSHA	ENERGY of:	ELEMENT	FUNCTION	IN BALANCE Dosha Promotes:	OUT OF BALANCE Dosha Triggers:	EFFECT OF SIX TASTES
VATA	Movement	Ether / Air	Respiration, heartbeat, muscles, blinking, cellular movement	CREATIVITY and FLEXIBILITY	FEAR, ANXIETY, ABNORMAL MOVEMENTS	↓ By sweet, sour, salty ↑ By pungent, bitter, astringent
PITTA	Transformation	Fire / Water	Metabolism, GI function, nutrition, body T°	UNDERSTANDING and INTELLIGENCE	ANGER, HATRED, JEALOUSY, INFLAMMATORY DISEASE	↓ By sweet, bitter, astringent ↑ By sour, salty, pungent
KAPHA	Lubrication & Structure	Water / Earth	Joint lubrication, skin moisture, immune system	LOVE, CALM, FORGIVENESS	GREED, POSSESSIVENESS, ATTACHMENT, CONGESTIVE DISORDERS	↓ By pungent, bitter, astringent ↑ By sweet, sour, salty

(Anjaria, Parabia, Dwivedi 2002; Lad 2002)

Pitta is the energy of transformation and is associated with metabolism. Visualize how fire transforms burning wood to produce heat, or how water carves its way through a *wadi* or riverbed, and you can understand the energy of pitta. In keeping with the flame analogy, pitta fire predominates in disease and results in aggressiveness and inflammatory emotions and disease. When it is in balance, pitta flows with understanding and intelligence.

Kapha is the energy of lubrication and structure; not surprisingly, it is simple to visualize the associated elements of water and earth. Kapha is the energy that binds the body together, particularly at the cellular level. Kapha governs joint lubrication, skin moisture, and immunity. In kapha balance, the individual is bathed in love, calm, and forgiveness. Out of balance, the individual's emotional state grinds to a halt like a machine without oil. Instead of kapha emotions flowing generously outward to generate positive karma and Prana, negative energy remains stagnant within the individual who becomes greedy, possessive, and prone to congestive disorders.

Each individual has a unique proportion of the three doshas that is determined by heredity, time, place, season, planetary alignment, as well as parental lifestyle and diet at our conception. Each doshic type has five subtypes (subdoshas). The unique psychophysiological makeup of each individual at conception is called *Prakruti. Vikruti* is the current doshic balance of the individual. If Prakruti equals Vikruti, there is health. However, the difference between doshic balance when prakruti and vikruti do not match is the basis for Ayurvedic diagnosis and treatment of disease.

In cases of extreme imbalance and chronic illness, the restorative technique known as *Panchakarma* may be applied. Panchakarma ("five actions") involves five purifying procedures to eliminate toxins from the body and restore doshic balance: emesis (*vamana*), purging (*virechana*), oil enema (*basti*), bloodletting (*rakta moksha,* usually with medicinal leech application), and nasal cleansing (*nasya*). However, in mild ailments the recommended treatment would include proper nutrition and herbs to restore balance to the doshas.

The Seven Dhatus

Ayurveda distinguishes seven body tissues (*Dhatus*). When toxic doshic energy enters a particular body tissue, it impacts the element of fire (*Dhatu Agni)* specific to that body tissue and the result is disease (Table 3-4). Every thought and emotion causes biochemical changes that impact any of the dhatus, although they affect primarily the *rasa* and *rakta dhatus.* Negative emotions diminish the quality of the doshas and cause disease-triggering doshic imbalance. Unresolved emotions may accumulate within the *asthi dhatu* and cause disease as well. Ayurveda teaches that the emotions are held in the lungs prior to being absorbed into the body and

Table 3-4: The Seven Dhatus and Their Characteristics

DHATU	BODY PARTS	ASSOCIATED DISORDERS
RASA	Plasma, leukocytes, lymph, cerebrospinal fluid	Fear, Anxiety, Anger, Hate, Depression, Sadness, Grief
RAKTA	Erythrocytes	Chronic fatigue syndrome, mononucleosis, HIV, Herpes
MAMSA	Muscle	Multiple sclerosis, paralysis, atrophy, myoma
MEDA	Adipose tissue	Hyperthyroidism, emaciation, hypertension, obesity, joint pain
ASTHI	Bone, cartilage	Osteoporosis, bone tumors, grinding teeth, dental disease, hair loss, hirsutism, osteoarthritis
MAJJA	Nervous system, bone marrow, connective tissue	Brain tumors, hydrocephalus, lethargy, anemia, insomnia, nightmares, neurological disease (e.g., Parkinson's, seizure disorders, autism, Attention Deficit Hyperactivity Disorder)
SHUKRA (Male) **ARTAVA (Female)**	Reproductive organs	Hypersexuality, impotence, prostatic disease, fear of sex, pain during sex (dyspareunia), perversion, sterility, ovarian cysts, uterine fibroids

(Anjaria, Parabia, Dwivedi 2002; Lad 2002)

spirit. We can inhale emotions around us that come from someone in the room or around the world. The importance of *pranayama*, yogic breath control techniques to regulate breathing, is relevant not only to assist in meditation but also to purify the body of toxic emotions.

To determine which dosha is disrupted, the doshas are qualified by twenty *Gunas* ("attributes" or "qualities") that serve as diagnostic tools (Table 3-5). The term "Guna" is also applied to three universal mental constitutions or qualities of consciousness, which also relate back to the five elements. *Sattva* is creative and includes qualities of clarity, alertness, love, compassion, and cooperation. Sattva is primarily associated with ether, but is influenced by air, fire, and water as well. Sattva is compared to potential energy, for example, the energy that infuses our bodies when we awake refreshed in the morning. *Rajas* is a maintenance state and is characterized by selfishness, restlessness, and egocentricity. It is associated with the elements air and fire. Rajas is kinetic energy, used as you plan your day. *Tamas* is destructive and has a tendency toward a dull, gloomy, depressed, sad, and lazy state. It is associated with water and earth and is comparable to inertia, or that feeling of post-prandial somnolence and lethargy.

There are seven possible combinations of vata, pitta, and kapha that determine seven psychophysiological constitutions. Each of these is described according to the relative rank of each dosha within each individual. For example, if an individual possesses equal amounts of vata and pitta, he or she would be described as $V_3P_3K_1$. If an individual is primarily kapha but has a moderate amount of pitta and a small amount of vata, the description would be $V_3P_2K_1$.

Table 3-5: Summary of the Doshas, Their Characteristic Gunas, and the Three Main Psychophysiological Body Types They Determine

DOSHA	VATA	PITTA	KAPHA
ELEMENTS	ETHER + AIR	FIRE + WATER	WATER + EARTH
GUNAS	DRY LIGHT COLD ROUGH SUBTLE MOBILE CLEAR	HOT SHARP LIGHT LIQUID MOBILE OILY	HEAVY SLOW/DULL COLD OILY LIQUID SLIMY/SMOOTH DENSE SOFT STATIC STICKY/CLOUDY HARD GROSS
DOSHIC PROFILE	Light, flexible body; Small, recessed eyes; brown complexion Delicate health; Infertility; Digestive disease; Short-lived Excitable, Anxious, Fearful, Spontaneous, Easily Bored, Seeks Constant Activity	Medium frame & weight; Prone to Balding; Eyes are bright but photosensitive; red complexion Average constitution and longevity; Big appetite but healthy weight is maintained; Libido may be low; Prefers sweets Judgmental, critical, perfectionist, compulsive,-irritable	Large, strong body; Often has thick, curly hair; Large eyes; pale complexion Robust constitution and long-lived; Loves to sleep, lounge, sit, eat; Steady appetite but slow metabolism predisposes to weight gain; Craves sweet and salty, prone to water retention Calm, steady mind, sharp memory

(Anjaria, Parabia, Dwivedi 2002; Lad 2002)

The Seven Chakras

The chakras are energy centers in the body, often associated with nerve plexus centers (Table 3-6). They can be explained as distinct cores of consciousness that connect the physical body with the spiritual plane. If energy blockages occur in the chakra, the individual will be impacted according to the chakra that is affected. Through meditation and living one's life in total awareness, *kundalini* (pure spiritual energy) awakens at the root chakra and moves upward through the chakras; eventually, the goal is to achieve *nirvana*, the state of pure existence and total bliss described by Buddha. The *kundalini chakra* system is similar to the ten *sefirot* of the *Kaballah*. These ten Divine Attributes, described by scholars of Jewish mysticism, also correlate to different body parts and metaphysical properties (see Appendix B, "Traditional Jewish Medicine: Parallels to Ayurveda and TCM.").

Table 3-6: The Seven Chakras and Their Significance

CHAKRA	NAME	LOCATION AND NEUROENDOCRINE CENTER	FUNCTION	STATE OF MIND
1	MULADHARA	ROOT CHAKRA (Base of Spine; Gonads)	Survival; Base Level of Existence	Instinct to survive; food, shelter
2	SVADHISHTHANA	PELVIC CHAKRA (Adrenals)	Procreation, Identity, Self-esteem, Sexual Love	Sex, self-actualization
3	MANIPURA	SOLAR PLEXUS (Pancreas)	Power, Ambition	Competition, Dominance, Control
4	ANAHATA	HEART CHAKRA (Thymus)	Compassion, Immune System	Bridge to higher consciousness; center of "I am"
5	VISHUDDHA	THROAT CHAKRA (Thyroid/Parathyroid)	Communication	Speaking the Truth (or not)
6	AJNA	THIRD EYE (Pituitary)	Intuition	Connection to the Cosmos, extra-sensory perception
7	SAHASRARA	CROWN CHAKRA (Pineal)	Bliss, Highest Level of Consciousness	Point at which the female and male energies merge into nirvana

(Anjaria, Parabia, Dwivedi 2002; Lad 2002)

Table 3-7: Ayurvedic Categories of Psychoneuropharmacological Herbs

AMNESICS	INTOXICANTS
Analgesics	Memory-enhancers
Anesthetics	Mind-soothing
Anti-aging	Mood-enhancers
Anticonvulsants	Narcotics
Antihypnotics	Neurohormones
Antipsychotics	Neurohumor-disrupting
Consciousness-restoring	Rejuvenating
Depressants	Sedatives
Intelligence-enhancers	Stimulants

(Vaidya 1997)

Ayurveda and Psychiatry

Classical Indian medicine has a long tradition in the diagnosis and classification of disease, including psychiatric disorders (Vaidya 1997). In fact, the Ayurvedic system identifies twenty categories of plants with specific CNS activity; among these, there are eighteen categories of psychoneuropharmacological herbs (Table 3-7). Psychiatric disorders were originally discussed in the *Bhuta Vidya* (demonology) as part of the *Ashtanga Ayurveda* (Rao 2000). Charaka, who introduced the doshic system around 1220 BC, also identified the psychological classification of the *manasika doshas*: Passion (*Rajas*) and Darkness (*Tamas*). More than 3,000 years ago, he realized the intimate connection between physical and psychological disease and *dis-ease*. He identified two types of insanity. The first type was attributed to endogenous factors and the second type to exogenous factors. Charaka describes four types of lives: Happy (*Sukha*), Unhappy (*Dukha*), Good (*Hita*), and Bad (*Ahita*). A life that is unaffected by psychological or physical disease and filled with vitality, pleasure, and success is *sukham ayuh*. Its opposite, filled with disease, depression, and misery, is the *asukham ayuh*. A person who is always honest, generous, charitable, ethical, honorable, respectful, and self-controlled has a life of *hitam ayuh*; the opposite is *ahitam ayuh*. Ayurvedic philosophy and practice promotes the concept of positive health of the body, mind, and spirit; the system aims to assist the individual in leading a long, happy, healthy, and balanced life (*Swastha vrutta*).

Ayurvedic herbs had significant influence on modern Western psychiatry and continue to be a source of inspiration and research. For example, *Rauwolfia serpentina* (Rauvolfia root, Serpentine root, *Candrika*, *Chotacard*) is a small shrub found across India that grows as high as 1.5 m. Its leaves are lanceolate, shiny, and smooth (Fig. 3-1). Axillary flowers are born on umbelliform panicles and are white with tinges of violet. The medicinal parts of the plant are the roots and

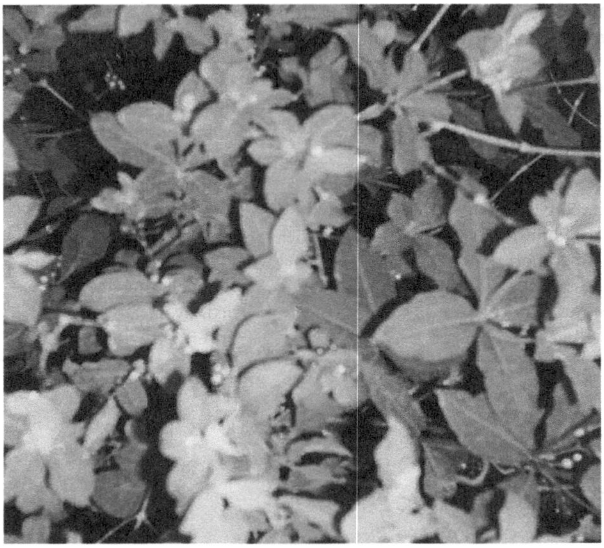

FIGURE 3-1. *Rauwolfia serpentina* is the source of reserpine, a widely used antipsychotic medication of the mid twentieth century. (Photo courtesy of Dr. Jayvir Anjaria)

leaves, which are used traditionally for their laxative, antihelminthic, diuretic, anticonvulsant, hypotensive, and sedative properties. It has vata and kapha properties. This plant is the source of reserpine, an early antipsychotic medication identified in 1958 and extensively used in Western psychiatry; it is now replaced with newer psychiatric compounds.

Ayurveda and Veterinary Behavior Medicine

Ayurveda applies to all animals. It does not arrive at a diagnosis by focus on anatomical signs as does Western medicine, nor does it treat symptomatically as does homeopathy. Ayurvedic principles hold true for veterinary medicine, and in fact, Ayurvedic medicine has a long history of application to veterinary practice. The Vedic Sutras, the *Mrig Ayurveda,* the *Ashwa Ayurveda*, and other texts mentioned above teach about health care for animals. They describe the traditional reverence for the cow and its treatment, as well as for animals of war such as the elephant (*hasti*) and horse (*ashwa* or *asva*), among many others.

Ayurvedic principles translate readily into veterinary medicine. Considering the major body types described according to the doshas, one can describe a St. Bernard or Great Dane as a "kapha," a German Shepherd or a Husky might be a "pitta," and an Italian Greyhound or Miniature Poodle could easily be a "vata." A

Greyhound or Saluki might have equal parts of Pitta and Vata ($P_1V_1K_3$) depending on temperament, for example. Among domestic cats, a large, placid Persian would be the Kapha cat, an average domestic cat would be the Vata, and a sensitive Abyssinian or Siamese would be consistent with the Pitta. A Maine Coon with an excitable temperament might be $P_1V_3K_1$.

Restoring balance to the three Doshas is relevant to veterinary behavior medicine as well. A consideration of the nutritional balance of the seven tastes also applies to veterinary medicine and is consistent with the importance of diet in well-being and health. Vatta imbalance is often associated with anxiety, fear, and nervousness; aggression and irritability with Pitta imbalance; possessiveness with over-attachment from Kapha. A fearful cat or anxious dog, for example, might respond well to restoring balance to Vatta. A distinction of the pet's state of mind is also relevant to its treatment. For example, a hyperthyroid cat that is agitated, irritable, and restless could be considered to be in the *Kshipta* state of mind. A dog with active and passive clinical signs of separation anxiety syndrome might be in *Vikshipta* mind if it paces anxiously or exhibits other agitated behaviors such as destructiveness, alternating with depression (e.g., lethargy and social withdrawal) (Schwartz 2003).

Approximately 1,250 plants are in current use in Ayurvedic preparations (Dev 1999). It is beyond the scope of this book to cover every one that is applied as a psychoactive medicinal. The primary rasayanas that appear to be most useful in veterinary behavior medicine follow and it is hoped that they will inspire the reader to learn more. Ayurvedic herbs common to other healing traditions, such as *Aconitum spp.* (*Bhugara*, *Vachnag*), *Valeriana spp.*, and *Cannabis sativa*, are discussed in detail elsewhere in this book.

"One can measure the greatness and the moral progress of a nation by looking at how she treats her animals" —*Mahatma Gandhi* (1869–1948)

References

Anjara J, Parabia M, Dwvedi S. Ethnovet Heritage: Indian Ethnoveterinary Medicine, An Overview. Pathik Enterprise Publishers; Ahmedabad, India.

Lad VD. Ayurveda: Textbook of Fundamental Principles. The Ayurvedic Press; Albuquerque, New Mexico. 2002.

Schwartz S. Separation anxiety syndrome in dogs and cats. JAVMA. 2003;222:1526-1532.

Vivekananda S. The Complete Works of Swami Vivekananda, Volumes 1-8. Advaita Ashrama, Kolkata, India. 2003

Albizzia lebbeck

The deciduous tree *Albizzia lebbeck* (Shirish, Shoedhanam, Sage-leaved alangium; family *Mimosaceae*) is native to India and may be found throughout tropical and subtropical regions of Asia and Africa. It is commercially cultivated for making

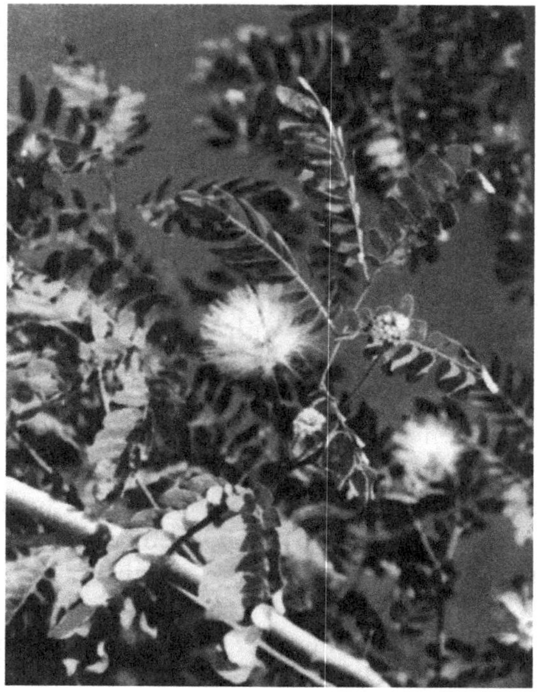

FIGURE 3-2. *Albizzia lebbeck* tree. (Photo courtesy of Dr. Jayvir Anjaria)

furniture, wood flooring, construction, and other industrial use. The tree grows 6 to 8 m high. It has a rough bark and an almost palm-like appearance because of the many paired and opposite leaflets (Fig. 3-2). Umbellate flower heads are cream colored and fragrant. The fruits of the tree are flat, pale-brown pods and contain four to twelve spherical seeds (Fig. 3-3). Medicinal parts of the plant are the leaf, flowers, seed, and bark (Anjaria, Parabia, Dwivedi 2002).

Traditional uses of *A. lebbeck* in Ayurveda include treatment of asthma, snake and scorpion bite, pruritus, leprosy, bronchitis, asthma, syphilis, gonorrhea, toothache, and excessive perspiration. *A. lebbeck* is thought to possess immunogenic, antihelminthic, aphrodisiac (flowers, seeds), and anti-inflammatory properties and is used as a brain tonic (seeds) (Anjaria, Parabia, Dwivedi 2002). Albizzia has also been used to treat allergic rhinitis and other allergies (Mills, Bone 2000). The tree's bark is fermented and distilled and has a mild sedative effect. The distillate may be taken orally (e.g., to treat paralysis) or applied topically to treat fungal or bacterial infection (Dr. Minoo Parabia, personal communication 2004).

A. lebbeck is considered to be astringent and bitter; it has a tridoshic effect, balancing vata, pitta, and kapha with a predominant effect on vata. Ingredients include tannins and saponins (Dr. Jayvir Anjaria, Dr. Arun Baxi and Dr. Minoo

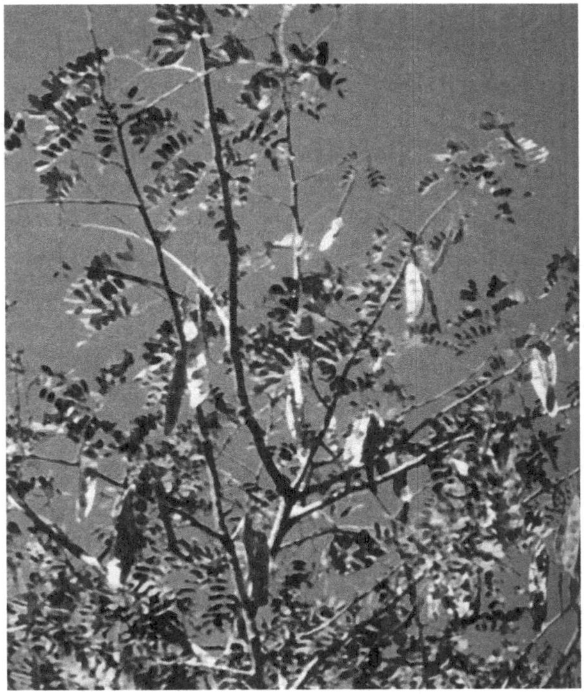

FIGURE 3-3. *Albizzia lebbeck* showing characteristic seedpods. (Photo courtesy of Dr. Jayvir Anjaria)

Parabia, personal communication 2004; Ueda, Tokunaga, Okazaki et al. 2003; Anjaria, Parabia, Dwivedi 2002).

In Traditional Chinese medicine (TCM), the bark and flowers of *A. julibrissin* are used for their sedative and analgesic properties in counteracting anger and depression (Kang, Jeong, Kim et al. 2000; Tierra 1998). In fact, the Chinese name He Huan Pi means "happiness bark." The recommended dosage is 10–15 gm (Tierra 1998). The flowers of *Albizzia julibrissin*, used in TCM, contain quercitrin and isoquercitrin, which were found to prolong barbiturate anesthesia in mice. This supports its traditional use as a sedative (Kang, Jeong, Kim et al. 2000) and suggests that similar compounds and effects may be found for *A. lebbeck*. In an earlier study, a decoction of *A. lebbeck* bark was found to inhibit mast cell degranulation and allergic reaction in rats, which supports its traditional use in the treatment of asthma and pruritic dermatopathy, including atopy (Tripathi, Sen, Das 1979).

CNS Effects

Recent evidence supports *A. lebbeck's* anticonvulsant and general CNS depressant effects (Kasture, Chopde, Deshmukh 2000; Kasture, Kasture, Pal 1996). This study also showed that *A. lebbeck* leaf extract potentiated barbiturate anesthesia and antagonized the behavioral effects of amphetamine. The extract was also GABAergic and serotonergic, but was found to be anxiogenic in action.

In another study, *A. lebbeck* leaf extract showed significant nootropic action on mice; however, brain concentrations of GABA and dopamine were inhibited and serotonin levels were increased (Chintawar, Somani, Kasture et al. 2002). Elsewhere, *A. lebbeck* leaf extract had a positive effect on anxiety and cognitive function; a GABAergic mechanism was suspected because the extract inhibited a $GABA_B$ agonist (Une, Sarveiya, Pal et al. 2001). Its nootropic effect could be related to similar effects attributed to potent antioxidant activity from a bark extract of its Asian relative *A. julibrissin* that was six times stronger compared to L-ascorbic acid (Jung, Chung, Kang et al. 2003).

An opioid mechanism may also be involved in its effects. The effect of loperamide was potentiated by *A. lebbeck* seed extract, and the opioid antagonist naloxone significantly inhibited the antidiarrheal activity of *A. lebbeck* seed extract (Besra, Gomes, Chaudhury et al. 2002).

Clinical Application in Veterinary Behavior Medicine

Albizzia lebbeck could be of use as an adjunct to other nootropic herbs such as *Gingko biloba*, *Bacopa monniera*, or *Withania somnifera*, among others. It is unclear whether it inhibits or enhances GABA mechanisms, although it does appear to have antidopaminergic, serotonergic, and opioid inhibiting effects. *A. lebbeck* deserves further investigation and may be of particular interest for its anxiolytic effect in mild to moderate cases of fear and anxiety.

References

Anjaria J, Parabia M, Dwivedi S. Ethnovet Heritage: Indian Ethnoveterinary Medicine, An Overview. Pathik Enterprise Publishers; Ahmedabad, India. 2002;190.

Besra SE, Gomes A, Chaudhury L et al. Antidiarrheal activity of seed extract of *Albizzia lebbeck* Benth. Phytother Res. 2002;16:529–533.

Chintawar SD, Somani RS, Kasture VS et al. Nootropic activity of *Albizzia lebbeck* in mice. J Ethnopharmacol. 2002;81:299–305.

Jung MJ, Chung HY, Kang SS et al. Antioxidant activity from the stem bark of *Albizzia julibrissin.* Arch Pharm Res. 2003;26:458–462.

Kang TH, Jeong SJ, Kim NY et al. Sedative activity of two flavonol glycosides isolated from the flowers of *Albizzia julbrissin* Durazz. J Ethnopharmacol. 2000;71:321–323.

Kasture VS, Chopde CT, Deshmukh VK. Anticonvulsive activity of *Albizzia lebbeck*, *Hibiscus rosa sinesis* and *Butea monosperma* in experimental animals. J Ethnopharmacol. 2000;71:65–75.

Kasture VS, Kasture SB, Pal SC. Anticonvulsant activity of *Albizzia lebbeck* leaves. Indian J Exp Biol. 1996;34:78–80.

Mills S, Bone K. Principles and Practice of Phytotherapy. Churchill Livingstone, Philadelphia, PA. 2000; 177; 210; 213; 216; 328–334.

Tierra M. The Way of Chinese Herbs. Pocket Books, New York, NY 1998;280–281.

Tripathi RM, Sen PC, Das PK. Studies on the mechanism of action of *Albizzia lebbeck*, an Indian indigenous drug used in the treatment of atopic allergy. J Ethnopharmacol. 1979;1:385–396.

Ueda M, Tokunaga T, Okazaki M et al. Albiziahexoside: a potential source of bioactive saponin from the leaves of *Albizzia lebbeck*. Nat Prod Res. 2003;17:329–335.
Une HD, Sarveiya VP, Pal SC et al. Nootropic and anxiolytic activity of saponins of *Albizzia lebbeck* leaves. Pharmacol Biochem Behav. 2001;69:439–444.

Asparagus racemosus

Asparagus racemosus (Shatavari, Satavar, Satavara, Satavari, Satamuli, Bojhidan, Shakakul, Chatavali, Hundred Husbands, Wild Asparagus; family *Liliaceae*) is a climbing, deciduous plant with spine-like leaves (color plate 3-1). After flowering, the white, fragrant blooms are followed by small, scarlet berries. The plant prefers higher elevations of tropical and subtropical forests of India, Africa, Java, and Australia but can also be found at elevations of up to 1,000 feet in the Himalayas (Anjaria, Parabia, Dwivedi 2002). Medicinal parts of the plant are the tuberous roots (Figure 3-4).

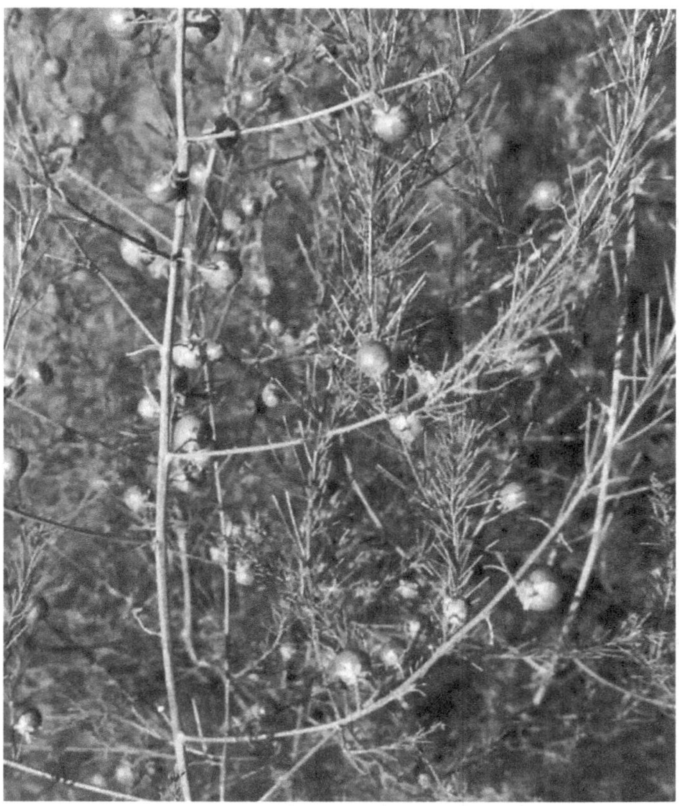

FIGURE 3-4. *Asparagus racemosus* showing berries. (Photo courtesy of Dr. Jayvir Anjaria)

A. racemosus is used for the treatment of digestive disorders (e.g., diarrhea, dysentery, ulcer), respiratory disease (e.g., cough, pneumonia), infertility, menopause, and rheumatism (Mills, Bone 2000). *A. adscendens* may be used as a substitute for *A. racemosus* in commercial preparations. *A. racemosus* affects the vata and kapha doshas (although it affects pitta as well) and is sheeta virya (Dr. Jayvir Anjaria, Dr. Arun Baxi, personal communication 2004).

In TCM, a related plant, *Asparagus cochinchinensis* (Tian men dong), is used as a yin tonic (Mills, Bone 2000). *Asparagus lucidus* is also used as a yin tonic to enhance fluid secretions throughout the body and vitalize the lungs. It is also mixed with honey and used to treat cough and bronchitis (Tillotson, Tillotson, Abel 2001).

Ingredients

Identified compounds include isoflavones (Saxena, Chourasia 2001) and phyto-ecdysteroids, which are similar to reptilian hormones (Dinan, Savchenko, Whiting 2001).

Miscellaneous Effects

In a comparison study between *A. racemosus* and metoclopramide (Reglan®) of gastric emptying in healthy human volunteers, no significant difference was found (Dalvi, Nadkarni, Gupta 1990). *A. racemosus* has proven and traditional use for its galactogogue, antispasmodic, immunogenic, anti-inflammatory, tonic, aphrodisiac, and antioxidant properties (Parihar, Hemnani 2004; Goyal, Singh, Lal 2003; Kamat, Boloor, Devasagayam et al. 2000). Its antitussive effect is comparable to that of codeine (Mandal, Kumar, Mohana Lakshmi et al. 2000).

A. racemosus also showed important antibacterial effects against *Escherichia coli, Shigella spp., Vibrio cholerae, Salmonella spp., Pseudomonas putida, Bacillus subtilis,* and *Staphylococcus aureus* (Mandal, Nandy, Pal et al. 2000).

Availability

A. racemosus is available as a powder or decoction but is best used in combination with other Ayurvedic herbs (Anjaria, Parabia, Dwivedi 2002). A popular commercial preparation containing equal parts (100 g each, taken as 1 tsp one half-hour following morning tea) of *A. racemosus* and *Withania somnifera* equal parts referred to as Rasayan-Plus is recommended as a tonic and to boost the immune system in people over 50 years of age; when powdered seeds of *Mucuna pruriens* are added to this combination, it may be used to treat Parkinsonian tremors (Dr. Jayvir Anjaria, personal communication 2004).

Clinical Application in Veterinary Behavior Medicine

There are no data to substantiate the psychotropic or neurologic effects of *A. racemosus* at this time; however, preliminary evidence of its antioxidant properties at least seem to support its traditional use in combination with other rasayanas to enhance their effect. *A. racemosus* is most often used in combination with other rasayanas for a presumed additive effect. Agitated or anxious patients such as hyperthyroid cats, or dogs with noise phobia, might respond to the Rasayan Choorna, an Ayurvedic polyherbal mixture containing *Asparagus racemosus*, *Withania somnifera*, *Tinospora cordifolia*, *Tribulus terrestris*, and *Phyllanthus emblica*. This balancing preparation is also recommended in people over 45 years of age to maintain vigor and boost the immune system (Dr. Jayvir Anjaria, personal communication 2004).

References

Anjaria J, Parabia M, Dwivedi S. Ethnovet Heritage: Indian Ethnoveterinary Medicine, An Overview. Pathik Enterprise Publishers; Ahmedabad, India. 2002;219.

Dalvi SS, Nadkarni PM, Gupta KC. Effect of *Asparagus racemosus* (Shatavari) on gastric emptying time in normal healthy volunteers. J Postgrad Med. 1990;36:91–94.

Dinan L, Savchenko T, Whiting P. Phytoecdysteroids in the genus Asparagus (*Asparagaceae*). Phytochemistry. 2001;56:569–576.

Goyal RK, Singh J, Lal H. Asparagus racemosus: An update. Indian J Med Sci. 2003;57:408–414.

Kamat JP, Boloor KK, Devasagayam TP et al. Antioxidant properties of *Asparagus racemosus* against damage induced by gamma-radiation in rat liver mitochondria. J Ethnopharmacol. 2000;71:425–435.

Mandal SC, Kumar CKA, Mohana Lakshmi S et al. Antitussive effect of *Asparagus racemosus* root against sulfur dioxide-induced cough in mice. Fitoterapia. 2000;71:686–689.

Mandal SC, Nandy A, Pal M et al. Evaluation of antibacterial activity of *Asparagus racemosus* wild root. Phytother Res. 2000;14:118–119.

Mills S, Bone K. Principles and Practice of Phytotherapy. Churchill Livingstone: Philadelphia, PA. 2000;156.

Parihar MS, Hemnani T. Experimental excitotoxicity provokes oxidative damage in mice brain and attenuation by extract of *Asparagus racemosus*. J Neural Transm. 2004;1111:1–12.

Saxena VK, Chourasia S. A new isoflavone from the roots of *Asparagus racemosus*. Fitoterapia. 2001;72: 307–309.

Sharma S, Ramji S, Kumari S et al. Randomized controlled trial of *Asparagus racemosus* (Shatavari) as a lactogogue in lactational inadequacy. Indian Pediatr. 1996;33:675–677.

Tillotson AK, Tillotson HSH, Abel R. The One Earth Herbal Sourcebook. Kensington Publishing, New York, NY 2001; 231–232.

Bacopa monniera

Bacopa monniera (Brahmi, Nira brahmi, Jalnavali, Sambranichatt, Water Hyssop, and Thyme-leaved greatiala; also known as *Bacopa monnieri*; family *Scrophulariaceae*) is a creeping, semi-succulent ground-covering herb that is widely distributed in tropical, moist habitats. Solitary axillary flowers are usually pale blue or purple with five ovate sepals (Figure 3-5). Oblong leaves measure about 1 cm by 0.4 cm and are arranged opposite each other along creeping stems. The entire plant is used in traditional preparations but the leaves and aerial portions are of particular interest (Anjaria, Parabia, Dwivedi 2002). In Ayurveda, it is a bitter substance (ushna virya) that balances vata and kapha with a predominant effect

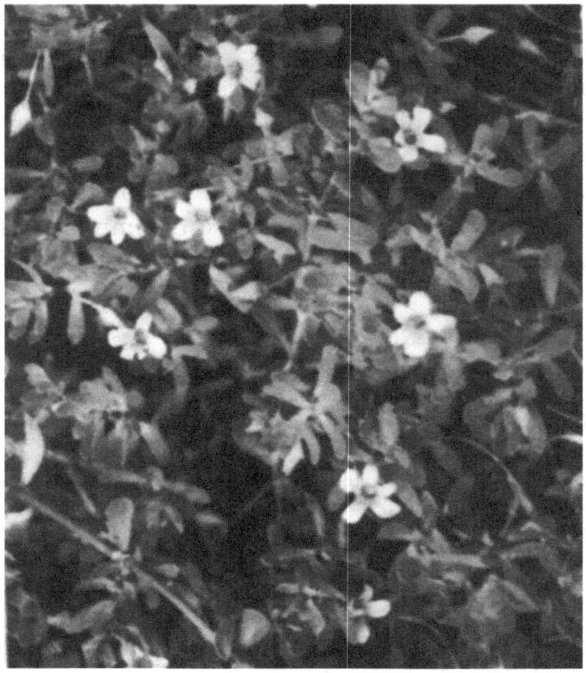

FIGURE 3-5. *Bacopa monniera* in bloom. (Photo courtesy of Dr. Jayvir Anjaria)

on vata (Dr. Jayvir Anjaria, Dr. Arun Baxi, Dr. Minoo Parabia, personal communication 2004).

In the United States, *Centella asiatica* and *B. monniera* are both sometimes referred to as Brahmi; however, *B. monniera* is more appropriately called Brahmi in reference to its Sanskrit name of Nira brahmi. Brahmi is first mentioned in Vedic scriptures as old as 5000 BC. The two plants are differentiated in later Ayurvedic texts; *C. asiatica* (Mandukaparni, Gotu kola) was considered of benefit to restore general mental health, whereas Brahmi (*B. monniera*) was considered more specific for "insanity" and epilepsy (Sivarajan 1994).

Traditional uses of *B. monniera* include treatment of digestive upset, anemia, arthritis and rheumatism, snakebite and scorpion sting, scabies, epilepsy, syphilis, and leprosy. It is reputed to have emetic, laxative, anti-ulcer, anti-inflammatory, antitumor, cardiac, and aphrodisiac effects. In particular, it has been used as a nervine tonic for the treatment of depression and "insanity." It is primarily advocated to improve memory, intelligence, and vitality (Anonymous 2004; Goel, Sairam, Babu et al. 2003; Anjaria, Parabia, Dwivedi 2002) and may be used alone or in combination with other botanical ingredients such as *Evolvulus nummularius* (*Shankhapushpi* also known as *Vishnukanta*) in polyherbal formulations thought to have an additive tonic action on the brain (Dr. Jayvir Anjaria, personal communication 2004).

Ingredients

Compounds isolated in *B. monniera* include glycosides (Chakravarty, Sarkar, Nakane et al. 2002), triterpene saponins (e.g., bacosides, bacopasides and bacopasaponins), flavonoid glycosides, phytosterols, and alkaloids (e.g., brahmine) (Hou, Lin, Cheng et al. 2002; Garai, Mahato, Ohtani et al. 1996; Rastogi, Pal, Kulshreshtha 1994). The bacosides A and B consistently emerge as the most biologically active components (Singh, Dhawan 1997).

Cognitive-Enhancing Effects

An accumulating body of data supports the traditional Ayurvedic usage of *B. monniera* to enhance cognitive function. In a study of the rat frontal cortex, striatum and hippocampus, *B. monniera* extract containing 82% bacoside A was orally administered in doses of either 5 or 10 mg/kg for 14 or 21 days (Bhattacharya, Bhattacharya, Kumar et al. 2000). Bacopa extract was compared to deprenyl, which is also recognized for its central antioxidant effect and control of canine and feline cognitive dysfunction syndrome. Results of this Indian study showed that both treatments increased oxidative free radical scavenging activity. Unlike deprenyl, however, *B. monniera* extract exerted significant activity in the hippocampus. In a study of mice, *B. monniera* extract (30 mg/kg) was compared to *Gingko biloba* extract (14, 30, and 60 mg/kg) (Das, Shanker, Nath et al. 2002). Both compounds showed significant antidementia effects but also showed a dose dependent inhibition of AChE. This suggests that the effects of *B. monniera* are modulated, at least in part, by cholinergic mechanisms.

Cognitive enhancement was also shown in healthy human subjects given *B. monniera* extract compared to placebo. Anxiety was also decreased (Stough, Lloyd, Clarke et al. 2001). In a double-blind, placebo controlled study of seventy-six adults between the ages of 40 and 65 years, *B. monniera* decreased the rate of forgetting new information. However, it did not affect attention, short-term memory, daily memory function, and retention of preexperimental information. Anxiety level was not affected (Roodenrys, Booth, Bulzomi et al. 2002). In a study of healthy people randomly assigned to either *B. monniera* (300 mg) or placebo treatment groups, cognitive function two hours after administration was unchanged compared to pretrial measures (Nathan, Clarke, Lloyd et al. 2001). This data suggests only that at the dose selected for study no acute cognitive effects were found.

In a placebo-controlled, double-blind study of 85 healthy people, a preparation containing a mixture of *Ginkgo biloba* (120 mg) and *B. monniera* (30 mg) was tested (Nathan, Tanner, Lloyd et al. 2004). No cognitive changes were determined; however, the herbal preparation was not administered over a sufficient period of time to make any conclusions. Elsewhere, daily dosages of 100 and 200 mg for four weeks were well tolerated and without adverse reactions in healthy male volunteers (Singh, Dhawan 1997). In a recent placebo-controlled Australian study, the acute effect of treatment with a combination of *Gingko biloba* (120 mg) and *B. monniera* (300 mg) was tested in 12 healthy, young adult volunteers (Maher, Stough, Shelmerdine et al. 2002). No significant neuropsychological changes were detected, although both herbs yield positive effects on cognition over time. The investigation of this herbal combination would be important to pursue.

Antidepressant Effects

The antidepressant effect of *B. monniera* extract (20 and 40 mg/kg IP SID) was compared to the tricyclic antidepressant imipramine in rats and was found to be comparable in its effects (Sairam, Dorababu, Goel et al. 2002). In an earlier rat study, Bacopa extract was compared to the benzodiazepine lorazepam (Bhattacharya SK, Ghosal 1998). Significant anxiolytic effects were associated with *B. monniera* at 10 and 20 mg/kg PO. Unlike lorazepam, which was accompanied by an anamnesic action, *B. monniera* was associated with improved cognitive function.

Miscellaneous Effects

The use of *B. monniera* for an antiepileptic effect may be more attributable to its antioxidant properties. It has been shown to reverse cognitive impairment caused by phenytoin without affecting antiseizure effects, suggesting that concomitant use may benefit epileptic patients (Vohora, Pal, Pillai 2000). In an *in vitro* experiment, *B. monniera* extract was shown to reduce withdrawal symptoms induced by morphine (Sumathi, Nayeem, Balakrishna et al. 2002). This not only suggests its clinical application in the treatment of addiction but also may point to the involvement of opioid systems in its mechanism of action.

Availability

Preparations include poultice application (e.g., bronchitis), liquid extract (4–12 ml), powder (5–10 g), dried (2–6 g) and infusion (8–18 ml). The juice of fresh leaves may be taken alone or mixed in a petroleum base for topical application (Anjaria, Parabia, Dwivedi 2002). In commercial preparations, it is available as the sole ingredient or in combination with *Ginkgo biloba* and *Panax ginseng*, also known to benefit cognitive function. Buyers should carefully verify the ingredients of commercial products labeled as "Brahmi" because it could contain *Centella asiatica* and not *B. monniera.*

Clinical Application in Veterinary Behavior Medicine

B. monniera may be of interest as an herbal supplement for pets suffering from feline or canine cognitive dysfunction syndromes. It may be useful combined with *Ginkgo biloba* or used alone; future clinical trials will better reveal its best application. It may also be helpful to epileptic pets as an adjunct to other anticonvulsant medication to minimize cognitive side effects of the drug or the seizure events. The use of *B. monniera* as a treatment of anxiety or depression is unclear based on current data. Possible cholinergic and opioid mechanisms suggest it may be of interest in the treatment of compulsive behaviors, but this has not yet been studied or reported.

References

Anjaria J, Parabia M, Dwivedi S. Ethnovet Heritage: Indian Ethnoveterinary Medicine, An Overview. Pathik Enterprise Publishers; Ahmedabad, India. 2002;223.

Anonymous. *Bacopa monniera*—Monograph. Altern Med Rev. 2004;9:79–85.

Bhattacharya SK, Bhattacharya A, Kumar A et al. Antioxidant activity of *Bacopa monniera* in rat frontal cortex, striatum and hippocampus. Phytother Res. 2000;14:174–179.

Bhattacharya SK, Ghosal S. Anxiolytic activity of a standardized extract of *Bacopa monniera*: an experimental study. Phytomedicine. 1998;5:77–82.

Chakravarty AK, Sarkar T, Nakane T et al. New phenylethanoid glycosides from *Bacopa monniera*. Chem Pharm Bull (Tokyo). 2002;50:1616–1618.

Das A, Shanker G, Nath C et al. A comparative study in rodents of standardized extracts of *Bacopa monniera* and *Ginkgo biloba*: anticholinesterase and cognitive enhancing activities. Pharmacol biochem Behav. 2002;73:893–900.

Garai S, Mahato SB, Ohtani K et al. Dammarane-type triterpenoid saponins from *Bacopa monniera*. Phytochemistry. 1996;42:815–820.

Goel RK, Sairam K, Babu MD et al. In vitro evaluation of *Bacopa monniera* on anti-*Helicobacter pylori* activity and accumulation of prostaglandins. Phytomedicine. 2003;10:523–527.

Hou CC, Lin SJ, Cheng JT et al. Bacopaside III, bacopasaponin G, and bacopasides A, B, and C from *Bacopa monniera*. J Nat Prod. 2002;65:1759–1763.

Maher BFG, Stough C, Shelmerdine A et al. The acute effects of combined adminstraiton of *Ginkgo biloba* and *Bacopa monniera* on cognitive function in humans. Hum Psychopharmacol Clin Exp. 2002;17:163–164.

Nathan PJ, Clarke J, Lloyd J et al. The acute effects of an extract of *Bacopa monniera* (Brahmi) on cognitive function in healthy normal subjects. Hum Phsychopharmacol. 2001;16:345–351.

Nathan PJ, Tanner S, Lloyd J et al. Effects of a combined extract of *Ginkgo biloba* and *Bacopa monniera* on cognitive function in healthy humans. Hum Psychopharmacol. 2004;19:91–96.

Rastogi S, Pal R, Kulshreshtha DK. Bacoside A3—a triterpenoid saponin from *Bacopa monniera*. Phytochemistry. 1994;36:133–137.

Roodenrys S, Booth D, Bulzomi S et al. Chronic effects of Brahmi (*Bacopa monniera*) on human memory. Neuropsychopharmacology. 2002;27:279–281.

Sairam K, Dorababu M, Goel RK et al. Antidepressant activity of standardized extract of *Bacopa monniera* in experimental models of depression in rats. Phytomedicine. 2002;9:207–211.

Singh HK, Dhawan BN. Neurophsychopharmacological effects of the Ayurvedic nootropic *Bacopa monniera* (Brahmi). Indian J Pharm. 1997;29:S359–S365.

Sivarajan VV. Ayurvedic Drugs and their Plant Sources. Lebanon, New Hampshire: International Science Publisher, 1994.

Stough C, Lloyd J, Clarke J et al. The chronic effects of an extract of *Bacopa monniera* (Brahmi) on cognitive function in healthy human subjects. Psychopharmacology (Berl). 2001;156:481–484.

Sumathi T, Nayeem M, Balakrishna K et al. Alcoholic extract of "*Bacopa monniera*" reduces the in vitro effects of morphine withdrawal in guinea-pig ileum. J Ethnopharmacol. 2002;82:75–81.

Vohora D, Pal SN, Pillai KK. Protection from phenytoin-induced cognitive deficit by *Bacopa monniera*, a reputed Indian nootropic plant. J Ethnopharmacol. 2000;71:383–390.

Centella asiatica

Centella asiatica (Mandukaparni, Brahmamanduki, Bhekaparni, Bheki, Gotu Kola, Brahmi, Karvana, Kodagam, Babassa, Tsubo-kusa, Luei gong gen, Tungchian, Indian Pennywort, Indischer Wassernable, Hydrocotyle asiatica; family *Apiaceae*) is a creeping, perennial ground cover native to moist, marshy, subtropical areas of India, southeast Asia, parts of China, the South Sea Islands, South Africa, the southeastern United States, Mexico, and parts of South America (Russo 2001; PDR 2000). Its most popular name in the Western world, "Gotu kola," is actually in the Sri Lankan language. In India, it is best known as Brahmamanduki, Mandukaparni, or simply as Centella.

The plant has circular, ribbed leaves with a crenate margin that averages between 2 and 3 cm in diameter (Figure 3-6). Axillary florets are pink, purple, or white. Medicinal parts of the plant are the aerial parts, and in particular the leaves and stems. These are gathered year-long and are sun dried (Anjaria, Parabia, Dwivedi 2002; Russo 2001; PDR 2000).

First reported in an ancient Vedic text dating back to around 500 BC, *C. asiatica* was recommended as a daily tonic to ensure longevity and good complexion

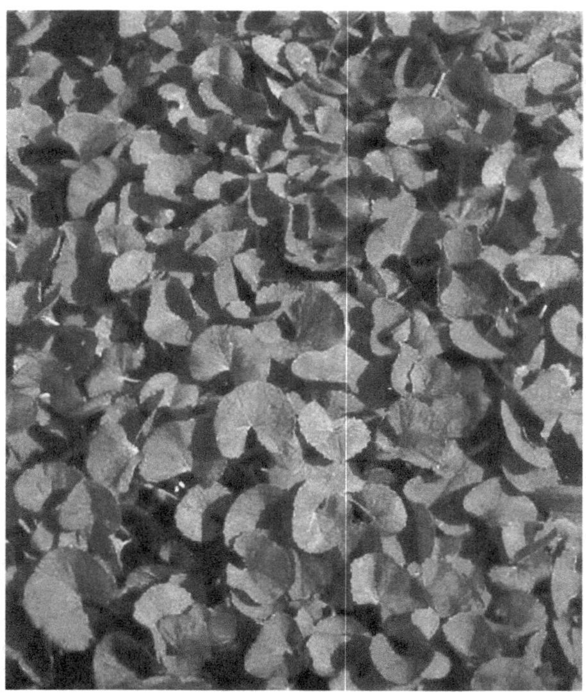

FIGURE 3-6. Leaves of *Centella asiatica.* (Photo courtesy of Dr. Jayvir Anjaria)

and to preserve memory and cognitive function. It is also used in Traditional Chinese Medicine (TCM). In Ayurveda, it is a bitter substance (*sheeta virya*) that regulates the tridosha but in particular affects kapha and pitta with a predominant effect on pitta (Dr. Jayvir Anjaria, Dr. Arun Baxi, and Dr. Minoo Parabia, personal communication 2004).

Traditional uses include the treatment of leprosy, epilepsy, syphilis, asthma, bronchitis, cystitis, dehydration, inappetance, and headache. It has been used as a soporific, diuretic, and carminative and to improve memory and mental clarity. It has proven anti-inflammatory, antitumor, and cytotoxic effects. In addition, it inhibits gastric ulceration, promotes wound healing (for example, by stimulating collagen synthesis and epithelialization), and may stimulate the immune system (Cheng, Guo, Luk et al. 2004; Coldren, Hashim, Ali et al. 2003; MacKay, Miller 2003; Wang, Dong, Zuo et al. 2003; Anjaria, Parabia, Dwivedi 2002; De Sanctis, Belcaro, Incandela et al. 2001; PDR 2000; Maquart, Bellon, Gillery et al. 1990). It is used in both Ayurveda and TCM to treat emotional disturbances such as anxiety and depressive symptoms (Bradwejn, Zhou, Koszycki et al. 2000; PDR 2000). It is also particularly helpful to relieve anxiety and stress in patients suffering from nonspecific illness (Dr. Minoo Parabia, personal communciation 2004).

Ingredients

C. asiatica contains no caffeine and is not related to the caffeine-containing nuts of the African cola tree. Active ingredients include triterpene acids (e.g., asiatic acid, madecassic acid) and triterpene acid esters (pseudosaponins) such as madegassoside and the asiaticosides (Russo 2001; PDR 2000). It also contains an essential oil, tannins, glucosides, and ascorbic acid (Anjaria, Parabia, Dwivedi 2002).

CNS and Neuroprotective Effects

Oxidative stress is a recognized element of Alzheimer's disease and senile cognitive impairment. In a rat model of Alzheimer's disease, *C. asiatica* aqueous extract (200 and 300 mg/kg) effectively prevented cognitive deficits and showed antioxidant effects (Veerendra Kumar, Gupta 2003).

An important neuroprotective effect of asiatic acid is drawing recent attention, and several of its derivatives seem to possess even more potent antioxidant properties. In fact, a major pharmaceutical company has patented it as a treatment for dementia and for cognitive enhancement (Lee, Kim, Sung et al. 2000). Aqueous extract of *C. asiatica* showed a beneficial effect on cognitive tests in a rat experiment testing learning and memory. The most effective doses were 200 and 300 mg/kg, although 100 mg/kg was also effective. An antioxidant mechanism was suspected (Veerendra Kumar, Gupta 2002).

Aqueous extract of *C. asiatica* (100 and 300 mg/kg) also showed potential as an adjuvant to antiepileptic drugs. A study of seizures in rats also demonstrated that the extract helped to prevent cognitive impairment that is associated with seizure activity, presumably due to its neuroprotective properties (Gupta, Veerendra Kumar, Srivastava 2003).

Earlier studies have suggested that *C. asiatica* increased intelligence in cognitively impaired children (Sharma, Jaiswal, Kumar et al. 1985; Appa Rao, Srinivasan, Koteswara 1977); unfortunately, follow-up investigations have not been pursued.

Psychological and Emotional Effects

Preliminary findings of a Canadian double-blind, placebo-controlled study suggest that *C. asiatica* possesses an anxiolytic effect in humans (Bradwejn, Zhou, Koszycki et al. 2000). In an earlier study of mice, its anxiolytic effect (50 mg/kg IP) was comparable to diazepam (4 mg/kg IP) (Diwan, Karwande 1991). Traditionally, *C. asiatica* has been used for the treatment of anxiety and depression but clinical data are lacking. Psychoactive properties have been attributed to affinity for *C. asiatica* extract to glycine and CCK_A receptors, but the mechanism remains to be clarified and its psychoactive application deserves further attention (Cott 1995).

Adverse Effects

The only known adverse reactions are reports of allergic contact dermatitis (Gonzalo Garijo, Revenga Arranz, Bobadilla Gonzalez 1996; Danese, Carnevali, Bertazzoni 1994).

Availability

C. asiatica is commercially available in capsules containing between 400 and 500 mg, in liquid, and in the form of dried leaves, which are prepared as an infusion three times a day. The recommended dose is 60 to 120 mg per diem (Russo 2001). Tablets of 30 mg and 60 mg are also available and have been used to treat hypertension and edema associated with varicose veins, apparently with some success. Traditionally, it is taken as a tea, cooked, or eaten as a fresh herb (Russo 2001; PDR 2000).

Clinical Application in Veterinary Behavior Medicine

C. asiatica may become an important alternative to other drugs currently marketed for the control of canine and feline cognitive dysfunction syndromes. Its comparison to diazepam's anxiolytic effects deserves investigation. Further research, including placebo-controlled, comparative clinical studies are warranted.

References

Anjaria J, Parabia M, Dwivedi S. Ethnovet Heritage: Indian Ethnoveterinary Medicine, An Overview. Pathik Enterprise Publishers; Ahmedabad, India. 2002;285.

Appa Rao MVR, Srinivasan K, Koteswara RTL. The effect of *Centella asiatica* on the general mental ability of mentally retarded children. Indian J Psychiatry. 1977;19:54–59.

Bradwejn J, Zhou Y, Koszycki D et al. A double-blind, placebo-controlled study on the effects of Gotu Kola (*Centella asiatica*) on acoustic startle response in healthy subjects. J Clin Psychopharmacol. 2000;20:680–684.

Cheng CL, Guo JS, Luk J et al. The healing effects of Centella extract and asiaticoside on acetic acid–induced gastric ulcers in rats. Life Sci. 2004;74:2237–2249.

Coldren CD, Hashim P, Ali JM et al. Gene expression changes in the human fibroblast induced by *Centella asiatica* triterpenoids. Planta Med. 2003;69:725–732.

Cott J. Medicinal plants and dietary supplements: sources for innovative treatment or adjuncts? Psychopharm Bull. 1995;31:131–137.

Danese P, Carnevali C, Bertazzoni MG. Allergic contact dermatitis due to *Centella asiatica* extract. Contact Dermatitis. 1994;31:201.

De Sanctis MT, Belcaro G, Incandela L et al. Treatment of edema and increased capillary filtration in venous hypertension with total triterpenic fraction of *Centella asiatica*: a clinical, prospective, placebo-controlled, randomized, dose-ranging trial. Angiology. 2001;52(Suppl 2):S55–59.

Diwan PV, Karwande I. Anti-anxiety profile of mandukaparni (*Centella asiatica*) in animals. Fitoterapia. 1991;62:253–257.

Gonzalo Garijo MA, Revenga Arranz F, Bobadilla Gonzalez P. Allergic contact dermatitis due to *Centella asiatica*: a new case. Allergol Immunopathol (Madr). 1996;24:132–134.

Gupta YK, Veerendra Kumar MH, Srivastava AK. Effect of *Centella asiatica* on pentylenetetrazole-induced kindling, cognition and oxidative stress in rats. Pharmacol Biochem Behav. 2003;74:579–585.

Lee MK, Kim SR, Sung SH et al. Asiatic acid derivatives protect cultured cortical neurons from glutamate-induced excitotoxicity. Res Commun Mol Pathol Pharmacol. 2000;108:75–86.

MacKay D, Miller AL. Nutritional support for wound healing. Altern Med Rev. 2003;8:359–377.

Maquart FX, Bellon G, Gillery P et al. Stimulation of collagen synthesis in fibroblast cultures by a triterpene extracted from *Centella asiatica*. Connect Tissue Res. 1990;24:107–120.

PDR for Herbal Medicines (2nd ed) Medical Economics Company Inc., Montvale, NJ 2000;359–361.

Russo E. Handbook of Psychotropic Herbs: A Scientific Analysis of Herbal Remedies for Psychiatric Conditions. The Haworth Press, Binghamton, NY 2001;153–157.

Sharma R, Jaiswal AN, Kumar S et al. Role of bhrahmi (*Centella asiatica*) in educable mentally retarded children. J Research Educ Indian Med. 1985;4:55–57.

Veerendra Kumar MH, Gupta YK. Effect of *Centella asiatica* on cognition and oxidative stress in an intracerebroventricular streptozotocin model of Alzheimer's disease in rats. Clin Exp Pharmacol Physiol. 2003;30:336–342.

Veerendra Kumar MH, Gupta YK. Effect of different extracts of *Centella asiatica* on cognition and markers of oxidative stress in rats. J Ethnopharmacol. 2002;79:253–260.

Wang XS, Dong Q, Zuo JP et al. Structure and potential immunological activity of a pectin from *Centella asiatica* (L.) Urban. Carbohydr Res. 2003;338:2393–2402.

Vitex negundo

Native to India, *Vitex negundo* is a small, slender tree with white or lavender flowers in the same family as *Verbena spp.* and *Vitex agnus-castus* (Chaste berry tree, Five-leaved chaste tree, Nirgundi, Nirkundi, Karunocci, Nagoda, Banna, Nisinda; family *Verbenaceae*) (Figure 3-7). *V. negundo* has been used traditionally to treat intestinal parasites, colds, rheumatism, headaches, and convulsions, and anxious or nervous patients (Anjaria, Parabia, Dwivedi 2002; Hobbs 1991). In Ayurveda,

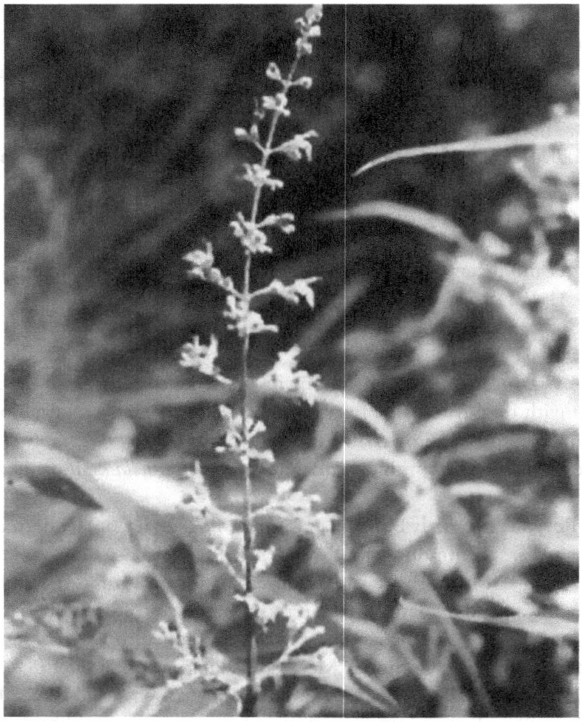

FIGURE 3-7. *Vitex negundo* in bloom. (Photo courtesy of Dr. Jayvir Anjaria)

the roots and leaves are used to balance conditions associated with vata, which may include dermatologic, digestive, and inflammatory illnesses (Dharmasiri, Jayakody, Galhena et al. 2003; Avadhoot, Rana 1991).

CNS Effects

A leaf extract of *V. negundo* significantly prolonged barbiturate anesthesia and extended the effects of diazepam and chlorpromazine in mice. It possesses analgesic properties, potentiates morphine, and produces a dose-dependent CNS depression (Gupta, Mazumder, Bhawal 1999). *V. negundo* also has anticonvulsant properties; it demonstrated significant protection against strychnine-induced convulsions (Gupta, Mazumder, Bhawal 1999).

Miscellaneous Effects

Laboratory evidence has indicated an anti-inflammatory, analgesic, and antibacterial effect, in support of traditional applications of the plant extract in Ayurvedic practices (Dharmasiri, Jayakody, Galhena et al. 2003; Perumal Samy, Ignacimuthu, Sen 1998).

Another study of *V. negundo* revealed a broad cytotoxic effect against human cancer cells by of one its isolates (Diaz, Chavez, Lee et al. 2003).

Vitex negundo seed extract was administered to castrated and intact adult dogs (10 mg/kg IP EOD) in an effort to determine its effect on testosterone levels. A reduction in androgen production was confirmed, suggesting that *V. negundo* seed extract exerts an antagonistic effect on testosterone (Bhargava 1989). Its antiandrogenic effect and suppression of sperm production may limit its clinical usefulness. Nevertheless, this finding may be of interest in veterinary medicine for the treatment of a variety of testosterone-sensitive ailments (e.g., benign prostatic hyperplasia).

Clinical Application in Veterinary Behavior Medicine

In veterinary behavior practice, *V. negundo's* antiandrogenic property could be of particular interest for the control of inappropriate urine marking or persistent sexual behavior in the cat. Cyproheptadine, an antihistamine with antiandrogenic effects, has also been helpful in this regard (Schwartz 1999a,b). This effect has not been studied in *V. agnus catus* but may be predicted based upon reports of its successful treatment of male acne (Mills, Bone 2000).

References

Anjaria J, Parabia M, Dwivedi S. Ethnovet Heritage: Indian Ethnoveterinary Medicine, An Overview. Pathik Enterprise Publishers; Ahmedabad, India. 2002;539.

Avadhoot Y, Rana AC. Hepatoprotective effect of *Vitex negundo* against carbon tetrachloride-induced liver damage. Arch Pharm Res. 1991;14:96–98.

Bhargava SK. Antiandrogenic effects of a flavonoid-rich fraction of *Vitex negundo* seeds: a histological and biochemical study in dogs. J Ethnopharmacol 1989;27:327–339.

Dharmasiri MG, Jayakody JR, Galhena G et al. Anti-inflammatory and analgesic activities of mature fresh leaves of *Vitex negundo*. J Ethnopharmacol. 2003;87:199–206.

Diaz F, Chavez D, Lee D et al. Cytotoxic flavone analogues of vitexicarpin, a constituent of the leaves of *Vitex negundo*. J Nat Prod. 2003;66:865–867.

Gupta M, Mazumder UK, Bhawal SR. CNS activity of *Vitex negundo* Linn. in mice. Indian J Exp Biol. 1999;37:143–146.

Hobbs C. The chaste tree: *Vitex agnus castus*. Pharm Hist. 1991;33:19–24.

Mills S, Bone K. Principles and Practice of Phytotherapy. Churchill Livingstone, Philadelphia, PA 2000; 328–334.

Perumal Samy R, Ignacimuthu S, Sen A. Screening of 34 Indian medicinal plants for antibacterial properties.J Ethnopharmacol. 1998;62:173–182.

Schwartz S. Use of cyproheptadine to control urine spraying in a castrated male domestic cat. JAVMA. 1999a;215:501–502.

Schwartz S. Use of cyproheptadine in the control of urine spraying and masturbation in a domestic cat. JAVMA. 1999b;214:369–371.

Withania somnifera

Withania somnifera (Ashwagandha, Aswagandha, Asoda, Amukkira, Amukkuram, Asgandh, Vagigandha, Indian Ginseng, and Winter Cherry; family *Sola-*

naceae) is an erect, perennial shrub that reaches heights of 70 to 150 cm. The ovate and pointed leaves can measure up to 8.5 cm long by 4.2 cm wide. Axillary flowers are small (1 cm), greenish-yellow, and hermaphrodite and are followed by red berries (color plate 3-2). *W. somnifera*, a member of the nightshade family, prefers dry habitat and grows wild or is cultivated. The tuberous roots are of primary medicinal value, but the leaves are also used (Anjaria, Parabia, Dwivedi 2002). Its Indian name (*Ashwa* means horse and *gandha* means scent or odor, translating as "smell and strength of a horse") refers to its aphrodisiac reputation (Mills, Bone 2000).

W. somnifera ranks high among the most valued rasayanas of Ayurvedic medicine and is used alone or in combination (e.g., with shilajatu or bitumen mineral pitch; Tillotson, Tillotson, Abel 2001) with other rasayanas. In Ayurveda, it is a bitter and astringent substance (ushna virya) that balances vata and kapha with a predominant effect on vata (Dr. Jayvir Anjaria, Dr. Arun Baxi and Dr. Minoobhai, personal communication 2004).

Traditional and proven uses of *W. somnifera* include treatment of fever, epilepsy, ulcers, edema, parasites, arthritis, fertility, impotence, inflammation, constipation, diuresis, debility, chronic fatigue syndrome, tumors, and premature aging. It is valued for its aphrodisiac effect as well as for the treatment of "nervous breakdown" and insomnia (Diwanay, Chitre, Patwardhan 2004; Leyon, Kuttan 2004; Jayaprakasam, Zhang, Seeram et al. 2003; Iuvone, Esposito, Capasso et al. 2003; Anjaria, Parabia, Dwivedi 2002; Davis, Kuttan 2002; Singh, Naidu, Gupta et al. 2002; Dhuley 2000; Mills, Bone 2000).

Ingredients

Primary components of *W. somnifera* include steroidal lactones (e.g., withaferin A), alkaloids (e.g., tropine, pseudotropine) and acylsteryl glucosides (e.g., sitoindosides) (Abou-Douh 2002; Mills, Bone 2000).

Neurological and CNS Effects

A GABAergic mechanism is suggested by evidence that *W. somnifera* root extract showed specific binding affinity to GABA receptor sites (Mehta, Binkley, Gandhi et al. 1991). It appears to be a highly effective antistress adaptogen, supported by studies in rodents that suggest at least part of this effect may be due to its antioxidant activity in the CNS (Bhattacharya, Muruganandam 2003; Kaur, Sharma, Mathur et al. 2003; Singh, Chandan, Gupta 2003; Bhattacharya, Ghosal, Bhattacharya 2001; Singh, Saxena, Chandan et al. 2001; Bhattacharya, Bhattacharya, Chakrabarti 2000).

Recently, *W. somnifera* has been shown to be effective in experimental models of cerebral ischemia, suggesting its potential in the treatment of stroke (Chaudhary, Sharma, Jagannathan et al. 2003; Adams, Yang, Mishra et al. 2002). This newly identified effect has been attributed to antioxidant properties that have been demonstrated (Gupta, Dua, Vohra 2003; Parihar, Hemnani 2003; Scartezzini, Speroni 2000).

In a prospective study of Parkinson's disease patients, an Ayurvedic remedy containing *W. somnifera* was found to be an effective treatment (Nagashayana, Sankarankutty, Nampoothiri et al. 2000).

W. somnifera also prevented the extrapyramidal side effects associated with the antipsychotic drug haloperidol; this was attributed to its antioxidant properties and suggests another clinical application (Naidu, Singh, Kulkarni 2003; Bhattacharya, Bhattacharya, Sairam et al. 2002). Recent results of a Japanese study show that withanolide A induced axon extension, and withanosides IV and VI extended dendrites (Kuboyama, Tohda, Zhao et al. 2002). The potential application in neurological disorders is exciting, and future research will confirm its clinical uses.

Behavioral and Psychological Effects

In an important study of the mood stabilizing effects of *W. somnifera*, an isolated extract of glycowithanolides (20 and 50 mg/kg PO) had comparable activity when tested against imipramine for its antidepressant activity and lorazepam for its anxiolytic effect (Bhattacharya, Bhattacharya, Sairam et al. 2000). This study supports its traditional use for the treatment of emotional disturbances but also calls attention to a need for further testing in other species. Although *W. somnifera* has been compared to *Panax ginseng* (hence the name of "Indian ginseng") for its adaptogenic properties, it is distinguished by its mild sedative action (hence the "somnifera").

Miscellaneous Effects

W. somnifera protects against the cytotoxic side effects of anticancer drugs such as cyclophosphamide (Davis, Kuttan 2000).

Adverse Effects

Other than increased appetite and weight gain, serious side effects are rarely reported for *W. somnifera* at therapeutic dosages (Aphale, Chhibba, Kumbhakarna et al. 1998; Grandhi, Mujumdar, Patwardhan 1994). It has generally been considered a safe compound (Singh, Chandan, Gupta 2003; Mishra, Singh, Dagenais 2000). However, renal lesions have been associated with its administration (Arseculeratne, Gunatilaka, Panabokke 1985).

W. somnifera may elevate thyroid hormone levels (Panda, Kar 1999, 1998). Although this effect has not been well studied, patients with hyperthyroid disease should probably avoid its use without careful and consistent monitoring.

W. somnifera extract appeared to inhibit libido and sexual performance in male rats (Ilayperuma, Ratnasooriya, Weerasooriya 2002); this, too, should be considered in people, or in pets used for breeding.

Clinical Application in Veterinary Behavior Medicine

W. somnifera in combination with *Asparagus racemosus* is recommended for the control of aggression, and in particular for dominance aggression in dogs, based on the understanding that this type of behavior relates to the Mudha mind. *W. somnifera* may also be effective in the treatment of masturbation or urine-spraying cats, given its impact on sexual behavior, anxiety, and restlessness. Preliminary data supporting its antidepressant and anxiolytic effects in comparison to conventional drugs make this one of the Ayurvedic herbs of greatest potential in veterinary behavior medicine. It may be useful used alone or in combination with other psychoactive herbs discussed in this book. Clinical investigation will reveal how it is best applied.

References

Abou-Douh AM. New withanolides and other constituents from the fruit of *Withania somnifera*. Arch Pharm (Weinheim). 2002;335:267–276.

Adams JD Jr, Yang J, Mishra LC et al. Effects of ashwagandha in a rat model of stroke. Altern Ther Health Med. 2002;8:18–19.

Anjaria J, Parabia M, Dwivedi S. Ethnovet Heritage: Indian Ethnoveterinary Medicine, An Overview. Pathik Enterprise Publishers; Ahmedabad, India. 2002;541.

Aphale AA, Chhibba AD, Kumbhakarna NR et al. Subacute toxicity study of the combination of ginseng (*Panax ginseng*) and ashwagandha (*Withania somnifera*) in rats: a safety assessment. Indian J Physiol Pharmacol. 1998;42:299–302.

Arseculeratne SN, Gunatilaka AA, Panabokke RG. Studies of medicinal plants of Sri Lanka. Part 14: Toxicity of some traditional medicinal herbs. J Ethnopharmacol. 1985;13:323–335.

Bhattacharya A, Ghosal S, Bhattacharya SK. Anti-oxidant effect of *Withania somnifera* glycowithanolides in chronic footshock stress-induced perturbations of oxidative free radical scavenging enzymes and lipid peroxidation in rat frontal cortex and striatum. J Ethnopharmacol. 2001;74:1–6.

Bhattacharya SK, Bhattacharya A, Chakrabarti A. Adaptogenic activity of Siotone, a polyherbal formulation of Ayurvedic rasayanas. Indian J Exp Biol. 2000;38:119–128.

Bhattacharya SK, Bhattacharya A, Sairam K et al. Anxiolytic-antidepressant activity of *Withania somnifera* glycowithanolides: an experimental study. Phytomedicine. 2000;7:463–469.

Bhattacharya SK, Bhattacharya D, Sairam K et al. Effect of *Withania somnifera* glycowithanolides on a rat model of tardive dyskinesia. Phytomedicine 2002;9:167–170.

Bhattacharya SK, Muruganandam AV. Adaptogenic activity of *Withania somnifera*: an experimental study using a rat model of chronic stress. Pharmacol Biochem Behav. 2003;75:547–555.

Chaudhary G, Sharma U, Jagannathan NR et al. Evaluation of *Withania somnifera* in a middle cerebral artery occlusion model of stroke in rats. Clin Exp Pharmacol Physiol. 2003;30:399–404.

Davis L, Kuttan G. Effect of *Withania somnifera* on CTL activity. J Exp Clin Cancer Res. 2002;21: 115–118.

Davis L, Kuttan G. Effect of *Withania somnifera* on cyclophosphamide-induced urotoxicity. Cancer Lett. 2000;148:9–17.

Dhuley JN. Adaptogenic and cardioprotective action of ashwagandha in rats and frogs. J Ethnopharmacol. 2000;70:57–63.

Diwanay S, Chitre D, Patwardhan B. Immunoprotection by botanical drugs in cancer chemotherapy. J Ethnopharmacol. 2004;90:49–55.

Grandhi A, Mujumdar AM, Patwardhan B. A comparative pharmacological investigation of Ashwagandha and Ginseng. J Ethnopharmacol. 1994;44:131–135.

Gupta SK, Dua A, Vohra BP. *Withania somnifera* (Ashwagandha) attenuates antioxidant defense in aged spinal cord and inhibits copper induced lipid peroxidation and protein oxidative modifications. Drug Metabol Drug Interact. 2003;19:211–222.

Ilayperuma I, Ratnasooriya WD, Weerasooriya TR. Effect of *Withania somnifera* root extract on the sexual behaviour of male rats. Asian J Androl. 2002;4:295–298.

Iuvone T, Esposito G, Capasso F et al. Induction of nitric oxide synthase expression by *Withania somnifera* in macrophages. Life Sci. 2003;72:1617–1625.

Jayaprakasam B, Zhang Y, Seeram NP et al. Growth inhibition of human tumor cell lines by withanolides from *Withania somnifera* leaves. Life Sci. 2003;74:125–132.

Kaur P, Sharma M, Mathur S et al. Effect of 1-oxo-5beta, 6beta-epoxy-with a-2-ene-27-ethoxy-olide isolated from the roots of *Withania somnifera* on stress indices in Wistar rats. J Altern Complement Med. 2003;9:897–907.

Kuboyama T, Tohda C, Zhao J et al. Axon- or dendrite-predominant outgrowth induced by constituents from Ashwagandha. Neuroreport. 2002;13:1715–1720.

Leyon PV, Kuttan G. Effect of *Withania somnifera* on B16F-10 melanoma induced metastasis in mice. Phytother Res. 2004;18:118–122.

Mehta AK, Binkley P, Gandhi SS et al. Pharmacological effects of *Withania somnifera* root extract on GABAA receptor complex. Indian J Med Res. 1991;94:312–315.

Mills S, Bone K. Principles and Practice of Phytotherapy. Churchill Livingstone: Philadelphia, PA. 2000;595–602.

Mishra LC, Singh BB, Dagenais S. Scientific basis for the therapeutic use of *Withania somnifera* (ashwagandha): a review. Altern Med Rev. 2000;5:334–346.

Nagashayana N, Sankarankutty P, Nampoothiri MR et al. Association of L-DOPA with recovery following Ayurveda medication in Parkinson's disease. J Neurol Sci. 2000;176;124–127.

Naidu PS, Singh A, Kulkarni SK. Effect of *Withania somnifera* root extract on haloperidol-induced orofacial dyskinesia: possible mechanism of action. J Med Food. 2003;6:107–114.

Panda S, Kar A. *Withania somnifera* and *Bauhinia purpurea* in the regulation of circulating thyroid hormone concentrations in female mice. J Ethnopharmacol. 1999;67:233–239.

Panda S, Kar A. Changes in thyroid hormone concentrations after administration of ashwagandha root extract to adult male mice. J Pharm Pharmacol. 1998;50:1065–1068.

Parihar MS, Hemnani T. Phenolic antioxidants attenuate hippocampal neuronal cell damage against kainic acid induced excitotoxicity. J Biosci. 2003;28:121–128.

Scartezzini P, Speroni E. Review on some plants of Indian traditional medicine with antioxidant activity. J Ethnopharmacol. 2000;71:23–43.

Singh A, Naidu PS, Gupta S et al. Effect of natural and synthetic antioxidants in a mouse model of chronic fatigue syndrome. J Med Food. 2002;5:211–220.

Singh B, Chandan BK, Gupta DK. Adaptogenic activity of a novel withanolide-free aqueous fraction from the roots of *Withania somnifera* (Part II). Phytother Res. 2003;17:531–536.

Singh B, Saxena AK, Chandan BK et al. Adaptogenic activity of a novel, withanolide-free aqueous fraction from the roots of *Withania somnifera*. Phytother Res. 2001;15:311–318.

Tillotson AK, Tillotson HSH, Abel R. The One Earth Herbal Sourcebook. Kensington Publishing, New York, NY. 2001;335, 338.

Miscellaneous Psychoactive Herbs of Ayurvedic Medicine

Abies pindrow is a well-known Indian coniferous tree (Talisapatra, West Himalayan fir) that belongs to the *Pinaceae* family. It grows between 50 and 75 ft high at maturity at altitudes of 2000 to 3000 m. It prefers partial shade and damp soil.

Intolerant of pollution, it is cultivated in Europe and North America as a landscape specimen.

The leaf of the tree is medicinal and known to contain glycosides, steroids, terpenoids, and flavonoids but is otherwise not well investigated (Singh, Nath, Goel et al. 1998). Another component (+)−pinitol (2.5–10 mg/kg IP) has shown a significant anti-inflammatory effect on paw edema in rats that was comparable to phenylbutazone at the highest dose tested (Singh, Pandey, Tripathi et al. 2001).

A leaf extract has shown an ability to stabilize mast cells and exerted an anti-ulcer effect in rats; it also had a bronchoprotective effect against histamine challenge in guinea pigs (Singh, Bhattacharya, Acharya 2000). The leaf extract also appears to have an anti-inflammatory and anti-ulcer effect. An antibacterial effect has not been demonstrated (Singh, Nath, Goel et al. 1998).

In a recent investigation of its leaf extract in rats, *A. pindrow* (50 and 100 mg/kg PO) demonstrated significant anxiolytic effects that was, however, not as potent as that of the benzodiazepine lorazepam (Kumar, Singh, Jaiswal et al. 2000). It also prolonged barbiturate anesthesia and appeared to exert a mild antidepressant activity (Singh, Nath, Goel et al. 1998). Further study will elucidate its clinical application, if any, to veterinary behavior medicine.

Cannabis sativa (Indian hemp, Bhang) grows wild in central Asia and throughout India and is a well-known herb used as an aphrodisiac, stimulant, analgesic, antispasmodic, sedative, laxative, diuretic, and tonic. Today, it is sold under government license in parts of India but continues to be used by indigenes for its traditional medicinal applications (Anjaria, Parabia, Dwivedi 2002).

Canscora diffusa (Zinku kariyatu, Chang bato) is a member of the *Gentianaceae* family. It grows erect or diffuse and has thin leaves and delicate, pale-purple flowers. It can be found throughout tropical Asia, Australia, and Africa. In Ayurveda, it is used traditionally as an antiepileptic, nerve tonic, and antimalarial. It is considered to be a treatment for insanity and nervous debility (Anjaria, Parabia, Dwivedi 2002). A search of the scientific literature did not reveal any data to substantiate its traditional Ayurvedic uses.

Celastrus paniculatus (Jyotishmati, Malkanguni, Avega, Agnimasha, Black Oil Tree) is a flowering woody climber and member of the *Celastraceae* family (Figure 3-8). Seed oil is of particular value, although the bark and leaf are also used. *C. paniculatus* is used traditionally as an aphrodisiac, stimulant, and tonic as well as in the treatment of rheumatism, leprosy, gout, paralysis, respiratory symptoms, and digestive complaints (Anjaria, Parabia, Dwivedi 2002). An earlier study indicated a tranquilizing effect (Sheth, Vaz, Deliwala et al. 1963). Antifungal (Vonshak, Barazani, Sathiyamoorthy et al. 2003) and analgesic (Ahmad, Khan, Rasheed 1994) properties have also been recognized.

C. paniculatus may show neuroprotective, anti-inflammatory, and antioxidant effects that are relevant to the treatment of a number of neurodegenerative diseases (Godkar, Gordon, Ravindran et al. 2003; Ahmad, Khan, Rasheed 1994). Its

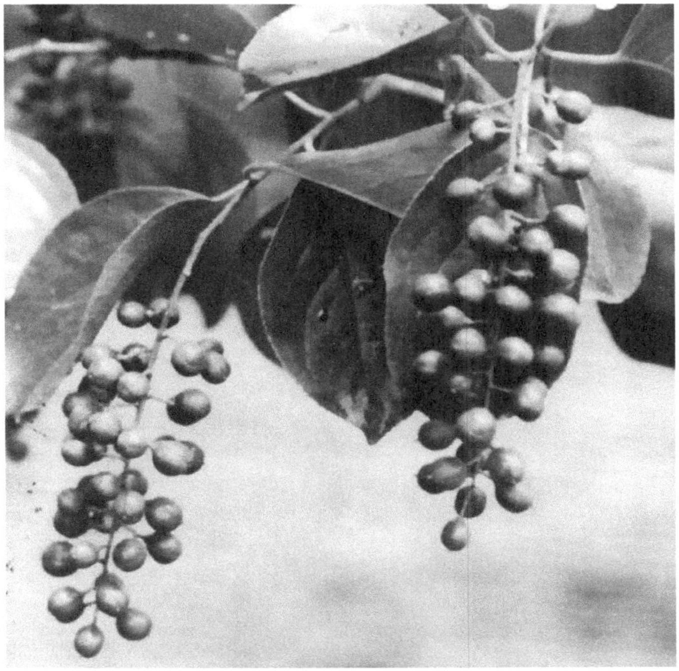

FIGURE 3-8. *Celastrus paniculatus* with fruit. (Photo courtesy of Dr. Jayvir Anjaria)

antioxidant property may explain its enhancement of cognitive function in rats at dosages of 200 to 300 mg/kg (Kumar, Gupta 2002). In an important study of its effects, Celastrus oil enhanced learning and memory in rats (Nalini, Karanth, Rao et al. 1995). This study also showed that all three CNS monoamines (norepinephrine, dopamine, and serotonin [5-HT]) had an overall decrease, suggesting their part in the mechanism of learning and memory. In rat studies, the enhancement of cognitive performance by aqueous extract of Celastrus seed was attributed to an antioxidant mechanism (Godkar, Gordon, Ravindran et al. 2003; Kumar, Gupta 2002). Celastrus seed oil was shown to reverse spatial memory impairment caused by central muscarinic blockade, although this was not thought to be a cholinergic action *per se* (Gattu, Boss, Terry et al. 1997).

Catharanthus roseus (Indian periwinkle) is a perennial ground cover and member of the family *Apocynaceae* (Figure 3-9). Also referred to as *Vinca rosea,* Sadabahar, Sangkhaphuli, Sadaphuli, Sadasuhagan, Barmasi, Anubhava Siddha Chikitsa, it is a common garden plant in India and around the world. The entire plant has medicinal purposes, not only in traditional Eastern medicine but also in modern pharmaceuticals. The flower is the source of the anticancer drugs vincristine and vinblastin. The roots contain the antipsychotic compound reserpine.

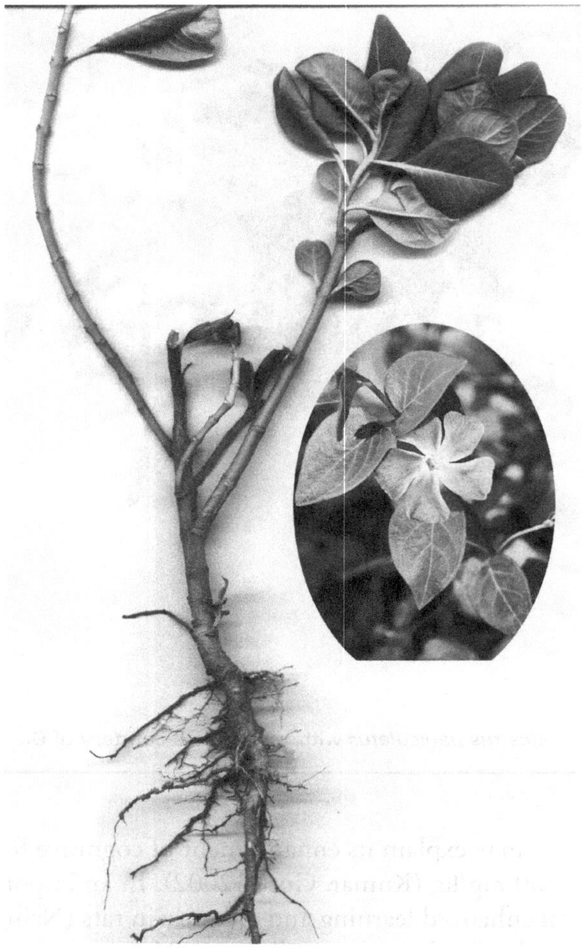

FIGURE 3-9. *Catharanthus roseus* flower, leaves, and root. (Photo courtesy of Dr. Jayvir Anjaria)

In Ayurveda, the leaves may be prepared as a tea after soaking in water overnight, for example, for the treatment of diabetes. The plant is also used for the treatment of depression and listlessness. An infusion of flowers is traditionally prepared by soaking the flowers in tea for one minute. It is recommended to drink the tea with periwinkle flowers two to three times a day for two days and then tapering to once a week, twice a month, once a month, and every six months as needed (Dr. Jayvir Anjaria, personal communication 2004; Nammi, Boini, Lodagala et al. 2003; Anjaria, Parabia, Dwivedi 2002; Duffin 2002; Vidyasagar, Ramanujam, Fernandes et al. 1999; Marmont, Damasio 1967).

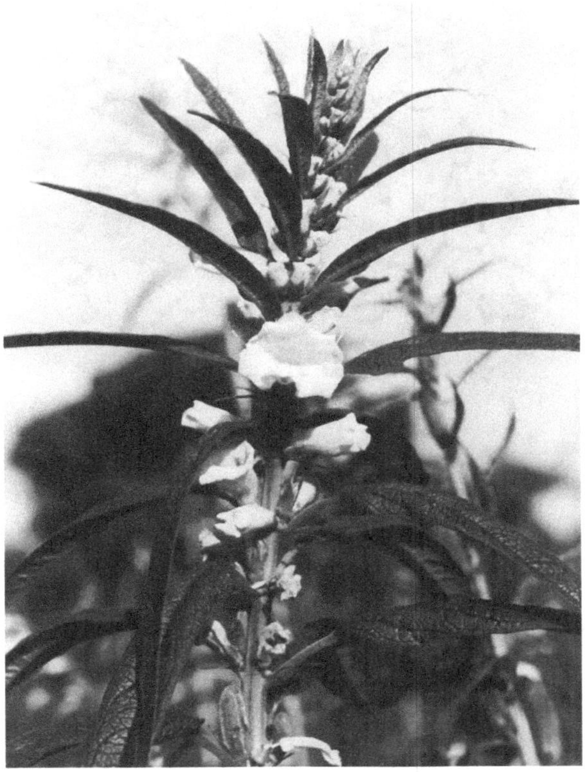

FIGURE 3-10. *Sesamum indicum* tree. (Photo courtesy of Dr. Jayvir Anjaria)

Other Ayurvedic herbs used to treat conditions of restlessness and hyperactivity such as *Sesamum indicum* (sesame seeds, *Hei zhi ma*; traditionally used as a *yin* tonic in TCM) (Figures 3-10, 3-11) and *Terminalia chebula* (Figure 3-12) have proven antioxidant effects that lend support to their traditional applications and suggest their investigation for clinical application in neurodegenerative and neoplastic disease (Hu, Xu, Chen et al. 2004; Cheng, Lin, Yu et al. 2003).

Valeriana wallichii (Indian valerian, synonym *V. pyrolaefolea*) is reviewed in context with *Valeriana officinalis* elsewhere in this book and should be considered with interest in veterinary behavior. Both *V. officinalis* and *V. wallichii* have been used in Ayurvedic practice for the treatment of hysteria, neurosis, and epilepsy (Chopra, Chopra, Handa et al. 1982).

Zingiber officinale (Ginger, Ardrakam, Adrak, Adu, Allamu, Ala, Ingi) is used to treat emotional and physical disorders in Ayurveda, as well as being a favorite condiment; it is discussed in detail in Chapter 4, which is devoted to Oriental psychoactive herbs.

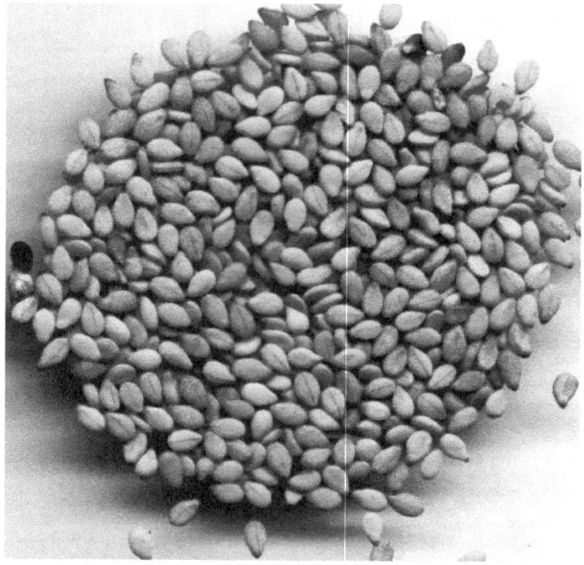

FIGURE 3-11. Sesamum indicum seeds (sesame seeds) are used in Ayurvedic and Traditional Chinese medicine. (Photo courtesy of Dr. Jayvir Anjaria)

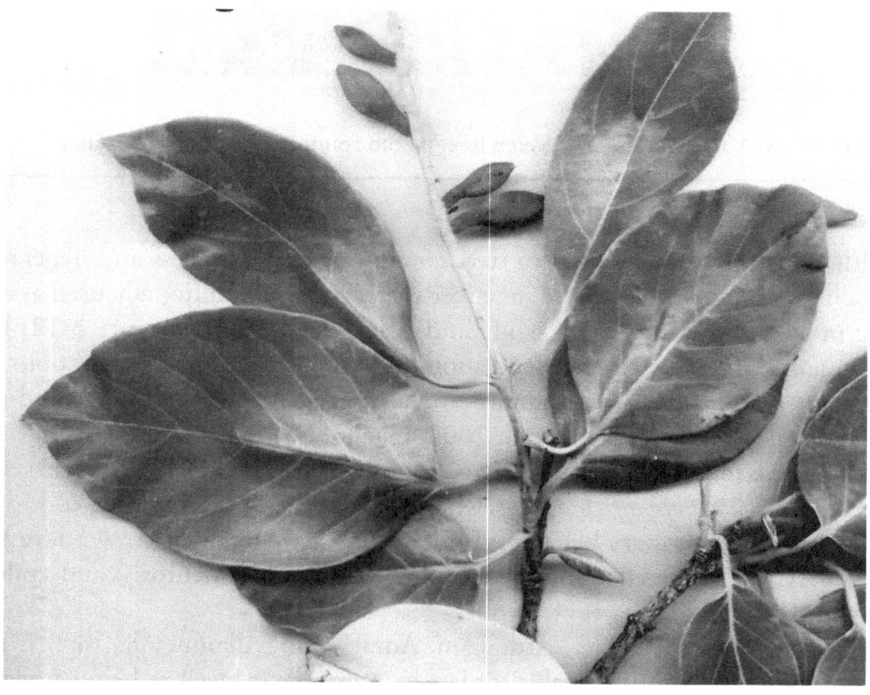

FIGURE 3-12. *Terminalia chebula* (fruit and leaves). (Photo courtesy of Dr. Jayvir Anjaria)

References

Ahmad F, Khan RA, Rasheed S. Preliminary screening of methanolic extracts of *Celastrus paniculatus* and *Tecomella undulata* for analgesic and anti-inflammatory activities. J Ethnopharmacol. 1994;42: 193–198.

Anjaria J, Parabia M, Dwivedi S. Ethnovet Heritage: Indian Ethnoveterinary Medicine, An Overview. Pathik Enterprise Publishers; Ahmedabad, India. 2002.

Cheng HY, Lin TC, Yu KH et al. Antioxidant and free radical scavenging activities of *Terminalia chebula*. Biol Pharm Bull. 2003;26:1331–1335.

Chopra RN, Chopra IC, Handa KL et al. Chopra's indigenous drugs of India. (2nd ed) Academic Publishers; Calcutta, India. 1982:253–255.

Dev S. Ancient-modern concordance in Ayurvedic plants: some examples. Enron Health Perspect. 1999; 107:783–789.

Gattu M, Boss KL, Terry AV et al. Reversal of scopolamine-induced deficits in navigational memory performance by the seed oil of *Celastrus paniculatus*. Pharmacol Biochem Behav. 1997;57:793–799.

Godkar P, Gordon RK, Ravindran A et al. *Celastrus paniculatus* seed water soluble extracts protect cultured rat forebrain neuronal cells from hydrogen peroxide-induced oxidative injury. Fitoterapia. 2003;74:658–669.

Hu Q, Xu J, Chen S et al. Antioxidant activity of extracts of black sesame seed (*Sesamum indicum* L.) by supercritical carbon dioxide extraction. J Agric Food Chem. 2004;52:943–947.

Kumar MH, Gupta YK. Antioxidant property of *Celastrus paniculatus willd.*: a possible mechanism in enhancing cognition. Phytomedicine. 2002;9:302–131.

Kumar V, Singh RK, Jaiswal AK et al. Anxiolytic activity of Indian *Abies pindrow Royle* leaves in rodents: an experimental study. Indian J Exp Biol. 2000;38:343–346.

Lad, VD. Ayurveda: Textbook of Fundamental Principles. The Ayurvedic Press; Albuquerque, New Mexico. 2002.

Marmont AM, Damasio EE. The effects of two alkaloids derived from *Vinca rosea* on the malignant cells of Hodgkin's disease, lymphosarcoma and acute leukemia in vivo. Blood. 1967;29:1–21.

Nalini K, Karanth KS, Rao A et al. Effects of *Celastrus paniculatus* on passive avoidance performance and biogenic amine turnover in albino rats. J Ethnopharmacol. 1995;47:101–108.

Nammi S, Boini MK, Lodagala SD et al. The juice of fresh leaves of *Catharanthus roseus Linn.* reduces blood glucose in normal and alloxan diabetic rabbits. BMC Complement Altern Med. 2003;3:4.

Rao AV. Depression in Indian History. J Indian Med Assoc. 2000;98:219–223.

Schwartz S. Separation anxiety syndrome in dogs and cats. JAVMA. 2003;222:1526–1532.

Sheth UK, Vaz A, Deliwala CV et al. Behavioural and pharmacological studies of a tranquilising fraction from the oil of *Celastrus paniculatus* (Malkanguni oil). Arch Int Pharmacodyn Ther. 1963;144:34–50.

Singh RK, Bhattachrya SK, Acharya SB. Pharmacological activity of *Abies pindrow*. J Ethnopharmacol. 2000;73:47–51.

Singh RK, Nath G, Goel RK et al. Pharmacological actions of *Abies pindrow Royle* leaf. Indian J Exp Biol. 1998;36:187–191.

Singh RK, Pandey BL, Tripathi M et al. Anti-inflammatory effect of (+)−pinitol. Fitoterapia. 2001;72: 168–170.

Vaidya ADB. The status and scope of Indian medicinal plants acting on central nervous system. Ind J Pharmacol. 1997;29:S340–S343.

Vidyasagar MS, Ramanujam AS, Fernandes DJ et al. Vincristine (Vinca-alkaloid) as a sclerosing agent for malignant pleural effusions. Acta Oncol. 1999;38:1017–1020.

Vonshak A, Barazani O, Sathiyamoorthy P et al. Screening South Indian medicinal plants for antifungal activity against cutaneous pathogens. Phytother Res. 2003;17:1123–1125.

CHAPTER

4

Oriental Psychoactive Herbs

"It matters not if medicine is old or new
so long as it brings about a cure.
It matters not if theories be Eastern or Western
so long as they prove to be true."
—*Jen-Hsou Lin, DVM, PhD* Taipei

Introduction

Eastern healing practices are becoming integral to Western medicine and culture. In the Americas and in Europe, there is growing popularity and appreciation of acupuncture, tai chi, yoga, and other methods of Eastern traditional medicine. Patients and the scientific community alike are becoming increasingly aware of the vast pharmacopoeias of medicinal herbs of Eastern traditions. Nonetheless, a substantial group of medicinal herbs appear to be strong candidates for application to veterinary behavior practice. As the international research community and clinical practitioners in both human and veterinary medicine continue to study the potential of herbs for healing, exciting new applications of traditional healing herbs and novel compounds derived from plants are anticipated. Caution is required, however, given that there is still insufficient scientific evidence to substantiate all herbal formulas; if herbs are used incorrectly, adverse effects even for "natural" remedies are possible.

Traditional Chinese Medicine (TCM) and Ayurveda remain the two major philosophies of healing and health to influence Asia to the present day. Distinct remedies of Japanese traditional medicine (*Kampo*) with potential for use in veterinary behavior medicine are also briefly mentioned. It would be impossible to truly appreciate the medicinal herbs that arise from Eastern cultures without some understanding of the philosophies from which they grow. The Chinese speak of *Qi* when Ayurveda teaches of *Prana*, but both great traditions embody principles of holistic healing and the healthy flow of energy within and surrounding us. The elegant Chinese concepts of yin and yang are no less astounding than the doshic principles of Ayurveda. Both traditions categorize energies within organ systems, concepts of heating and cooling energy, five tastes in TCM and six flavors in Ayurveda, and five elements (*Maha Bhutas* of Ayurveda and *Wu Xing* in TCM). Ayurveda and TCM are in agreement on the ultimate importance of balance and moderation in life. There are parallels between TCM and Ayurveda, but there are differences, too. The fundamental doctrines of TCM and Ayurveda will be presented. The reader is encouraged to study further, and the reference lists at the end of each chapter or section are a good place to start.

Historical Perspective of Traditional Chinese Medicine

The Yellow Emperor Huangdi (*Huang Ti*; circa 2600 BC) was a great innovator; among other things, he originated the cycle of the animal-based Chinese Zodiac and is thought to have constructed the Great Wall of China. The earliest Chinese teachings of medicine have also been attributed to the Yellow Emperor, although several scholars likely compiled them over time based on the oral tradition (Anonymous 2004, 2000; Tierra 1998). Completed around the year 200 BC, the classic is known as the *Huangdi Neijing* (*Huang-di Ni Ching*, The Yellow Emperor's Canon of Medicine). Despite the uncertainty of its date, all agree that this work is the founding text of Traditional Chinese Medicine (TCM). One volume contains details of anatomy, physiology, and acupuncture. The other presents a philosophy of medicine and life. The *Huangdi Neijing* incorporates the concepts of yin-yang, the five elements, and basic principles of Taoism. In 1974, his tomb was discovered and revealed more than 7,000 terra cotta life-sized warriors. Huangdi's influence was so grand, reaching almost mythical proportions, that some proclaim him a founder of Taoism along with Lao Tzu even though they lived centuries apart.

Lao Tzu and Confucius, the founder of Confucianism, were contemporaries during sixth and fifth centuries BC. The philosophy of TCM integrates both Taoism and Confucianism. Lao Tzu, thuoght by some to have never really existed, is thought to be the author of the famous *Ijing* (*I Ching*, Book of Changes), dated to 1250 BC, in which the concept of *yin* ("shady side of the mountain") and *yang* ("sunny side of the mountain") are formalized (Table 4-1). Principles of Buddhism, emanating from India and surrounding regions and incorporating the teachings of Ayurvedic Medicine, later reached into China and Japan. These principles continue to influence medical practice across Asia and beyond.

The Emperor Shennong (*Shen Nung;* circa 2700 BC) is considered to be the true Father of Chinese Medicine; his wife is credited with the discovery of silk production). Although some consider him to be a mythical figure, he is generally thought to have revolutionized agriculture in ancient China and is said to have personally tested hundreds of plants for their medicinal value. This was done at great personal risk, given the toxic effects of many botanicals that he is said to have

Table 4-1. Qualities Associated with the Traditional Chinese Concepts of Yin and Yang

Yin	Yang
Female, dark, passive, receiving, below, front	Male, bright, active, giving, above, back
Earth (Centripetal, Condenses)	Heaven (Centrifugal, Expands)
Moon (Dark)	Sun (Bright)
Water	Fire
Winter (Cold; Slow Metabolism, low T°)	Summer (Hot; High Metabolism, high T°)
Vegetable (Immobile)	Animal (Mobile)
Form (Material)	Energy (Immaterial)
Rest (Patience)	Activity (Driven)
Space	Time
Psychological	Physiological
Right/Descending	Left/Ascending
Receptive (Feminine)	Aggressive (Masculine)
Introvert, Sensitive, Dull	Extrovert, Rigid, Motivated
Parasympathetic Nervous System (associated with reproduction and maintenance); "kidney yin"	Sympathetic Nervous System (associated with stress and danger); "kidney yang"
Bitter, Salty, and Sour Tastes (Cooling)	Sweet and Spicy Tastes (Heating)
Heart, lungs, spleen, liver, pancreas, kidneys, adrenal glands (organic disorders or internal ailments)	Intestines, stomach, gallbladder, bladder, skin, muscle (functional imbalance of hollow organs or external ailments)
Moist	Dry
Chronic	Acute
Dark colors, Dark herbs	Bright colors, brightly colored herbs

(Mills, Bone 2000; Tierra 1998; Zhong, Wiseman, Ellis 1996)

experienced himself. His survival apparently was due at least in part to his ability to produce timely antidotes. The *Shennong Bencao* (*Shen Nung Pen T'sao)* or Shennong's Materia Medica describes 365 medicinal preparations; 100 medicines were from plants and the remainder was derived from animals and minerals. It remains possible that this text was a compilation of several authors. The Emperors Huangdi and Shennong have been deified and called the fathers of the Han Chinese (Huaxia) race.

The golden age of Chinese medicine occurred during the Han dynasty (206–220 AD). Huato (100–207 AD) performed the first surgery under anesthesia; tragically, a paranoid and mistrusting patient who was a powerful general executed him. In his text (*Mai Jing,* The Pulse Classics), Wan Shu Ho (180–270 AD) described 24 pulse patterns associated with illness. The greatest physician of this time was Zhang Zhongjing (*Chang Chung-ching,* 150–219 AD) who has been called the Hippocrates of China. Inspired by a devastating plague, he was the author of *Shanghanlun* (Treatise on Colds and Fevers), another classic of Chinese medicine that included many herbal formulas still in use today. In his classic text *Bencao Jingjizhu,* the physician Tao Hung Ching (452–536 AD) added another 365 medicinal herbs to the botanical material medica.

During the Tang dynasty (618–907 AD), Sun Si Miao (581–682 AD) recognized the role of nutrition and diet in maintaining health and treating disease. He produced two major medical works *Qianjin Yaofang* (Prescriptions Worth a Thousand Pieces of Gold) and later *Qianjin Yifang* (Supplement to Prescriptions Worth a Thousand Pieces of Gold).

Qian Yi (*Chien-yi,* 1032–1113 AD) wrote *Xiaoer Yaozheng Zhijue* (Key to Therapeutics of Children's Diseases), the first text of pediatric medicine. Sung Tzu wrote the first text of forensic pathology (*Hsi Yun Lu,* "Washing Away the Wrong") in 1247 AD. During the Ming dynasty (1368–1644), it took Li Shizhen (*Li Shih-chen;* 1518–1593 AD) 27 years to complete the great pharmacopoeia of *Bencao Kangmu* (*Pen ts'ao kang mu,* The Great Herbal), which details no fewer than 1892 medicines and their applications. In his book (*Wen Yilun*; Acute Epidemic Febrile Diseases Treatise), Wu Youxing (*Wu Yu Hsing;* 1582–1652 AD) was the first to present the concept of transmissible disease. Wang Qingren (*Wang Chin Ren;* 1768–1831 AD) emphasized the importance of understanding anatomy in medical practice and the concept of "blood stasis" in the treatment of many illnesses.

Basic Principles of TCM

Qi

Chinese philosophy has one absolute law, the Law of Change (Mills, Bone 2000; Tierra 1998; Zhong, Wiseman, Abel 1996a). It states that nothing is fixed; everything is in a constant state of flux, transformation, and dynamic change. Stasis is abnormal and blocks the flow of the life force. *Qi* (*chi*) is the energy of all forms of life including animals, plants, and minerals. Plants have characteristic qi reflected in their color, growth rate, and form. Minerals, although not alive, possess their own infinitesimal rate of change and also contain qi. The flow of a human or nonhuman animal's qi is determined by health and age. An individual's qi is reflected in his or her digestion, virility or femininity, immune system, and level of energy. Disease occurs when qi is deficient, stagnant, or blocked. Qi assumes a number of forms within the body. *Original qi* (*yuanqi*) includes *organ qi,* which is specific to each organ, as well as *ancestral qi (zongqi),* which enters the airways and dwells within the heart to become the force of circulating qi, blood, pulse, body temperature, and movement. In Ayurvedic philosophy, *prana* is the equivalent to qi. In Kabbalah, there are at least three levels of the Divine or Life Force (*koach, chayut, ohr*), which is also believed to be omnipresent and permeating all things (see Appendix B, "Traditional Jewish Medicine").

Yin and Yang

The concepts of *yin* and *yang* are ancient principles of Chinese philosophy that are intrinsic to the Chinese perspective of life as a whole and integral to the Chinese art of healing. Yin is the female essence. It is the receptacle of the yang, which is the active male energy of the body; it generates heat and maintains circulation. Together, the yin and yang compose the vital force of qi. Introduced in the *Ijing*, yin-yang duality signifies continual evolution and transformation. The forces of *yinqi* and *yangqi* both attract and repel each other. One of them must always predominate because nothing remains neutral for long. When yin peaks, it changes into yang and vice versa. Everything, including disease and death, involves a dynamic equilibrium between yin and yang. Moderation is always wise in life and in health. The infinite cycles of the universe reflect the constantly revolving polarity of yin and yang and their transformation into each other. Changes in season, day to night, relationships between people, and balance within us are all dependent upon yin-yang dynamics. Yin and yang are continually mingling yet never achieve homogeneity. The bipolar qualities that characterize yin and yang are summarized in Table 4-1. Qualities of feminine and masculine energy are also discussed in the Kaballah (see Appendix B, "Traditional Jewish Medicine").

Zang and Fu

Chinese philosophy teaches that all physical forms are composed of yang at the surface and yin at the center. For example, superficial anatomical structures are viewed as yang and internal structures as yin. Furthermore, the upper half (and, lengthwise, the dorsal section) of the body is yang; the lower half (and ventral section) is yin. The *zang* ("solid viscera": spleen, heart, lung, liver, kidney) are yin; the *fu* ("hollow bowels": stomach, small and large intestine, bladder, gallbladder, triple warmer) are yang. Each of these structures also has a yin and yang polarity (e.g., heart yin and heart yang). The *zang-fu* are arranged in mutually supporting yin-yang organ pairs (Table 4-2). Energy systems between body parts are also discussed in Kaballistic scriptures of Judaism (see Appendix B).

Disease reflects the body's attempt to correct or compensate for imbalance; Chinese medicine attempts to enhance yin (yin tonic) in conditions when yin is low, or to boost yang (yang tonic) when yang is low. If the overall pattern of symptoms suggests yang excess, for instance, the treatment would require heat-draining, cold and bitter yin agents. Most yang excesses are relative conditions and due primarily to either yin deficiency (treatment is aimed at increasing yin) or stasis (e.g., Liver Stasis with Yang Rising; treatment would be aimed at removing the stasis and downbearing yang). When either yin or yang is out of balance in excess or in depletion, it will eventually drain the energy of the other. Yin deficiency exists in all wasting disease accompanied by agitation and nervousness (yang qualities include heat, activity, restlessness); excess yang is the consequence of yin deficiency. Overeating and overindulgence in anything that brings pleasure may result in yang deficiency; yin domination will be manifested by feelings of lethargy and heaviness. Post-prandial somnolence following a large and rich meal is an example of yin excess. Yin deficiency will appear as excessive yang and is called "defi-

Table 4-2. The Five ´Elements *(Wu Xing)* of Traditional Chinese Medicine and a Partial Listing of Their Attributes

Attributes of the 5 Elements	Fire	Water	Earth	Wood	Metal
Yin Organ (*Zang*)	Heart/Pericardium	Kidneys, Endocrine System	Spleen, Pancreas	Liver	Lungs
Yang Organ (*Fu*)	Small Intestine	Bladder	Stomach	Gallbladder	Large Intestine
Function	Governs xue (Blood), origin of joy and social skills, stores shen	Governs birth and reproduction, stores jing (Essence, Reproductive secretions), source of yin/yang	Governs digestion and transformation, stores qi	Governs distribution of body's resources, stores xue	Governs self-defense and rhythm, produces qi
Planet	Mars	Mercury	Saturn	Jupiter	Venus
Direction	South/Heat	North/Cold	Center/Dampness	East/Wind	West/Dryness
Season/Weather	Summer	Winter	Indian summer	Spring	Autumn
Color	Red	Black	Yellow	Green-Blue	White
Sense/Sensory Organ	Speech/Tongue	Hearing/Ears, anus, lower urinary tract	Taste/Mouth	Vision/Eyes	Smell/Nose
Taste	Bitter	Salty	Sweet	Sour	Spicy, Acrid
Emotion	Happiness, Joy (*Shen*)	Fear, Paranoia (*Zhi*)	Worry, Sympathy (*Yi*)	Anger (*Hun*)	Sorrow, Grief (*Po*)
Dynamic	Visionary	Will	Thinking, Intellectual	Spirituality	Vitality
Action	Walk	Stand	Sit	See	Recline
Animal Symbol	Fowl	Pig	Ox	Sheep	Dog

(Mills, Bone 2000; Tierra 1998; Zhong, Wiseman, Ellis 1996)

ciency heat." The manifestation of yang deficiency manifested by apparent yin excess is known as "deficiency cold."

Chronic problems are most often caused by deficiencies (of qi, blood, or jing) or stasis (of Qi or blood). Conditions of excess usually stem from external attack by the six *Xie* ("evils" of damp, cold, wind, heat, summerheat, dryness). Other causes of excess include trauma and parasites that usually invade a weakened body. Heat Excess, for example, dries or "burns off" blood, fluids, and yin. Its treatment calls for releasing the surface and expelling heat and must also include building yin, blood, or fluids as appropriate to the case.

Males are predisposed to qi ailments and women tend more toward *xue* (blood) problems. The dynamic balance between yin and yang in the course of disease may vary. In addition, each individual has a characteristic equilibrium of yin-yang. In general, yang symptoms are characterized by restless, extroverted, agitated attitudes and behaviors; yin symptoms tend toward passive, lethargic, and introverted patterns of mood and activity.

The Five Tastes

TCM identifies Five Tastes (Tables 4-1, 4-2). Spicy and sweet tastes are associated with yang and ascend in the body; bitter, sour, and salty tastes are primarily yin and flow downward. Each taste corresponds to an organ function: Heart (bitter), Spleen (sweet), Lungs (spicy), Kidney (salty), and Liver (sour). By virtue of the upward and downward circulation of ingested tastes, other target organs may be adversely or positively affected by excessive or conflicting tastes. For example, the spleen routes salty tastes to the kidneys and sour tastes to the liver. Both are yin tastes and spread downward in the body. The spleen directs bitter tastes downward to the Heart but keeps sweet to itself before sweet moves upward to nourish other parts of the body. The rising yang of spicy tastes moves through the Spleen into the Lungs. These are believed to move the qi and open the pores to expel pathogens such as Cold and Wind (common references to respiratory ailments in TCM). Wind, Cold, Fire, Summerheat, Dampness, and Dryness are the predominant external body-invading pathogens known as the External Evils (Exogenous Pathogenic Factors; *Wai Xie*).

The Five Elements

The Yellow Emperor first described the Five Elements (*Wu Xing*) in the *Huangdi Neijing* (Table 4-2). Much like the Ayurvedic elements, the Chinese five elements include Wood, Fire, Earth, Metal, and Water. They reflect the orderly Confucian influence and serve to classify illness and direct appropriate treatment. The elements, or phases as they are often called, interact with each other according to four cycles that are either inhibitory or enhancing in nature. Each of the five elements corresponds to an organ: Liver/Wood, Heart/Fire, Spleen/Earth, Lung/Metal, and Kidney/Water. Each of the five elements also corresponds to a yin-yang organ pair (Table 4-2). The theme of yin and yang emerges in the "husband-wife" paired organ system in which there is an association of a yin organ (*zang*) with a yang organ (*fu*) within the same elemental category: Wood (Gallbladder/Liver), Fire (Small intestine/Heart), Earth (Stomach/Spleen), Metal (Large Intestine/ Lung), and Water (Bladder/Kidney).

Each main Yin organ (Heart, Spleen, Lung, Kidney, Liver) has a corresponding Spirit or Emotion, so herbs that target these organs will also influence the spirit of the organ and in that sense will have "psychotropic" effects. The Triple Warmer (yang) is paired with the Pericardium (yin); these are also associated with Fire. The Triple Warmer (*San Jiao*) concept encompasses the coordination of three sections of the body: Upper Warmer (heart, pericardium, lung, throat, head); middle warmer (spleen, stomach, gallbladder); and Lower Warmer (liver, kidney, bladder, intestines, genitalia). The pericardium represents circulation, sex, and the emotional aspects of Heart and sexuality. Colors associated with each element also emerge in the practice of *Fung Shui*, which teaches that the placement of furnishings and even the color of the clothing we wear impact our sense of well-being, fortunes, mood, and qi.

According to the *Wu Xing* doctrine, the Heart governs the flow of blood and has a direct connection to the mind and verbal communication. A person with manic behavior (note the associated action is the most active one, walking) or uncontrollable giggling is under the influence of an imbalance in Heart qi and the Fire element. In traditional Chinese philosophy, the Heart is the source of emotional and cognitive function. A diseased Heart results in a restless spirit and results in symptoms of nervousness, neuroses, irritability, insomnia, and other clinical findings. Extreme Fear will impact the Heart (palpitations, insomnia; think of the physiological response to danger in the "fight or flight" phenomenon, for example). On the other hand, excessive indulgence in pleasures ("Joy" or "Happiness" in Table 4-2 refer to hedonistic extremes) will also tax the heart and result in mood swings, hysteria, insanity, insomnia, and cognitive dysfunction.

The Heart and Spleen have a very close, sometimes overlapping relationship. The Spleen is the source of qi and blood production and also controls what a person is thinking. Prolonged worrying, overwork, long hours of study and stress (sitting is the activity associated with the Earth element) deplete Spleen qi and may cause Earth-related symptoms such as obesity, fatigue, and digestive complaints (e.g., stress-related inflammatory bowel disease and peptic ulcers).

The organs of Metal (Lung and Large Intestine) are both responsible for eliminating bodily waste, or negative emotions. If these organs become imbalanced or blocked, the result could be asthma, constipation, or depression. The Lung governs the intake of qi through respiration; however, it is the Kidney that ensures qi absorption. A key function of Kidney is to capture Lung qi. If the Kidneys are diseased, ancestral qi is rapidly depleted because the Lungs cannot function alone. The Lungs also work in conjunction with the Spleen to distribute phlegm and with the Heart to distribute blood. Sadness depletes Heart and Lung qi, causing respiratory ailments (e.g., asthma), fatigue, depression, and decreased resistance to respiratory infections. Grief can also impact the lungs and cause chronic or acute respiratory illness.

The connection between the Water element and the Kidney is easy enough to understand from the Western perspective; however, in TCM it is deeper than that. There is *kidney yin* (parasympathetic nervous system) and *kidney yang* (sympathetic nervous system) and even *kidney qi* (will power). The kidneys are considered to govern life and are the source of yin and yang within each individual. Fears and phobias are signs of Water imbalance, manifested by the act of standing (think of the expression "frozen with fear"). Fear affects the kidneys because it causes qi to rise from the lower warmers; think of cases of submissive urination, urinary incontinence, or separation-related inappropriate urination. The Kidney will also be impacted in prolonged states of shock and extreme fear (e.g., night sweats).

Finally, the Liver is the seat of the soul and opens directly into the eyes. The Liver directs movement because of the connection to vision; however, it is the gall bladder (the Liver's yang organ) that makes the decisions and provides the courage to act. Imbalance in Liver is expressed as anger and frustration (think of inflammatory emotions corresponding to burning wood), whereas gall bladder imbalance results in submissiveness and indecision (think of "wooden" as in immobile). Anger causes qi to rise and concentrate in the upper warmers, causing hypertension, mental confusion, dizziness, and emotional signs including several forms of aggression, foul mood, and frustration. The free-flow of Liver qi is particularly important not only to the organ's own function but also to consequent emotional disturbance. Obstruction or stagnation of Liver qi must be considered in the diagnosis of behavioral disruptions and psychological disturbance.

Every individual possesses his or her own characteristic *jing* (essence) or *essential qi*. Jing implies whatever is essential to the maintenance of life. It is the result of "pre-heaven" or congenital essence (inherited potential) with "post-heaven" or acquired essence (influence of nourishment following birth). Kidney essence, for example, is the result of both these essences combined with the individual's inborn constitution. Inborn jing transforms into yuanqi and is exhaustible. It is used in the production of ova and spermatozoa and is depleted by excessive sexual behavior. On the other hand, acquired jing flows through the body's channels and can be stored in reserve in case of emergency. These concepts are to some extent similar to the Ayurvedic theories of *Prakruti*, *Vikruti*, and the individual's doshic balance discussed elsewhere in this section.

In TCM theory, qi, blood, jing, and fluids comprise the fundamental elements of the body. Along with yin and yang, these are believed to flow in twelve channels or meridians and eight secondary vessels through the body. Yin and yang pathways transmit nourishment and warming energies to link every part of the body. TCM aims to detect and resolve any blockages or deficiencies in qi and/or imbalance in yin and yang by methods that include the administration of healing herbs, acupuncture, moxibustion (a form of heat therapy using preparations of mugwort (*Artemisia vulgaris*), steam heat, hot wax, or electrocautery applied to acupuncture points, active and passive exercise (e.g., *tai chi* and *qi gong*), meditation, massage (*tui'na*), and nutritional therapy.

It is impossible to investigate the complexities of TCM principles fully in a single chapter. The central beliefs summarized here will help the reader to appreciate the impressive knowledge that is necessary for the practice of Chinese healing and to provide a point of reference as the Chinese herbs of interest in veterinary behavior medicine are investigated. The art of TCM requires the practitioner to acquire an exquisite understanding of the delicate balance that is normal for the individual patient and to restore that patient to health with appropriate herbal prescriptions. If an external pathogen has invaded, it must be expelled. If excess (*Shi*) is diagnosed, treatment requires that the excess be drained away (*Xie*), and is memorized with the instructive expression "in *Shi* use *Xie.*" If deficiency (*Xu*) is diagnosed, treatment requires that the deficiency be tonified, supplemented, or nourished (*Bu*), recalled in the expression "in *Xu* use *Bu.*" Stagnation, stasis or blockage calls for restoring the flow of qi and/or blood. Similarly, accumulation or stasis of fluids or Water would suggest the use of diuretics and/or purgatives. TCM focuses on balancing imbalances and accomplishes this by focusing on the function rather than the structure of the diseased parts.

Use of Herbs in TCM

According to Chinese philosophy, plants, too, possess *yinqi* and *yangqi*. Therefore, consuming plants impacts the individual's qi as well. Yang plants stimulate and boost the body's metabolism; yin plants are calmative and subdue metabolism. Furthermore, a plant's characteristic flavor influences the body's metabolism. In general, Sweet (e.g., sugar) and Spicy (e.g., ginger, cinnamon) tastes have a warming energy, not unlike adding fuel to the body's furnace. Cooling flavors such as Sour (e.g., citrus), Salty (e.g., NaCl, seaweed) or Bitter (e.g., gentian, rhubarb) calm the heat and energy of yang and balance the yin. In TCM, medicinal herbs are selected in part based upon their effect on the patient's qi and/or blood imbalance, and also according to the energy channel or meridian that conducts energy flow through the affected organ system. For instance, depression is viewed as the toxic effect on the body and neurotransmitters governing mood by the energy transformation of unrealized desires or frustrated goals.

The Liver is responsible for the free flow of qi and blood; it also regulates the free flow of emotion and thinking. Emotional disturbances imply an obstruction or stasis of the flow of qi and/or blood and a need to regulate Liver qi and/or blood. The classic Chinese herb *Bupleurum chinense* is used alone or in combination with other herbs to enhance the flow of Liver qi and relieve depression; this herb is discussed in depth later in this section. In general, Chinese herbs with potential use as psychotropic agents act to calm the Shen, nourish the Heart and ease the mind, open the orifices to restore consciousness, relieve blood and qi obstruction, and calm the Liver and Liver/Fire.

Herbal remedies are designed to combat four types of deficiency corresponding to the *Four Treasures*: yang, qi, yin, and blood. Yang deficiency is characterized by poor circulation, cold, low libido, and a submerged pulse and might respond to *Cinnamomum cassia* (cinnamon bark, *Rou gui*) or *Aconitum carmichaeli* (*Fu zi*). Deficient qi is associated with low energy, anxiety, sweating, weak pulse, and other physical signs and might be treated with formulas that contain qi-enhancing herbs such as *Panax ginseng* (*Ren shen*), *Astragalus membranaceus* (*Huang qi*), or *Codonopsis pilosula* (*Dang shen*). Yin deficiency's signs of Heat, restlessness, insomnia, night sweats, and rapid pulse might respond to *Panax quinquefolium* (American ginseng) or other herbs. Blood deficiency manifested by paleness, dizziness, agitation, nightmares, and irregular menstrual cycles in women might respond, for example, to *Angelica sinensis* (*Dang gui*).

Chinese medicinal plants are usually used in combination with others in polyherbal formulas. This is done to provide a synergy between the herbs, for example, or to minimize any toxic effects. Many, if not all, herbs are potentially toxic if the dose is wrong or if the body's adaptive and metabolic functions are compromised at the time of administration. Used properly by trained herbalists, reports of adverse reactions to TCM preparations are uncommon.

In the formulation of TCM polyherbal recipes, different herbs play different roles. For instance, the *emperor* herb (king or sovereign herb) is the primary therapeutic herb. It is assisted by the *minister* herb, which takes care of secondary symptoms or plays a supportive role. The *messenger* herb (*envoy*) may help to transmit the remedy to the target organ or helps to propel it along specific channels or meridians. Finally, the *assistant* herb (*harmonizer*) helps to counteract any harmful side effects of components of the mixture, or to attenuate the effects of the emperor in complex formulas aimed at treating complicated illness (personal communication Dr. Phil Rogers, 2004; Tierra 1998). For example, in the Four Nobles formula (*Si Jun Zi Tang*) used for low vitality and depression associated with illness as a general qi tonic, *Panax ginseng* (*Ren shen*) or *Codonopsis pilosula* (*Dang shen*) is the emperor herb; *Atractylodes macrocephala* (*Cang zhu*) is the minister herb; *Poria cocos* (*Fu ling*) is the assistant herb; and *Glycyrrhiza glabra* (*Gan cao,* Licorice) is the messenger herb frequently used to harmonize medicinal mixtures. Ingredients of some TCM formulas mentioned below are provided in Tables 4-3 and 4-4, although this list cannot be considered exhaustive by any means. To assist in deciphering the Chinese names of traditional herbal formulas, common pinyin prefixes and suffixes are presented in Table 4-5.

In TCM, qi or blood stasis or stagnation will cause local blood stasis and could result in Liver/Spleen blockage; this produces blood and phlegm stasis, which in

Table 4-3. Ingredients and Actions of Spirit-Quieting formulas of Traditional Chinese Medicine Relevant to Veterinary Behavior Medicine[1]

SPIRIT-QUIETING FORMULAS	INGREDIENTS	ACTIONS
Tian Wang Bu Xin Dan (Celestial Emperor Heart-Supplementing Elixir)	Rehmannia, Ginseng, Asparagus, Ophipogon, Scrophularia, Salvia (Dan shen), Poria, Polygala, Tangjuei, Schisandra, Biota see, Spiny Jujube, Platycodon, Cinnabar	Enriches yin and nourishes the Blood; treats yin-blood insufficiency and Disquieted Heart Spirit in the form of Vexation, Palpitation, Insomnia, Poor Memory, Dry Stool, Night Sweats
Huang lian e- jiao tang (Coptis and Ass Hide Glue Decoction)	Coptis, Scutellaria, Ass Hide Glue, White Peony, Egg Yolk	Enriches yin, cools Heart Heat; treats Vexation, Insomnia, Heat in the palms and soles, dry mouth and throat
Gan mai da-zao tang (Licorice, Wheat and Jujube Decoction)	Licorice, Light Wheat Grain, Jujube	Nourishes the Heart and calms the spirit; treats visceral upset accompanied by sadness, tearfulness, emotional upheaval and mood swing, vexation, agitation

[1]The TCM materia medica includes animal and mineral ingredients that are part of many medicinal formulations. These ingredients are not advocated for use by this author primarily because of animal welfare and environmental concerns, as well as the risk of transmissible disease. In this recipe, Ass Hide Glue (gelatin) may be substituted with *Zyzyphus jujube* (Da zao) and *Salvia miltiorrhiza* (Dan shen) in emotional conditions due to a Blood Deficiency with a concomitant Heart Blood or Heart Yin Deficiency; substitute with Zyzyphus alone if the problem stems from an external evil stress on the Heart (Dr. Ihor Basko, personal communication 2004; Zhong, Wiseman, Ellis 1996).

turn blocks the Heart channel and the mind. Consequences of Liver/Spleen stagnation include depression (*dian*). Treatment for symptoms of depression calls for removal of phlegm and relief of the blockage by regulating Liver qi and/or strengthening Spleen qi. Helpful polyherbal formulas include *Xiao Yao San*, *Di Tan Tang*, *Er Chen Tang*, *Yang Xin Tang*, *Si Jun Zi Tang*, and *Di Tang*.

Manic, aggressive, hyperreactive, and irritable symptoms (*kuang*) are consistent with excessive yang or yin deficiency and overactive Fire, although qi and blood stagnation may also be involved. Chinese herbal prescriptions for these diagnoses might include *Er Yin Jian* and *Ding Zhi Wan* to enhance yin and reduce Fire to calm the mind. Relevant formulas to improve qi or blood stasis include *Dian Kuang Meng Xing Tang* and *Tao Hong Si Wu Tang*. Other formulations used in TCM to treat mental and emotional symptoms include *Tian Wang Bu Xin Tang* for the regulation of Heart and Kidney Yin Deficiency, and *Wen Dan Tang* and *Huang Lian Jie Du Tang* for the relief of excess Fire.

The TCM formula *Xiao Huo Luo Dan* (Minor Invigorate the Collateral Circulation Pill) has been suggested as a treatment for pet behavior problems such as compulsive disorders (Wynn, Marsden 2003). However, it is not advised for long-term administration, which limits its clinical usefulness; it is more appropriately intended for use as a treatment of joint stiffness, rheumatism, and painful joints (Wynn, Marsden 2003; Tierra 1998; Bensky, Gamble 1993). Considering that many of the compulsive disorders in pets are characterized by restlessness and agitation, a formula that is meant to promote further motion might even be considered contraindicated for the treatment of problem behaviors. From a TCM perspective, this formula is meant to restore the circulation, and there is some basis for its recommendation, although other formulas seem more appropriate. Similarly, *Zhen Gan Xi Feng Tang* (Subdue the Endogenous Liver Wind Decoction) has been suggested for the treatment of compulsive pets. It is used to treat unsettled Liver yang accompanied by dizziness, headache, movement progressive motor dysfunction, and mental confusion (Bensky, Gamble 1993). Its use seems limited, in part because this description of its function seems inconsistent with most misbehavior in pets from a Western perspective, but also from the Chinese perspective, which teaches that Heart and Spleen would be of primary consideration. In particular, alternative formulas are advised because its ingredients require the sacrifice of other animals (Table 4-4).

Xue Fu Zhu Yu Tang (Blood Mansion Expel Blood Stasis Decoction) could be of interest in the treatment of a variety of behavior disorders in pets. It is traditionally used to treat depression, chronic chest pain, palpitations, restlessness, irritability, mood swings, and headaches. It invigorates the Blood and resolves Blood stasis in the upper warmer. Among other components, it contains *Angelica sinensis* and Bupleurum root, both of which are discussed in detail later in this chapter (Schoen, Wynn 1998). This formula could be useful in the control of compulsive behavior, agitated forms of separation anxiety syndrome, and irritable aggression in pets.

Long Dan Xie Gan Tang (Gentian Drain Liver Decoction) has been suggested to treat compulsive behavior in pets (Wynn, Marsden 2003). However, it seems more appropriate for the treatment of house-soiling pets accompanied by agitated moods. This formula clears Liver Gallbladder Heat and is traditionally used to treat urinary dysfunction, headache, dizziness, irritability and anger, and Internal Dampness. Nonetheless, urine-marking pets suffering from separation anxiety syndrome or triggered by territorial conflict between house pets might benefit from this remedy.

Tian Wang Bu Xin Dan (Celestial Emperor Heart-Supplementing Elixir) is a leading candidate among Chinese polyherbal recipes for the treatment of pet misbehavior. It contains Ginseng, Codonopsis, Angelica, Schisandra, and Jujube, ground to a fine powder and blended with honey. The formula is based on TCM principles aimed at supplementing the Heart, which is at the root of most emotional dysfunction according to TCM philosophy. It also soothes the spirit and resolves yin-blood insufficiency. The recommended dose is 6 to 9 g twice a day or once at bedtime (Zhong, Wiseman, Ellis 1996b). Clinical trials are warranted.

Individual Chinese herbs of greatest interest to veterinary behavior medicine are discussed below. Miscellaneous Chinese herbs are briefly presented later in this section. Herbs that are common to other ethnobotanical traditions such as Ayurveda are mentioned in other relevant sections. *Scutellaria baicalensis* (*Huang*

Table 4-4. Ingredients of Polyherbal Formulas of Traditional Chinese Medicine Relevant to Veterinary Behavior Medicine[1]

TCM Formula	Ingredients	Reference
Banxia Houpu	*Pinellia ternata, Poria cocos, Magnolia officinalis, Perilla frutescens, Zingiber officinale*	Luo, Nong Wang, Kong et al 2000
Di Dang Tang (Dead-On Decoction)	Leech (Shui zhi), Tabanus (Meng chong), Rhubarb, (Da huang), Peach kernel (Tao ren)	Zhong, Wiseman, Ellis 1996
Er Chen Tang (Two Ancient Herb Decoction)	Pinellia (Ban Xia) Ju Hong (pericarpium citri erythrocarpae), Poria (Fu ling), Licorice (Gan Cao)	Bensky, Gamble 1993
Huang Lian Jie Du Tang (Coptis Resolve Toxin Decoction)	Coptis (Huang lian), Phellodendron (Huang bo), Gardenia (Shan zhi zi), Scutellaria (Huang qin)	Zhong, Wiseman, Ellis 1996
Long Dan Xie Gan (Gentian Drain Liver Decoction)	Long Dan Cao (Gentian), Huang Qin (Scutellaria), Zhi Zi (Gardenia fruit), Mu Tong (Akebia stem), Che Qian Zi (Plantago seed), Ze Xie (Alisma tuber), Chai Hu (Bupleurum root), Sheng Di Huang (Rehmannia root), Dang Gui (Angelica root), Gan Cao (Licorice root);	Schoen, Wynn 1998; Bensky, Gamble 1993
Si Jun Zi Tang	Ginseng (Ren shen) or Codonopsis (Dang shen), Atractylodes (Cang zhu), Poria (Fu ling), Licorice (Gan cao)	Tierra 1998
Tao Hong Si Wu Tang (Peach Kernel and Carthamus Four Agents Decoction)	Peach kernel (Tao ren), Carthamus (Hong hua), Tangkuei (Dang gui), Rehmannia (Shou di huang), White peony (Bai shao yao), Ligusticum (Chuan xiong)	Zhong, Wiseman, Ellis 1996)
Tian Wang Bu Xin Dan (Celestial Emperor Heart-Supplementing Elixir)	Rehmannia (Sheng di huang), Ginseng (Ren shen), Asparagus (Tian men dong), Ophiopogon (Mai men dong), Scrophylaria (Xuan shen), Savlia miltiorrhiza (Dan shen), Poria (Fu ling), Plygala (Yuan zhi),	Zhong, Wiseman, Ellis 1996
Tian Wang Bu Xin Tang *is the decoction of this formula*	Tangkuei (Dang gui), Schisandra (Wu wei zi), Biota seed (Bo zi ren), Jujube (Suan zao ren), Platycodon (Jie geng) and Cinnabar (Zhu sha)	
Wen Dan Tang (Warm the Gallbladder Decoction)	Pinellia (Ban xia), Tangerine pell (Chen pi), Poria (Fu ling), Licorice (Gan cao), Bamboo shavings (Zhu ru), Unripe Bitter orage (Zhi shi), Ginger (Sheng jiang) and Jujube (Da zao)	Zhong, Wiseman, Ellis 1996
Xiao Huo Luo Dan	Zhi Cao Wu (radix aconiti kusnezoffii praeparata), Zhi Chuan Wu (radix aconiti carmichaeli praeparata), Tian Nan Xing (rhizoma arisaematis), Mo Yao (Myrrhe), Ru Xiang (Frankincense), Di Long (lumbricus)	Bensky, Gamble 1993
Xiao Yao San (Free Wanderer Powder)	Bupleurum (Chai hu), Ovate Atractylodes (Bai zhu), Tangkuei (Dang gui), White peony (Bai shao yao), Poria (Fu ling), Mint (Bo he), Licorice (Gan cao), Ginger (Sheng jiang)	Zhong, Wiseman, Ellis 1996

Xue Fu Zhu Yu Tang (Blood Mansion Expel Blood Stasis Decoction)	Tao Ren (Persica seed), Hong Hua (Carthamus), Dang Gui (Chinese Angelica root), Chuan Xiong (Ligusticum rhizome), Chi Shao (Red Peony root), Niu Xi (Achyranthes root), Chai Hu (Bupleurum root), Jie Geng (Platycodon root), Zhi Qiao (Bitter Orange), Sheng Di Huang (Rehmannia root), Gan Cao (Licorice root)	Schoen, Wynn 1998; Bensky, Gamble 1993
Yang Xin Tang (Nourish the Heart Decoction)	Codonopsis (Dang shen), Astragalus (Huang qi), Tangkuei (Dang gui), Root Poria (Fu shen), Poria (Fu ling), Cinnamon bark (Rou gui), Biota seed (Bo zi ren), Spiny Jujube (Suan zo ren), Polygala (Yuan zhi), Ligusticum (Chuan xiong), Schisandra (We wei zi), Pinellia (Ban xia), Licorice (Gan cao)	Zhong, Wiseman, Ellis 1996
Zhen Gan Xi Feng Tang (Subdue Endogenous Liver Wind Decoction)	Huai Niu Xi (Achyranthis root), Zhi Shi (haematitum), Long Gu (Dragon bone), Mu Li (Oyster shell), Gui Ban (Tortoise plastrum), Xuan Shen (Scrophularia), Tian Men Dong (Asparagus tuber), Bai Shao (Peony root), Yin Chen Hao (Capillaris), Chuan Lian Zi (Toosendan fruit), Mai Ya (Barley sprout), Gan Cao (Licorice root)	Bensky, Gamble 1993

[1]Although not tabulated, the TCM formulas *Dian Kuang Meng Xing*, *Tang Ding Zhi Wa*, *Er Yin Jian*, and *Di Tan Tang* may also be of interest.

Table 4-5. Common Pinyin Prefixes and Suffixes in Traditional Chinese Herbal Prescriptions[1]

Pinyin Prefix	Significance or Meaning	Example	Pinyin Suffix
Chao	Stir-fried	Chao bai shao (White Peony)	
Gan	Dried root or rhizome	Gan jiang (dried ginger); Gan di huang (dried rehmannia root); Gan cao (dried licorice root)	
Sheng	Fresh, raw	Sheng mai san; Sheng jiang (Fresh Ginger root)	
Zhi	Honey-baked, fried	Zhi gui zhi (Cinnamon); Zhi gan cao (Licorice)	
	Elixir	Tian wang bu xin dan	***Dan***
	Root	Houpo gen (Magnolia)	***Gen***
	Flower	Houpo hua (Magnolia)	***Hua***
	Bark, peel	Rou gui pi (Cinnamon bark)	***Pi***
	Seed	Huma ren (Sesame);	***Ren***
	Powder	Xiao yao san; Sheng mai san	***San***
	Root (Radix); also signifies Spirit or Mind	Dan shen; Dang shen, Ren shen; Hong shen	***Shen***
	Decoction	Long dan xie gan tang; Chai hu gui zhi tang; Wen Dan Tang	***Tang***
	Pill	Shen qi wan; Ci zhu wan	***Wan***
	Solution, liquid	Sheng mai ye	***Ye***
	Leaf	Yin xing ye (Ginkgo)	***Ye***
	Drink, liquid	Sheng mai yin	***Yin***
	Oil	Rou gui you (Cinnamon oil)	***You***
	Fruit, seed, berry	Sha yuan zi (Astragalus)	***Zi***

[1] Compiled with the assistance of Dr. Phil Rogers, MRCVS, Dublin, Ireland.

qin, Chinese Scullcap), for example, is discussed in context with *Scutellaria lateriflora* in the section on Native American herbal medicine.

References

Anonymous. Chinese Medicine History. http://www.taijichinesemedicine.com/TCMhistory.htm, 2004.

Anonymous. Classics of Traditional Chinese Medicine. National Library of Medicine Online, History of Medicine Division, http://www.nlm.nih.gov/hmd/chinese/emperors.html, 2000.

Mills S, Bone K. Principles and Practice of Phytotherapy. Churchill Livingstone, Philadelphia, PA 2000; 5–10.

Schoen AM, Wynn SG. Complementary and Alternative Veterinary Medicine: Principles and Practice. Mosby Inc., Philadelphia, PA. 1998;420–421, 433.

Tierra M. The Way of Chinese Herbs. Pocket Books, New York, NY. 1998;2–28.

Wynn SG, Marsden S. Manual of Natural Veterinary Medicine: Science and Tradition. Mosby Inc, Philadelphia, PA. 2003;62, 373.

Zhong YX, Wiseman N, Ellis A. Fundamentals of Chinese medicine. Paradigm Publications; Brookline, MA. 1996a;1–48; 1996b;399.

Angelica sinensis

Angelica sinensis (*Dang gui*, Tangkuei, Angelicae Sinensis Radix, Chinese Angelica, Dong quai, Toki) is a perennial member of the *Apiaceae* (*Umbelliferae*) family, which also includes *Centella spp.*, *Bupleurum spp.*, and carrots. *A. sinensis* is indigenous to Asia. It grows 0.5 to 1 m tall and has fragrant white flowers born on umbels.

The medicinal root has a head, body, and tail. In TCM, the head is considered to be particularly tonic whereas the tail is prized as a Blood mover. *A. sinensis* is considered to be Warm in energy and Sweet and Bitter in flavor. It affects the Heart, Liver, and Spleen channels and is considered a Blood tonic. It is traditionally used as an analgesic and to treat menstrual problems, headache, dizziness, and other symptoms of Blood deficiency (vacuity).

A close relative, *Angelica archangelica* grows in the wild in many parts of Eastern Europe, although it may be indigenous to Syria, Holland, or Poland (Mills, Bone 2000; PDR 2000). Native Americans were familiar with a variety of Angelica species (Moerman 2002). The majority was used for alleviating physical ailments, although the Lolahnkok tribe used it as a love medicine and the Mendocino applied a poultice of Angelica root to treat recurrent nightmares.

Ingredients

Identified compounds include phytosterols (e.g., angelicone, angelol) and essential oil (Mills, Bone 2000).

Clinical Efects

A. sinensis is often found in products marketed for use as aphrodisiacs; however, there is no evidence to support this effect (Mills, Bone 2000). In a recent clinical trial in Israel, 55 post-menopausal women participated in a study of a commercial preparation marketed for use as an alternative treatment for hot flashes (Kupfersztain, Rotem, Fagot et al. 2003). The group treated with a combination of *Matricaria chamomilla* (Chamomile) and *A. sinensis* reported a 90% reduction in symptoms compared with 10% reduction reported in the control group. However, other studies do not support *A. sinensis* as an alternative treatment of menopausal symptoms (Huntley, Ernst 2003).

One study on rats determined a slight improvement in learning acquisition following treatment with a traditional Chinese formula containing *A. sinensis* (*Dang gui shao yao san)* (Lu 2001). Unfortunately, studies of polyherbal formulations cannot make fair conclusions about the effectiveness of a single ingredient.

Availability

A. sinensis is prepared as a medicinal wine or is available in pills and powders (*Dang gui san*), which may be made into a paste for topical application. Other formulas include *Dang gui liu huang wan* (Angelica, Astragalus, Coptis mixture for the treatment of agitated and hyperactive conditions such as hyperthyroid disease characterized by deficiency of yin and Blood and Hyperactivity of Fire) and *Dang gui shao yao san* (*A. sinensis* with Peony for the treatment of abdominal bloating and gestational discomfort associated with Internal Dampness and stagnation of qi and

Blood due to Liver Deficiency). *A. sinensis* is one of the ingredients in Tangkuei, Gentian, and Aloe Pill (*Dang gui long hui wan*, used for the treatment of constipation and hypertension, for example, as it relieves Liver Fire) and Tangkuei Six Yellows Decoction (*Dang gui liu huang tang*), used to treat yin deficiency fire, "Vexing Heat in the Five Hearts" and enrich yin (Zhong, Wiseman, Abel 1996).

Clinical Application in Veterinary Behavior Medicine

There does not appear to be any firm scientific evidence to support a behavioral or psychological effect of *A. chinensis*. However, many herbs are best applied in polyherbal formulas for a synergistic effect. Based upon TCM principles and anecdotal reports of success, *Dang gui liu huang wan* might be helpful in the treatment of feline hyperesthesia syndrome. *Tangkuei Six Yellows Decoction* also contains *Scutellaria baicalensis* and *Astragalus membranaceus*, among other ingredients, and could be of value in treating pet behaviors characterized by aggressive conflicts between pets, or aggression directed toward the pet's guardian. Future clinical investigation will authenticate or refute these suggestions.

References

DSM-IV (Diagnostic and Statistical Manual of Mental Disorders) 4th ed. American Psychiatric Association, Washington, DC. 1994;715–718.

Huntley AL, Ernst E. A systematic review of herbal medicinal products for the treatment of menopausal symptoms. Menopause. 2003;10:465–476.

Kupfersztain C, Rotem C, Fagot R et al. The immediate effect of natural plant extract, *Angelica sinensis* and *Matricaria chamomilla* (Climex) for the treatment of hot flashes during menopause. A preliminary report. Clin Exp Obstet Gynecol. 2003;30:203–206.

Lu MC. Danggui shaoyao san improves colchichine-induced learning acquisition impairment in rats. Acta Pharmacol Sin. 2001;22:1149–1153.

Mills S, Bone K. Principles and Practice of Phytotherapy. Churchill Livingstone, Philadelphia, PA. 2000; 350–353.

Moerman DE. Native American Ethnobotany. Timber Press, Portland, OR. 2002;73–76.

PDR for Herbal Medicines. (2nd ed) Medical Economics Company Inc., Montvale, NJ. 2000;32–34.

Zhong YX, Wiseman N, Ellis A. Fundamentals of Chinese medicine. Paradigm Publications; Brookline, MA. 1996;347, 368.

Astragalus membranaceus

Astragalus membranaceus (*Huang qi,* Astragali radix, Membranous Milk Vetch, Tragacanth, Bei qi, Ougi, Ogi) is one of the major herbs of Oriental medicine. A member of the pea family (*Leguminosae*), *A. membranaceus* grows in the north and south of China, Japan, and Korea. The hardy perennial grows 1.5 to 2.0 m tall. Pinnate leaves have numerous leaflets and soft hairs. Small, bluish-purple flowers are followed by seedpods that are characteristically square in cross-section. The medicinal part of the plant is the impressively long root that grows at least 20 to 30 feet into the ground; there are also many lateral roots (Mills, Bone 2000; PDR

2000). *A. membranaceus* (*Huang qi*) should not be confused with *Scutellaria baicalensis* (*Huang qin*, Chinese Scullcap), which is described along with *S. lateriflora*, its Western and Native American herbal counterpart.

Other Astragalus species, such as *A. australis* and *A. canadensis* among many others, were well known to Native Americans and used medicinally for the treatment of respiratory ailments, fever, digestive disorders, and skin infection. Astragalus species were also used as analgesia and as food for both people and livestock. The Chippewa used *A. crassicarpus* (Groundplum Milkvetch) as a stimulant and tonic; the Omaha and Ponca used it as a ceremonial item (Moerman 2002). Some species, such as *A. lusitanicus*, are referred to as the "locoweeds" because they contain high concentrations of selenium that may cause cardiotoxicity, respiratory depression, and neuromuscular effects. *A. membranaceus* is not among the species associated with selenium toxicity (Mills, Bone 2000; PDR 2000).

Traditionally, it is considered to be an adaptogenic, diuretic, antioxidant, immunostimulant, and tonic medicine but is not recommended for treatment of acute illness (Mills, Bone 2000).

Ingredients

Active compounds of *A. membranaceus* include tragacanth, phytosterols, fatty acids (e.g., linolenic acid), amino acids (e.g., GABA, canavanine), saponins (e.g., astragalosides, chycloastragenol, chyclocanthosides), isoflavonoids (e.g., astrasieversianin) and triterpene glycosides (e.g., brachyosides, astrachrysosides, cyclocephalosides) (PDR 2000; Hirotani, Zhou, Rui et al. 1994).

Seasonal fluctuations and plant maturity influence the chemical components of *A. membranaceus* (Ma, Shi, Duan et al. 2002). This is an important consideration in the quality control of most, if not all, herbal medicinal preparations.

CNS and Neuroprotective Effects

A. membranaceus has emerged as a candidate for treating cognitive impairment. In separate studies, an aqueous extract of *A. membranaceus* (Hong, Qin, Huang 1994) and *A. membranaceus* as an ingredient in a polyherbal formula (Liu, Yang, Zheng 1993) improved memory-related cognitive function in mice; a cholinergic mechanism was suggested. An antisenility effect was determined for *Shou xing bu zhi*, a polyherbal remedy containing *A. membranaceus* (Chen 1989); however, with thirteen herbs in the formula, it is impossible to determine what effect if any could be attributed to any single component. Another herbal mixture containing 84% *A. membranaceus* (*Bu yang huan wu tang*; Tillotson, Tillotson, Abel 2001) showed an antioxidant neuroprotective effect in the brain.

Miscellaneous Effects

Chinese studies show that *A. membranaceus* stimulates sperm motility (Hong, Ku, Wu 1992) and antibody response (Zhao KS, Mancini C, Doria 1990). Laboratory and clinical findings support its traditional use. In TCM, *A. membranaceus* enters through the Lung and Spleen channels and is therefore ideal to boost associated organs and diseases. It has a warming, detoxifying effect that enhances qi and yang qi and balances the flow of fluids. It is contraindicated in cases of "Yin Deficiency with Yang Exuberance" because, as is true of *Codonopsis pilosula* (*Dang shen*), *Panax ginseng* (*Ren shen*) and *Zingiber officinale* (dried Ginger, *Gan jiang*), *A. membranaceus* stimulates yang (Zhong, Wiseman, Ellis 1996).

A. membranaceus is a major ingredient of the Kampo herbal formula *Ougi-Keishi-gomotsu-to*. Scientific investigation has revealed evidence to support its efficacy in the treatment of cancer (Cheng, Hou, Zhang et al. 2004; Cui, He, Wang et al. 2003), herpes virus (Sun, Yang 2004), osteoporosis (Kim, Ha, Lee et al. 2003), inflammation (Zhang, Hufnagl, Binder et al. 2003), ischemic cardiomyopathy (Lei, Gao, Li 2003), hepatic cirrhosis (Tan, Yin, Yu 2001; Zhang, Wen, Liu 1990), antioxidant (Toda, Yase, Shirataki 2000), and cerebral ischemia (Quan, Du 1998).

Availability

A. membranaceus is combined with *Panax ginseng* (*Ren shen*) to make *Bu zhong yi qi tang*, a classic vitality booster, and may also be mixed with *Dang shen* (*Salvia miltiorrhiza*). A combination of *A. membranaceus* and *Angelica sinensis* known as "Dang-Gui Decoction for Enriching the Blood" is used for stimulating erythropoiesis and as a cardiotonic agent (Yim, Wu, Pak et al. 2000).

A. membranaceus is administered orally in the form of a decoction, paste, pill, or powders. It may also be stir-fried with honey to boost qi and blood stagnation (*bi*); however, it is also used raw to expel toxins from the body (Zhong, Wiseman, Ellis 1996). It is often added to polyherbal formulas to boost their potency and is an ingredient of the general qi-boosting remedy known as the Four Gentlemen Decoction (Four Nobles Decoction, *Si jun zi tang*) (Zhong, Wiseman, Ellis 1996).

Daily human dosage is 10 to 30 g of the dried root by decoction and 4 to 8 ml of standard liquid extract, although larger doses may be prescribed depending on the severity of the symptoms (Mills, Bone 2002).

Clinical Application in Veterinary Behavior Medicine

A. membranaceus has promising evidence for its application in senile cognitive dysfunction and may be of value in treating canine and feline cognitive dysfunction syndromes. It may best be applied in polyherbal preparations with other neuroprotective and antioxidant herbs. Further investigation is warranted.

References

Chen J. An experimental study on the anti-senility effects of shou xing bu zhi. Zhong Xi Yi Jie He Za Zhi. 1989;9:226–227, 198.

Cheng XD, Hou CH, Zhang XJ et al. Effects of Huangqi (Hex) on Inducing Cell Differentiation and Cell Death in K562 and HEL Cells. Sheng Wu Hua Xue Yu Sheng Wu Wu Li Xue Bao (Shanghai). 2004;36:211–217.

Cui R, He J, Wang B et al. Suppressive effect of *Astragalus membranaceus* Bunge on chemical hepatocarcinogenesis in rats. Cancer Chemother Pharmacol. 2003;51:75–80.

Hirotani M, Zhou Y, Rui H et al. Cycloartane triterpene glycosides from the hairy root cultures of *Astragalus membranaceus*. Phytochemistry. 1994;37:1403–1407.

Hong CY, Ku J, Wu P. *Astragalus membranaceus* stimulates human sperm motility in vitro. Am J Chin Med. 1992;20:289–294.

Hong GX, Qin WC, Huang LS. Memory-improving effect of aqueous extract of *Astragalus membranaceus* (Fisch.) Bge. Zhongguo Zhong Yao Za Zhi. 1994;19:687–688, 704.

Kim C, Ha H, Lee JH et al. Herbal extract prevents bone loss in ovariectomized rats. Arch Pharm Res. 2003;26:917–924.

Lei Y, Gao Q, Li YS. Study on effects of astragalus, angelica and their combination on vascular endothelial cell proliferation in vitro. Zhongguo Zhong Xi Yi Jie He Za Zhi. 2003;23:753–756.

Liu ZY, Yang YG, Zheng B. Effect of improving memory and inhibiting acetylcholinesterase activity by invigorating-qi and warming-yang recipe. Zhongguo Zhong Xi Yi Jie He Za Zhi. 1993;13:675–676, 646.

Ma XQ, Shi Q, Duan JA et al. Chemical analysis of Radix Astragali (Huangqi) in China: a comparison with its adulterants and seasonal variations. J Agric Food Chem. 2002;50:4861–4866.

Mills S, Bone K. Principles and Practice of Phytotherapy. Churchill Livingstone, Philadelphia, PA. 2000;273–279.

Moerman DE. Native American Ethnobotany. Timber Press, Portland, OR. 2002;112–114.

PDR for Herbal Medicines. (2nd ed) Medical Economics Company Inc., Montvale, NJ. 2000:54–57.

Quan J, Du G. Protective effect of *Astragalus membranaceus* (Fisch.) Bge. and *Hedysarum polybotrys* Hand.-Mazz. on experimental model of cerebral ischemia in rats. Zhongguo Zhong Yao Za Zhi. 1998;23:371–373.

Sun Y, Yang J. Experimental study of the effect of Astragalus membranaceus against herpes simplex virus type 1. Di Yi Jun Yi Da Xue Xue Bao. 2004;24:57–58.

Tan YW, Yin YM, Yu XJ. Influence of *Salvia miltiorrhizae* and *Astragalus membranaceus* on hemodynamics and liver fibrosis indexes in liver cirrhotic patients with portal hypertension. Zhongguo Zhong Xi Yi Jie He Za Zhi. 2001;21:351–353.

Tierra M. The Way of Chinese Herbs. Pocket Books, New York, NY 1998;67.

Tillotson AK, Tillotson HSH, Abel R. The One Earth Herbal Sourcebook. Kensington Publishing, New York, NY 2001;102–104.

Toda S, Yase Y, Shirataki Y. Inhibitory effects of Astragali Radix, crude drug in Oriental medicines on lipid peroxidation and protein oxidative modification of mouse brain homogenate by copper. Phytother Res. 2000;14:294–296.

Yim TK, Wu WK, Pak WF et al. Myocardial protection against ischaemia-reperfusion injury by a *Polygonum multiflorum* extract supplemented "Dang-Gui decoction for enriching blood," a compound formulation, ex vivo. Phytother Res. 2000;14:195–199.

Zhao KS, Mancini C, Doria G. Enhancement of the immune response in mice by *Astragalus membranaceus* extracts. Immunopharmacology. 1990;20:225–233.

Zhang WJ, Hufnagl P, Binder BR et al. Antiinflammatory activity of astragaloside IV is mediated by inhibition of NF-kappaB activation and adhesion molecule expression. Thromb Haemost. 2003;90: 904–914.

Zhang ZL, Wen QZ, Liu CX. Hepatoprotective effects of astragalus root. J Ethnopharmacol. 1990;30: 145–149.

Zhong YX, Wiseman N, Ellis A. Fundamentals of Chinese medicine. Paradigm Publications; Brookline, MA. 1996;197, 346.

Bupleurum chinense

Bupleurum chinense (Chai hu, Bupleurum Root, Chinese Thoroughwax, Thorowax, Hare's Ear) is a wild perennial plant of China, Japan, and central Europe and a member of the carrot family (*Umbelliferae*). It grows approximately 40 to 80 cm tall. The plant's marginal-veined leaves, which are arranged in spirals, are the inspiration for its English name of Hare's Ear. The stem is hollow, branched, and gnarly. The medicinal part of the plant is the dried root. Those who collect the plant must be especially careful not to confuse it with *B. longiradiatum*, which is poisonous (Mills, Bone 2000; PDR 2000; Tierra 1998). *Bupleurum chinense* is the variety best known in China. *Bupleurum falcatum var. komarowi* is of Japanese origin but is now cultivated for use elsewhere, including China and Taiwan. *Bupleurum kaoi* is the species indigenous to Taiwan (Lin, Yen, Chen et al. 1991).

In TCM philosophy, the shape or color of the plant provides insight into its medicinal action. This "Doctrine of Signatures" alludes to the divine clues provided by the plant's physical traits that guide the application of the plant's medicinal use. In the case of *B. chinense*, for example, the symbolism of the free-flowing shape of its branches is thought to stimulate the unblocking of stagnating energy and excessive emotion so that energy flows smoothly, is evenly distributed throughout the individual's being, and balance is restored (Tillotson, Tillotson, Abel 2001).

In TCM, *B. chinense* is considered to be Cool in energy with pungent and bitter flavors. It affects the Liver and Gallbladder and is considered to be a triple warmer that raises the yang, clears Heat, and adjusts stagnant Liver qi (Tierra 1998). Symptoms associated with stagnant Liver qi include depression, menstrual irregularity and dysmenorrhea, and chest pain (Zhong, Wiseman, Ellis 1996). *B. chinense* is said to warm up cold extremities caused by tension, to reduce psychological stress, release anxiety, boost the immune system, stimulate bile, protect the liver, and improve digestion overall (Tillotson, Tillotson, Abel 2001).

Ingredients

B. chinense contains polyynes (e.g., saikodiines), triterpenes saponins (e.g., saikosides, saikosaponins, saikogenins); polysaccharides (e.g., bupleurans); and phytosterols (e.g., spinasterol, stigmasterol) (Liu, Liang, Zhao et al. 2001; Mills, Bone 2000; PDR 2000; Liang, Zhao, Bai et al. 1998; Ebata, Nakajima, Hayashi et al. 1996) (Fig. 4-1).

CNS Effects

In an interesting comparative study on children between the ages of 7 and 14 years with a diagnosis of minimal brain dysfunction including symptoms of hyperactivity, the standard treatment of Western medicine (Ritalin®) was compared

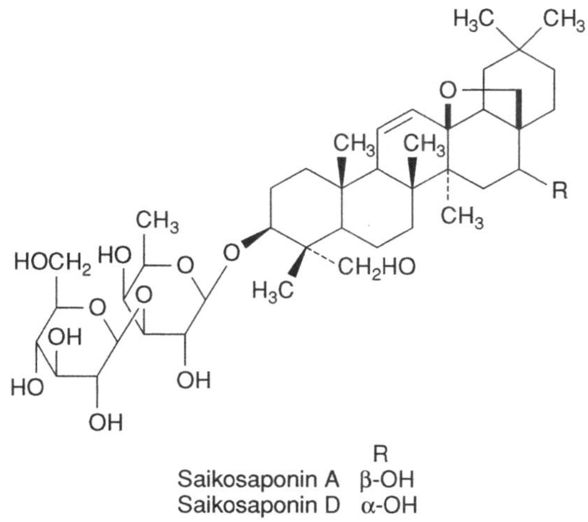

FIGURE 4-1. Active compounds of *Bupleurum chinense.* (Mills, Bone 2000)

to a TCM formula containing *B. chinense, Scutellaria baicalensis*, and *Astragalus membranaceus* among others (Zhang, Huang 1990). Results showed no significant difference between the two treatment groups except that there were fewer side effects, greater improvement to measures of IQ, and enuresis in the TCM group. An early Japanese study indicated that *B. falcatum* had a central depressant activity (Takagi, Shibata 1969). *B. chinense* has also shown a sedative effect in some patients (Mills, Bone 2000; PDR 2000).

Miscellaneous Effects

Clinical evidence of medicinal Bupleurum species supports their anti-inflammatory, antitussive, antihypertensive, anti-ulcerative (Matsumoto, Sun, Hanawa et al. 2002), immunogenic (Guo, Matsumoto, Kikuchi et al. 2000), and analgesic properties. There is also evidence to support the hepatoprotective effects suggested by TCM. In particular, Minor Bupleurum Decoction (*Xiao chai hu tang*; see Table 4-6) was particularly effective in reducing histopathological changes and serum biochemical changes associated with hepatic injury (Yen, Lin, Chuang et al. 1991).

Availability

B. chinense is available alone or in a variety of polyherbal formulations. For example, *Xiao Yao Wan* (Bupleurum Sedative Pills) is a commercial preparation marketed as a sedative and mood stabilizer that is considered particularly effective for conditions such as premenstrual dysphoric disorder (PMDD) and the less severe premenstrual syndrome (PMS) (DSM IV, 1994). *B. chinense* is more typically used in polyherbal formulas recommended to treat fever, jaundice, gynecological

Table 4-6. Summary of Ingredients in Harmonizing Formulas Containing *Bupleurum chinensis* (*Chai hu*)

Harmonizing Formula	Ingredients	Actions
Minor Bupleurum Decoction (*Xiao chai hu tang*)	Bupleurum, Scutellaria, Pinellia, Fresh Ginger, Ginseng, Licorice, Jujube	Harmonizes the Lesser Yang; eliminates Evils; treats Vexation, bitter taste in the mouth
Bupleurum and Cinnamon Twig Decoction (*Chai hu gui-zhi tang*)	Bupleurum, Pinellia, Scutellaria, Fresh Ginger, Ginseng, Cinnamon Twig, Peony, Licorice, Jujube	Harmonizes the Lesser Yang and Greater Yang; treats aversion to cold, joint pain, oppressive distention below the Heart
Major Bupleurum Decoction (*Da chai hu tang*)	Bupleurum, Scutellaria, Pinellia, Unripe Bitter Orange, Rhubarb, White Peony, Fresh Ginger, Jujube	Harmonizes the Lesser Yang; treats constipation, abdominal pain
Bupleurum Liver-Coursing Powder (*Chai hu shu gan san*)	Bupleurum, White Peony, Licorice, Bitter Orange, Lgusticum, Cyperus, Tangerine Peel	Clears the Liver and quickens the Blood; resolves depression; boosts Liver qi
Free Wanderer Powder (*Xiao yao san*)	Bupleurum, Ovate Atractylodes, Tangkuei, White Peony, Poria, Mint Licorice, Roasted Ginger	Clears the Liver and nourishes the Blood; treats Liver depression, headache, dizziness, menstrual disorders, liver disease

(Zhong, Wiseman, Ellis 1996)

disorders, nausea, vomiting, chest pain, headache, dizziness, malaria, and deafness (PDR 2000; Zhong, Wiseman, Ellis 1996). It is one of the ingredients consistently found in Minor Bupleurum Decoction (*Xiao chai hu tang*); Bupleurum and Cinnamon Twig Decoction (*Chai hu gui-zhi tang*); Major Bupleurum Decoction (*Da chai hu tang*); Bupleurum Liver-Coursing Powder (*Chai hu shu gan san*); and Free Wanderer Powder (*Xiao yao san*), collectively known as the Harmonizing Formulas summarized in Table 4-6 (Zhong, Wiseman, Ellis 1996).

The daily human dosage of *B. chinense* decoction is 2.4 to 4.5 g. It is also available in pills and powdered form (1 to 4 g per day) and as crude herb (3 to 12 g per day). Dosage may be higher if used in polyherbal formulas (Tillotson, Tillotson, Abel 2001; Mills, Bone 2000; Zhong, Wiseman, Ellis 1996).

Adverse Effects

B. chinense is not recommended during pregnancy, although side effects are not expected and drug interactions have not been reported so far (Tillotson, Tillotson, Abel 2001; Mills, Bone 2000; Zhong, Wiseman, Ellis 1996).

There is evidence for the risk of serious side effects associated with the use of Minor Bupleurum Decoction (e.g., interstitial pneumonitis) and mild to moderate digestive upset with *B. chinense* root alone (Mills, Bone 2000). Toxicological studies have also pointed to problems associated with Kampo formulas containing B. falcatum such as Sho-saiko-to and Saiko-keishi-to (Ikegami, Fujii, Ishihara et al. 2003).

Clinical Application in Veterinary Behavior Medicine

Despite its reputation and traditional use for alleviating anxiety and mood, little data was found to substantiate these claims. *B. chinense* products for the treatment of behavior problems in pets should be cautiously used, if at all, pending confirmation of their psychoactive benefits and accompanying risk of adverse effects.

References

Ebata N, Nakajima K, Hayashi K et al. Saponins from the root of *Bupleurum falcatum*. Phytochemistry. 1996;41:895–901.

Guo Y, Matsumoto T, Kikuchi Y et al. Effects of a pectic polysaccharide from a medicinal herb, the roots of *Bupleurum falcatum* L. on interleukin 6 production of murine B cells and B cell lines. Immunopharmacology. 2000;49:307–316.

Ikegami F, Fujii Y, Ishihara K et al. Toxicological aspects of Kampo medicines in clinical use. Chem Biol Interact. 2003;145:235–250.

Liang H, Zhao Y, Bai Y et al. A new saikosaponin from *Bupleurum chinense* DC. Yao Xue Xue Bao. 1998;33:282–285.

Lin CC, Yen MH, Chen JY et al. Anatomical and histological studies of Bupleuri radix. Am J Chin Med. 1991;19:265–274.

Liu QX, Liang H, Zhao YY et al. Saikosaponin v-1 from roots of *Bupleurum chinense* DC. J Asian Nat Prod Res. 2001;3:139–144.

Matsumoto T, Sun XB, Hanawa T et al. Effect of the antiulcer polysaccharide fraction from *Bupleurum falcatum* L. on the healing of gastric ulcer induced by acetic acid in rats. Phytother Res. 2002;16:91–93.

Mills S, Bone K. Principles and Practice of Phytotherapy. Churchill Livingstone, Philadelphia, PA. 2000;313–318.

PDR for Herbal Medicines. (2nd ed) Medical Economics Company Inc., Montvale, NJ. 2000;187.

Takagi K, Shibata M. Pharmacological studies on *Bupleurum falcatum* L. I. Acute toxicity and central depressant action of crude saikosides. Yakugaku Zasshi. 1969;89:712–720.

Tierra M. The Way of Chinese Herbs. Pocket Books, New York, NY 1998;165–166.

Tillotson AK, Tillotson HSH, Abel R. The One Earth Herbal Sourcebook. Kensington Publishing, New York, NY. 2001;110–112.

Yen MH, Lin CC, Chuang CH et al. Evaluation of root quality of Bupleurum species by TLC scanner and the liver protective effects of "xiao-chai-hu-tang" prepared using three different Bupleurum species. J Ethnopharmacol. 1991;34:155–165.

Zhang H, Huang J. Preliminary study of traditional Chinese medicine treatment of minimal brain dysfunction: analysis of 100 cases. Zhong Xi Yi Jie He Za Zhi. 1990;10:278–279, 260.

Zhong YX, Wiseman N, Ellis A. Fundamentals of Chinese medicine. Paradigm Publications; Brookline, MA. 1996;268, 296–297, 374-375.

Corydalis yanhusuo

Corydalis yanhusuo (Yan hu suo, Corydalis cava, Squirrel Corn, Corydale à bulbe creux) is a European perennial that has been integrated into the traditional Chinese system of healing. It has become an important herb in TCM, influencing its name change, and is therefore included in this section. *C. yanhusuo* has brownish-red flowers resembling foxglove blooms that appear only after four years of growth. The plant grows as high as 30 cm and is a member of the *Fumariaceae*

(*Papaveraceae*) family. The tuberous rhizome is the medicinal part of the plant, which is collected either during fall dormancy or just prior to blooming in the spring. The rhizome becomes hollow as the season progresses (PDR 2000; Tierra 1998).

North American varieties include *Corydalis canadensis* (Turkey Corn) and *Corydalis aurea* (Scrambledeggs). Native Americans also used Corydalis species for a variety of purposes. For example, the Navajo used *C. aurea* as an antidiarrheal, disinfectant, analgesic, and antispasmodic. The Ojibwa used smoke from the root to revive patients and to clear the head (Moerman 2002).

In TCM, Yan hu suo is Warm in energy and considered to be Pungent and Bitter in flavor. It affects the Heart, Liver, Lung, and Stomach channels and is classified as a Blood-rectifying herb. Yan hu suo is used as an analgesic, to invigorate the Blood, and to circulate qi. Traditionally, *C. yanhusuo* was used for the treatment of traumatic injury, dysmenorrhea, postpartum complications and complaints, chest pain, intestinal spasm, hyperactivity, menstrual disorders, internal parasites, and skin infection (PDR 2000; Tierra 1998; Zhong, Wiseman, Ellis 1996).

Ingredients

Compounds include a complex mixture of at least forty isoquinoline alkaloids (e.g., corytuberin, corydalin, bulbocapnine), which are typical of the *Papaveraceae* (PDR 2000; Preininger, Thakur, Santavy 1976). A neuroactive alkaloid DL-tetrahydropalmatine (tetrahydropalmatine, THP) has become of particular interest in research.

CNS Effects

The mechanisms of action of *Corydalis spp.* remain unclear, although a number of neurotransmitter systems appear to be affected. In one study, *C. yanhusuo* demonstrated a significant impact on morphine withdrawal symptoms in rats, suggesting an opioid mechanism and its potential benefit in the treatment of morphine addiction (Yang, Kwok 1986). An opioid mechanism was also suggested by its modulation of enkephalins (Reimeier, Schneider, Schneider et al. 1995).

In a recent Turkish study (Orhan, Sener, Choudhary et al. 2004), *Corydalis solida* showed potent inhibition of butylcholinesterase and suggests the potential of a cholinergic mechanism in *C. yanhusuo.*

Aqueous extracts derived from *C. yanhusuo* were shown to enhance adrenaline levels; *Eschscholzia californica*, another member of the *Papaveraceae* family, extract inhibited the degradation of catecholamines. The combination of these two herbs is thought to result in a synergistic mechanism that maintains high catecholamine levels and explains the sedative, antidepressant and hypnotic activities of this herbal formula (Kleber, Schneider, Schafer et al. 1995).

Protoberberine type 2 alkaloids, but not protoberberine type 1 alkaloids, were recently shown to possess a selective affinity in binding to the $GABA_A$ receptor (Halbsguth, Meissner, Haberline 2003). GABAergic mechanisms characterize benzodiazepine activity as well and may shed additional light on the anxiolytic effects claimed for *C. yanhusuo*.

C. yanhusuo is now recognized as a mild sedative, hypnotic, spasmolytic, and hallucinogenic herb that is used to treat neuroses, mild depression, emotional disturbances, and Parkinson's-like symptoms (PDR 2000). A commercial preparation, marketed in Europe for the treatment of anxiety and insomnia and containing *C. yanhusuo* (20%) and *Eschscholzia californica* (80%), has confirmed sedative properties (Schafer, Schafer, Schneider et al. 1995).

Tetrahydropalmatine (THP) has been isolated from a variety of Corydalis species, including *Corydalis ambigua*, as well as from other herbs (*Stephania spp.*). It has analgesic, sedative, tranquilizing, and hypnotic effects by dopamine pathways (Zhu 1991). THP may also have anticonvulsant properties through inhibition of amygdaloid dopamine release (Lin, Wang, Young 2002; Chang, Lin 2001). THP demonstrated an anxiolytic effect in mice that was attributed to benzodiazepine sites at the $GABA_A$ receptor (Leung, Zheng, Huen et al. 2003). Tetrahydropalmatine also has antioxidant effects (Ng TB, Liu F, Wang 2000; Yang, Jiang, Tang et al. 2000) and possesses an antithyroid effect comparable to that of propylthiouracil, possibly through inhibition of the pituitary's release of thyroid-stimulating hormone (TSH) (Hsieh, Wu 1996).

Adverse Effects

Corydalis yanhusuo is traditionally contraindicated for use during pregnancy (Tierra 1998; Zhong, Wiseman, Ellis 1996), but serious side effects have been clinically reported. Chronic intake in adults results in hepatotoxicity. Adverse effects include neurological, respiratory, and cardiac depression (Lai, Chan 1999; Horowitz, Feldhaus, Dart et al. 1996).

Tetrahydropalmatine has become more popular as a recreational drug. A purified, concentrated preparation of THP containing between 500 and 1700 mg of THP has been associated with at least one suicide and numerous pediatric poisonings. THP is classified as a controlled substance and is banned by the U.S. Food and Drug Administration, as well as in other countries (Lai, Chan 1999; Horowitz, Feldhaus, Dart et al. 1996).

C. yanhusuo should be used with caution in patients diagnosed with hypothyroid disease.

Availability

The daily human dose is 3 to 9 g of dried Corydalis root in decoction, powders, and pills (Tierra 1998; Zhong, Wiseman, Ellis 1996).

It may be used raw to stimulate Blood stasis or stir-fried with vinegar to move qi and relieve abdominal pain (Tierra 1998; Zhong, Wiseman, Ellis 1996).

Clinical Application in Veterinary Behavior Medicine

C. yanhusuo is of interest for its anxiolytic properties in cases of mild to moderate anxiety. It has traditionally been used to treat hyperactivity and sleeplessness and so may find use in controlling agitation associated with anxiety (e.g., active forms of separation anxiety syndrome or compulsive behavior) or nonspecific agitation (e.g., nighttime activity in young pets). However, it may be best used in combination with other herbs in traditional recipes. The practice of concocting polyherbal formulas in Eastern medicine has the distinct advantage of minimizing the levels of potentially toxic components such as THP and, therefore, the risk of toxic effects.

References

Chang CK, Lin MT. DL-Tetrahydropalmatine may act through inhibition of amygdaloid release of dopamine to inhibit an epileptic attack in rats. Neurosci Lett. 2001;307:163–166.

Halbsguth C, Meissner O, Haberlein H. Positive cooperation of protoberberine type 2 alkaloids from *Corydalis cava* on the GABA(A) binding site. Planta Med. 2003;69:305–309.

Horowitz RS, Feldhaus K, Dart RC et al. The clinical spectrum of Jin Bu Huan toxicity. Arch Intern Med. 1996;156:899–903.

Hsieh MT, Wu LY. Inhibitory effects of (+/−)−tetrahydropalmatine on thyrotropin-stimulating hormone concentration in hyperthyroid rats. J Pharm Pharmacol. 1996;48:959–961.

Kleber E, Schneider W, Schafer HL et al. Modulation of key reactions of the catecholamine metabolism by extracts from *Eschscholtzia californica* and *Corydalis cava.* Arzneimittelforschung. 1995;45: 127–131.

Lai CK, Chan AY. Tetrahydropalmatine poisoning: diagnoses of nine adult overdoses based on toxicology screens by HPLC with diode-array detection and gas chromatography-mass spectrometry. Clin Chem. 1999;45:229–236.

Leung WC, Zheng H, Huen M et al. Anxiolytic-like action of orally administered dl-tetrahydropalmatine in elevated plus-maze. Prog Neuropsychopharmacol Biol Psychiatry. 2003;27:775–779.

Lin MT, Wang JJ, Young MS. The protective effect of dl-tetrahydropalmatine against the development of amygdala kindling seizures in rats. Neurosci Lett. 2002 March 8;320:113–136.

Moerman DE. Native American Ethnobotany. Timber Press, Portland, OR. 2002;181.

Ng TB, Liu F, Wang ZT. Antioxidative activity of natural products from plants. Life Sci. 2000;66:709–723.

Orhan I, Sener B, Choudhary MI et al. Acetylcholinesterase and butyrylcholinesterase inhibitory activity of some Turkish medicinal plants. J Ethnopharmacol. 2004;91:57–60.

PDR for Herbal Medicines. (2nd ed) Medical Economics Company Inc., Montvale, NJ. 2000;226–227.

Preininger V, Thakur RS, Santavy F. Isolation and chemistry of alkaloids from plants of the family *Papaveraceae* LXVII: *Corydalis cava* (L.) Sch. et K. (*C. tuberosa* DC). J Pharm Sci. 1976;65:294–296.

Reimeier C, Schneider I, Schneider W et al. Effects of ethanolic extracts from *Eschscholtzia californica* and *Corydalis cava* on dimerization and oxidation of enkephalins. Arzneimittelforschung. 1995;45: 132–136.

Schafer HL, Schafer H, Schneider W et al. Sedative action of extract combinations of *Eschscholtzia californica* and *Corydalis cava.* Arzneimittelforschung. 1995;45:124–126.

Tierra M. The Way of Chinese Herbs. Pocket Books, New York, NY 1998;228.

Tillotson AK, Tillotson HSH, Abel R. The One Earth Herbal Sourcebook. Kensington Publishing, New York, NY 2001;102–104.

Yang G, Jiang C, Tang Y et al. Effects of L-tetrahydropalmatine on neuron apoptosis during acute cerebral ischemia-reperfusion of rats. J Tongji Med Univ. 2000;20:106–108.

Yang MM, Kwok JS. Evaluation on the treatment of morphine addiction by acupuncture Chinese herbs and opioid peptides. Am J Chin Med. 1986;14:46–50.
Zhong YX, Wiseman N, Ellis A. Fundamentals of Chinese medicine. Paradigm Publications; Brookline, MA. 1996;323–324.
Zhu XZ. Development of natural products as drugs acting on central nervous system. Mem Inst Oswaldo Cruz. 1991;86(Suppl 2):173–175.

Eleutherococcus senticosus

Eleutherococcus senticosus (Ci wu jia, Shikoga, Siberian ginseng, Devil's shrub, Wild pepper, Eleuthero, Eleutherococ; family *Araliaceae*) is a small, dioecious shrub that is native to Siberia, Korea, Japan, Manchuria, and northern China (Russo 2001; PDR 2000; Hikino, Takahashi, Otake et al. 1986). Although it has been referred to as "Siberian ginseng," *E. senticosus* is not a ginseng at all. Reaching a height of between 1 to 3 m, *E. senticosus* has thorny branches and leaves. The bioactive compounds are found in the woody root and root bark, which are often ground, dried, and brewed in the form of a tea. An alcohol extract is also prepared from the underground parts of the plant (Russo 2001; PDR 2000).

In TCM, *E. senticosus* has been used as an adaptogenic substance for many thousands of years. It is used to boost the male aspect, or yang, and balance the qi (Russo 2001). It is a popular tonic to counteract the effects of fatigue, promote convalescence, and improve cognitive and physical function. It is also used to treat complaints related to the urinary tract; arthritic or nonspecific pain, weakness in the joints; to stimulate the immune system and appetite; impotence; and insomnia (PDR 2000).

Ingredients

Active components include: hydroxycoumarins; caffeic acid derivatives; steroids (e.g., daucosterol, eleutheroside A); lignans; phenylacrylic acid derivatives (eleutheroside B); polysaccharides (e.g., eleutheranes A-G possess immunostimulating properties); and triterpene saponins (e.g., eleutherosides I, K, L, M) (PDR 2000). The compounds collectively referred to as the eleutherosides (A through M) are a heterogeneous group, in contrast to the true ginsenosides that are classified in the same group (Russo 2001; PDR 2000). Pharmacological properties may be attributed to lignans and iridoid glycosides (Deyama, Nishibe, Nakzawa 2001).

Clinical Effects

A liquid extract from *E. senticosus* has shown strong antiviral activity against human rhinovirus (HRV), respiratory syncytial virus (RS), and influenza A virus (Glatthaar-Saalmuller, Sacher, Esperster 2001). Some of the eleutherosides have been shown to induce interleukin-1 and interleukin-6, but the presence of eleutherosides B and E seem to counteract this effect (Steinmann, Esperester, Joller 2001).

Components of *E. senticosus* have been shown to possess anti-inflammatory, antipyretic, antibacterial, and antioxidant properties (Davydov, Kirkorian 2000; Yu, Kim, Lim et al. 2003). Evidence supports its effect in counteracting depression, fatigue, and stress as well as in boosting the immune system (Deyama, Nishib, Nakazawa 2001; Panossian, Davtyan, Gukassyan et al. 2002).

E. senticosus has been identified as an adaptogen. This term, coined by the Soviets in the late 1950s, is used to describe a substance that corrects any dysfunction in both sick and healthy individuals without adverse effects (Davydov, Kirkorian 2000). This definition has much in common with the placebo effect. Nonetheless, pharmacological properties demonstrated in *E. senticosus* compounds suggest that its primary activity may be as antioxidant protection against free radicals. For example, some evidence suggests a weak radioprotective property against gamma-irradiation; however, it is not as strong as the protection shown by *Panax ginseng* (Chinese ginseng) (Ben-Hur, Fulder 1981).

At least some of the effects of *E. senticosus* may be due to enzyme inhibition rather than enzyme induction (Medon, Ferguson, Watson 1984). Recently, a biphasic effect resulting from affinity for stress hormone receptors and a feedback mechanism including adrenergic inhibitory enzymes has been suggested to explain a paradoxical effect for *E. senticosus* as well as for *Panax ginseng*. These plants have been associated with both an increase and decrease in the catecholamine stress response (Gaffney, Hugel, Rich 2001a,b).

Behavioral and Psychological Effects

E. senticosus has been popular in Russia for decades. Studies in the Russian scientific literature point to a positive effect on cognitive and physical performance, psychological response to stress, and blood glucose; however, these were not well designed and are not decisive (Russo 2001). In a double-blind, placebo-controlled study of *E. senticosus* on athletic performance in distance runners, the data did not support any benefit on metabolic, performance, or psychological parameters measured (Dowling, Redondo, Branch et al. 1996). In rodent studies, aggressive behavior and duration of sleep were increased, whereas physical endurance and longevity were not impacted (Anonymous 1996).

Adverse Effects

Drug interactions have been reported. *E. senticosus* may potentiate the effects of digoxin (McRae 1996), insulin and other antidiabetic drugs (Hikino, Takahashi, Otake et al. 1986), barbiturates (Medon, Ferguson, Watson 1984), and anticoagulants or antithrombotics. There have also been rare reports of fatigue or drowsiness (Anonymous 1996). However, in a recent study of the impact of standardized *E. senticosus* extract on cytochrome P450, probe substrates dextromethorphan (possessing CYP2D6 activity) and alprazolam (with CYP3A4 activity) were not inhibited. This data suggest no drug interaction between *E. senticosus* and the probed medications (Donovan, DeVane, Chavin et al. 2003).

Availability

The daily human dosage of *E. senticosus* root bark is 9 to 15 gm. Daily dosage of the dried root is 9 to 27 gm. The liquid extract is dosed at 0.3 to 0.5 gm TID. *E. senticosus* preparations must be stored away from humidity and light (PDR 2000). It is sold alone or in combination with other ginsengs. A recent analysis of 25 commercial products containing *Panax ginseng* or *E. senticosus* confirmed that products are accurately labeled regarding plant species but that there was significant variation in the concentrations of active ingredient (Harkey, Henderson, Gershwin et al. 2001).

The popular name of "Siberian ginseng" may be misleading. *E. senticosus* and *Panax ginseng* are unrelated and their constituent compounds are distinct. Although some of their effects overlap, reference to both as a ginseng may lead to confusion with dosage, product labeling, and standardization. It has been suggested that "Siberian ginseng" be discontinued in favor of Eleutherococcus (Davydov, Kirkorian 2000), or perhaps Eleuthero might become an attractive alternative. Reference to Eleutherococcus as a ginseng should be reconsidered.

Clinical Application in Veterinary Behavior Medicine

As a traditional adaptogen, *E. senticosus* might be helpful to help pets overcome stressful events, such as moving to a new home or adjusting to life with a new family. Other indications consistent with traditional use include debilitated, diabetic, obese, or anxious pets with a history of coping poorly with stress. If an antiandrogenic effect is confirmed, it could be clinically applied to pets displaying persistent sexual activity such as masturbation. However, indications that it might trigger aggression in laboratory animals are of concern. Further investigation is warranted.

References

Anonymous. Eleutherococcus. Lawrence Rev Nat Products 1996; May;1–4.

Ben-Hur E, Fulder S. Effect of *Panax ginseng* saponins and *Eleutherococcus senticosus* on survival of cultured mammalian cells after ionizing radiation. Am J Chin Med. 1981;9:48–56.

Donovan JL, DeVane CL, Chavin KD et al. Siberian ginseng (*Eleutherococcus senticosus*) effects on CYP2D6 and CYP3A4 activity in normal volunteers. Drug Metab Dispos. 2003;31:519–522.

Dowling EA, Redondo DR, Branch JD et al. Effect of *Eleutherococcus senticosus* on submaximal and maximal exercise performance. Med Sci Sports Exerc. 1996;28:482–489.

Gaffney BT, Hugel HM, Rich PA. *Panax ginseng* and *Eleutherococcus senticosus* may exaggerate an already existing biphasic response to stress via inhibition of enzymes which limit the binding of stress hormones to their receptors. Med Hypotheses. 2001a;56:567–572.

——. The effects of *Eleutherococcus senticosus* and *Panax ginseng* on steroidal hormone indices of stress and lymphocyte subset numbers in endurance athletes. Life Sci. 2001b;70:431–442.

Glatthaar-Saalmuller B, Sacher F, Esperester A. Antiviral activity of an extract derived from roots of *Eleutherococcus senticosus*. Antiviral Res. 2001;50:223–228.
Harkey MR, Henderson GL, Gershwin et al. Variability in commercial ginseng products: an analysis of 25 preparations. Am J Clin Nutr. 2001;73:1101–1106.
Hikino H, Takahashi M, Otake K et al. Isolation and hypoglycemic activity of A,B,C,D,E,F, and G: glycans of *Eleutherococcus senticosus* roots. J Nat Prod. 1986;49:293–297.
McRae S. Elevated serum digoxin levels in a patient taking digoxin and Siberian ginseng. CMAJ 1996; 155:293–295.
Medon PJ, Ferguson PW, Watson CF. Effects of *Eleutherococcus senticosus* extracts on hexobarbital metabolism in vivo and in vitro. J Ethnopharmacol. 1984;10:235–241.
Mills S, Bone K. Principles and Practice of Phytotherapy. Churchill Livingstone, Philadelphia, PA 2000; 456–464.
Panossian A, Davtyan T, Gukassyan N et al. Effect of andrographolide and Kan Jang—fixed combinations of extract SHA-10 and extract SHE-3–on proliferation of human lymphocytes, production of cytokines and immune activation markers in the whole blood cells culture. Phytomedicine. 2002;9: 598–605.
PDR for Herbal Medicines. (2nd ed) Medical Economics Company Inc., Montvale, NJ. 2000;693–694.
Russo E. Handbook of Psychotropic Herbs: A Scientific Analysis of Herbal Remedies for Psychiatric Conditions. The Haworth Press, Binghamton, NY. 2001;195–198.
Steinmann GG, Esperester A, Joller P. Immunopharmacological in vitro effects of *Eleutherococcus senticosus* extracts. Arzneimittelforschung. 2001;51:76–83.
Yu CY, Kim SH, Lim JD et al. Intraspecific relationship analysis by DNA markers and in vitro cytotoxic and antioxidant activity in *Eleutherococcus senticosus*. Toxicol In Vitro. 2003;17:229–236.
Yun-Choi HS, Kim JH, Lee JR. Potential inhibitors of platelet aggregation from plant sources, III. J Nat Prod. 1987;50:1059–1064.

Ginkgo biloba

Ginkgo biloba (Ginkgo, Maidenhair tree, Ginkgoblatter, Tempeltrae, arbre aux quarante écus) is a native of China, Japan, and Korea and is also found in the United States and across Europe. The dioecious, deciduous tree grows as tall as 40 m and can live hundreds of years. Male trees are broader compared to the female trees, which are more pyramidal in shape. Light-greenish-yellow seeds 2.5 to 3 cm long appear on the female trees and have a noxious odor (color plate 4-1). This may explain why landscapers in North America tend to plant male Ginkgo trees; however, in Asia, female trees predominate (personal communication, Prof. George Ellmore, 2004). The edible nut contained in the seed must be boiled or roasted and is considered a delicacy in Asia. The leaves of *G. biloba* have a unique and characteristic fan shape and turn a stunning sunny yellow in the fall (Fig. 4-2). The two-lobed leaves (biloba) are unique in shape and have no central rib or network of cross-venation (PDR 2000; Mills, Bone 2000). The medicinal parts of the tree are the seeds and the fresh or dried leaf. The trees do not flower before at least 20 years of age and are now cultivated in commercial plantations. At springtime harvest, the leaves are dried and pressed into balls from which a dry extract is processed (Russo 2001; PDR 2000).

Japanese names for *G. biloba* include Icho ("tree"), Ginnan ("fleshy seed"), and

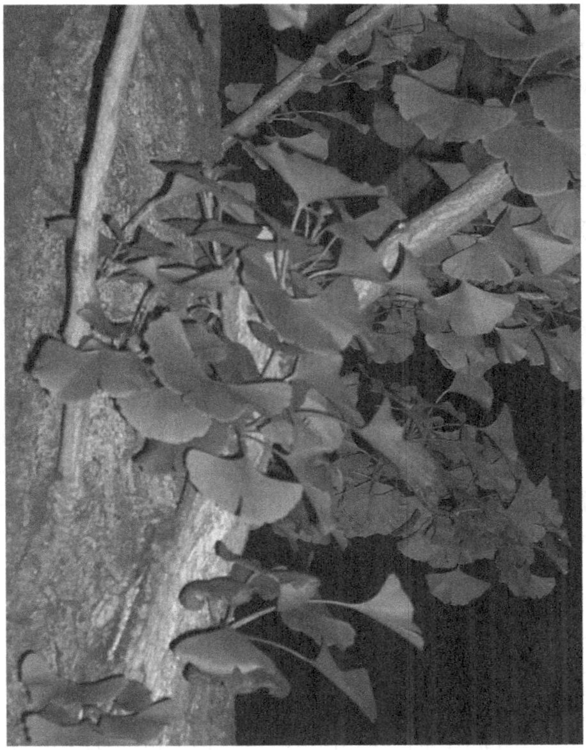

FIGURE 4-2. Characteristic leaves and bark of the *Ginkgo biloba* tree. (Photo courtesy of Daniel Wallace)

Yin-kuo. *G. biloba* is also known in Chinese as Ya chio, Yin hsing, and Kung sun shu. The name *Ya chio* means "duck's foot" in Chinese and refers to the shape of the leaf. Over time, the name *Yin hsing* (silver apricot) arose, referring to the popularity of the fruity seeds, which continue to be used in Chinese cooking and are believed to aid in digestion and reduce the intoxicating effects of wine. *Kung sun shu* means grandfather-grandson tree and refers to the long interval between planting and harvest (Russo 2001; Mills, Bone 2000).

Historical Perspective

G. biloba is the sole survivor of the Ginkgo genus (family *Ginkgoaceae*) dating back to the Jurassic period. In China, *G. biloba* specimens more than 3,000 years old have been identified (Russo 2001; Pang, Pan, He 1996). It has been determined that the species survived the ice age in sheltered mountain regions of eastern China (Li 1956). The Chinese may also have helped to preserve the tree by planting it around their temples. It remains a popular tree throughout Asia and beyond. For example, the proportion of *G. biloba* to other shade trees in Seoul, Korea, was 43.2% in 1998 (Yun, Ko, Park et al. 2000). Its survival became the stuff of legend when a normal *G. biloba* tree grew in the spring near the epicenter of the nuclear bomb site at Hiroshima (Russo 2001; Mills, Bone 2000; Schulz, Hansel, Tyler 1998).

Despite its 150- to 200-million-year-old prehistoric roots, *G. biloba* has been used medicinally only for the past 1,000 years (Russo 2001; Mill, Bone 2000). It was first mentioned in the eleventh century during the Sung Dynasty. Famous Chinese herbal references (notably the *Shih wu Bencao (Shih Wu Pen Ts'ao)*, the *Jijung Bencao* (*Jih Jung Pen Ts'ao*), and the *Bencao Kangmu* (*Pen Ts'ao Kang Mu*) report the use of *G. biloba* nuts for cardiopulmonary ailments. The tree spread throughout Europe following its initial import by a German enthusiast who had visited Japan in the late seventeenth century. By the end of the eighteenth century, it had made its way to the United States. Fossilized Jurassic specimens can be found around the world, including in the Ginkgo Petrified Forest State Park of Washington State (Russo 2001).

Ingredients

G. biloba components include the flavonoids (e.g., quercetin compounds, kaempferol, isorhamnetin, methylmyristicin), biflavonoids (e.g., bilobetin, ginkgetin, isoginkgetin, amentoflavone), proanthocyanidins, trilactonic diterpenes (ginkgolides A, B, C and J), and trilactonic sesquiterpene bilobalides (PDR 2000; Tang, Lou, Wang et al. 2001) (Fig. 4-3). Quercetin and kaempferol, for instance, are excreted as glucuronides in human urine (Wang, Yao, Zeng 2003) and may be the most potent extract components in the treatment of the neurotoxic effects of Alzheimer's disease (Smith, Luo 2003).

Standardized extracts of *G. biloba* EGb 761 and LI 1370 were an innovation of German scientists who first determined its hemodynamic properties. Both these

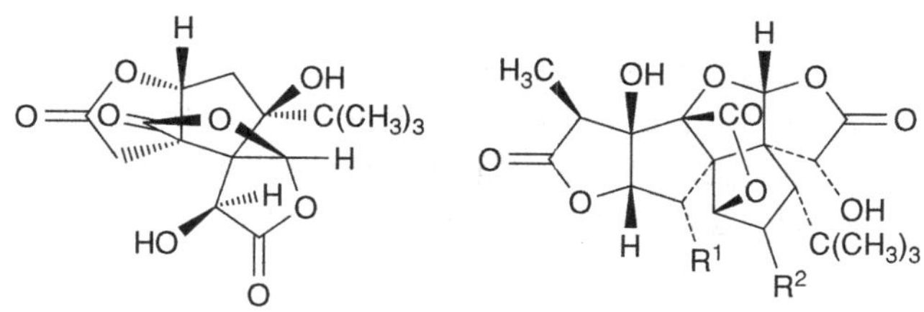

Bilobalide **Ginkgolides**

	R^1	R^2
Ginkgolide A	H	H
Ginkgolide B	OH	H
Ginkgolide C	OH	OH
Ginkgolide J	H	OH

FIGURE 4-3. Active compounds of *Gingko biloba.* (Mills, Bone 2000)

preparations contain 50:1 extracts containing 22–27% flavonoid glycosides, 3% ginkgolides, and 3% bilobalide and other components (Biber 2003; Russo 2001; Mills, Bone 2000; PDR 2000).

As is true of other phytomedicines, components of *G. biloba* extract are thought to have a synergistic effect, and individual components have been shown to possess specific actions. For example, the ginkgolide B demonstrated significant neuroprotective effects, and bilobalides appear to serve as an antibacterial for the tree itself (Russo 2001; Zhu, Wu, Gao et al. 1997; Itil, Martorano 1995). Flavonoid compounds, found in *G. biloba* and many plants discussed elsewhere in this volume, are recognized free radical scavengers and known to reduce oxidative reactions in brain tissue that are part of the age-related decline of CNS function (Schulz, Hansel, Tyler 1998; Oyama, Fuchs, Katayama et al. 1994).

CNS Effects

G. biloba extract demonstrated high affinity for $GABA_A$, $GABA_B$, and CCK_A receptors (Cott 1995). This may explain an anticonvulsant property associated with bilobalide, a primary component of *G. biloba* leaves, in a recent murine study; other components, such as the ginkgolides and flavonoids, are also likely involved (Smith, Maclennan, Darlington 1996). Bilobalide's anticonvulsant property has been attributed to a bilobalide potentiation of glutamic acid decarboxylase and its effect on GABA levels (Sasaki, Hatta, Wada et al. 2000). Elevated GABA levels in the hippocampus are also associated with the therapeutic benefit to memory in dementia patients (Russo 2001; Sasaki, Hatta, Haga et al. 1999).

Bilobalide's inhibition of glutamate and aspartate release may help to explain its neuroprotective mechanism (Davies, Hohns, Jones 2003; Klein, Weichel, Hilgert et al. 2003). Bilobalide is a less potent glycine inhibitor. However, ginkgolides and in particular bilobalide both inhibit $GABA_A$ receptors. Together, glycine and GABA receptors mediate the major inhibitory pathways of the CNS (Ivic, Sands, Fishkin et al. 2003). In Australia, scientists have determined that bilobalide antagonized the direct action of GABA on recombinant alpha1beta2gamma2L $GABA_A$ receptors (Huang, Duke, Chebib et al. 2003).

Amentoflavone, a component of *G. biloba* and other medicinal herbs such as *Hypericum perforatum*, is known to bind to benzodiazepine receptors and is a negative modulator at $GABA_A$ receptors (Hanrahan, Chebib, Davucheron et al. 2003). Most recently, researchers at Columbia University in New York City determined a potent, selective antagonism of glycine receptors by most ginkgolides (Ivic, Sands, Fishkin et al. 2003).

A *G. biloba* fraction extracted from both dried and fresh leaves was found to inhibit MAO_A and MAO_B in an American study of the rat brain (White, Scates, Cooper et al. 1996). It was suggested that MAO inhibition might help to explain reports of *G. biloba's* antistress and anxiolytic properties. Other studies of *G. biloba* extract EGb 761 showed no inhibition of MAO and concluded that mechanisms other than MAO inhibition were responsible for the CNS effects of *G. biloba* (Fowler, Wang, Volkow et al. 2000; Porsolt, Roux, Drieu 2000).

Laboratory strains of MAO_A deficient mice have elevated levels of serotonin (5-HT) and norepinephrine and display increased aggression (Shi, Chen, Ridd et al. 2000). These mice were treated with *G. biloba* extract EGb 761 and showed a significant reduction in conflicts between resident-intruder pairs that was attributed to a binding effect via $5\text{-}HT_{2A}$ receptors in the frontal cortex. *G. biloba* standardized extract EGb 761 may also impact serotonergic systems (Winter, Timineri 1999).

Studies in rats have shown that *G. biloba* extract EGb 761at 50 mg/kg targeted the frontoparietal somatosensory cortex, nucleus accumbens, cerebellar cortex, and pons (Duverger, DeFeudis, Drieu 1995); these findings are supported by clinical trials in people (Haguenauer, Cantenot, Koskas et al. 1986). Bilobalide in particular may be effective in the control of psychomotor seizures given its anticonvulsant property (Sasaki, Hatta, Wada et al. 2000).

Ginkgolide B, bilobalide, and *G. biloba* extract provide neuroprotection against ischemic brain injury (Chandrasekaran, Mehrabian, Spinnewyn et al. 2003; Mills, Bone 2000; Zhu, Wu, Gao et al. 1997). This has been attributed in part to *G. biloba's* inhibitory action on nitric oxide formation (Calapai, Crupi, Firenzuoli et al. 2000). Bilobalide and ginkgolides have been shown to interfere with Cl^- conductance and, therefore, with the function of membrane proteins (Muller, Chatterjee 2003). Specifically, the stabilization or protection of mitochondrial function may be the common denominator among the behavioral effects associated with EGb 761 (Muller, Chatterjee 2003).

Cognitive Effects

G. biloba EGb 761 appears to protect mitochondria from oxidative stress, which is thought to be an important part of the pathology of Alzheimer's disease (Eckert, Keil, Kressmann et al. 2003). The deposit of beta-amyloid protein plaques and neuronal destruction in the cortex and hippocampus characterize Alzheimer's disease (DeLaGarza 2003; Stackman, Eckenstein, Frei et al. 2003). Cholinergic neurons are particularly affected and, despite the risk of cholinergic side effects, acetylcholinesterase (AChE)–inhibiting drugs (e.g., donepezil, rivastigmine, and glantamine) have been the most effective thus far (DeLaGarza 2003). *G. biloba* extract has shown a significant anticholinesterase property (Das, Shanker, Nath et al. 2002).

In a rigorous meta-analysis of fifty studies of *G. biloba* in the treatment of Alzheimer's disease (Oken, Storzbach, Kaye 1998), pooled data of the final four studies strongly supported a clinical benefit to patients suffering from Alzheimer's disease. In a six-month, double-blind, placebo-controlled multicenter clinical trial of 244 patients suffering from uncomplicated Alzheimer's disease or multi-infarct dementia, those treated with 40 mg TID of EGb 761 showed modest improvement in cognitive function and social behavior without adverse effects (Le Bars, Kieser, Itil 2000). In a more recent study of Alzheimer patients, EGb 761 treatment was attributed with significant improvement in cognitive function (Kanowski, Hoerr 2003).

In a murine study of chemically induced dementia, *G. biloba* enhanced cognitive function at doses of 30 and 60 mg/kg (Das, Shanker, Nath et al. 2002). In another rodent study, researchers investigated the neuroprotective effects of EGb 761 components (Ahlemeyer, Krieglstein 2003). They found evidence to support the neuroprotective property of EGb 761 and discovered that bilobalide was the most potent. In a recent transgenic mouse model study of Alzheimer's disease that displays a mutant form of human beta-amyloid precursor protein accompanied by age-related cognitive decline, mice treated with *G. biloba* (70 mg/kg/day in water) retained cognitive ability despite the accumulation of protein plaques (Stackman, Eckenstien, Frei et al. 2003).

Administration of EGb 761 to pregnant rats results in an increase in the number of hippocampal neurons. This neurotropic effect was shown to impact genes including insulin growth factor and binding protein 2, testosterone-repressed prostate message-2, glutathione-dependent dehydroascorbate reductase, lipoprotein lipase, and DNA binding protein Brn-2 (Li, Trovero, Cordier et al. 2003), providing important new insight into the mechanism of *G. biloba*.

Another important part of *G. biloba's* mechanism of action in stabilizing memory function can be attributed to its beneficial effects on brain glucose metabolism and energy metabolism. Acetylcholine synthesis is dependent on acetyl CoA, which is a by-product of glucose breakdown. In addition, insulin controls the activity of AChE transferase. Therefore, damage to glucose metabolism, particularly at the level of the CNS, directly impacts normal memory function such as that seen in Alzheimer's disease (Hoyer 2003). *G. biloba* extract EGb 761 has been shown to decrease glucose utilization in the frontoparietal somatosensory cortex, nucleus accumbens, cerebellar cortex, and pons, a finding that may help to explain reports of its therapeutic effect in the treatment of vertiginous syndromes affecting vigilance and vestibular mechanisms (Duverger, DeFeudis, Drieu 1995).

A number of electroencephalographic studies of healthy subjects as well as patients with dementia have shown a benefit from *G. biloba* treatment (Itil, Eralp, Tsambis et al. 1996; Halama 1990; Kanowski, Herrmann, Stephan et al. 1996). In a recent British study, *G. biloba* and *Panax ginseng* significantly reduced frontal "eyes closed" theta and beta activity although the effects were more pronounced in *Panax ginseng* (Kennedy, Scholey, Drewery et al. 2003).

G. biloba has shown an advantage in the treatment of senile dementia when compared with tacrine (Cognex®); it may be at least as effective and is less costly than donepezil (Aricept®). These drugs are approved for the treatment of dementia in the United States (Russo 2001). In an important placebo-controlled double-blind study of 309 senile dementia patients, the EGb 761 group did not suffer the cognitive deterioration reported in the control group (Le Bars et al. 1997). The treatment group remained stable and appeared to improve cognitive functioning. However, in a meta-analysis of drugs used to improve cognitive impairment in patients with dementia, German researchers were challenged by the lack of standard procedures in studies of cognitive changes and could not draw any conclusions despite findings of cognitive improvement in some neuropsychological tests of patients treated with *G. biloba* EGb 761 (Ihl 2003).

In a study of 66 healthy subjects over a four-week period, *G. biloba* extract EGb 761 was associated with improved cognitive function in normal subjects without cognitive dysfunction (Cieza, Maier, Poppel 2003). No serious adverse effects were reported. In contrast, a recent Swedish study could not demonstrate a significant effect of *G. biloba* (or *Panax ginseng*) on memory performance in a placebo-controlled study (Persson, Bringlov, Nilsson et al. 2003).

The effects of *G. biloba* in cognitively impaired patients remain somewhat controversial. Some data support *G. biloba's* therapeutic benefit, whereas others minimize or even negate its clinical value. A recent study may be helpful in that it suggests there may be individuals who are responders or nonresponders (Canter, Ernst 2003). Patients diagnosed with dementia often show behavioral and psychological signs. The ideal treatment should reduce these symptoms as well as improve cognitive ability. In a recent study, EGb 761 significantly improved cognitive impairment as well as behavioral and psychological signs in dementia patients (Hoerr 2003).

Behavioral and Psychological Effects

Interest in the emotional effects of *G. biloba* has begun to increase in recent years. Preliminary evidence of its impact on stress is promising. In an important Japanese study, the anxiolytic effects of *G. biloba* extract and ginkgolides A, B, C and bilobalide were evaluated (Kuribara, Weintraub, Yoshihama et al. 2003). *G. biloba* extract showed a significant anxiolytic effect, which was attributed to ginkgolide A, the only other constituent to demonstrate an anxiolytic effect. *G. biloba* extract was also shown to reduce caffeine-induced stimulation and prolonged pentobarbital-induced sleep, effects not associated with ginkgolide A.

G. biloba EGb 761 successfully suppressed stress-induced detrimental changes in cognitive performance and plasma stress hormone concentration (epinephrine, norepinephrine, and corticosterone) in young and old rats (Rapin, Lamproglou, Dieu et al. 1994). *G. biloba* extract EGb761 at a dose of 50 to 100 mg/kg/day has been shown to facilitate behavioral adaptation and to decrease stress-related hormones under stressful environmental conditions in young and old rats (Rapin, Lamproglou, Drieu et al. 1994). However, in a Dutch study, administration of *G. biloba* at 150 mg/kg significantly prevented a corticosterone stress response in rats but did not improve their behavioral stress adaptation (Markus, Lammers 2003).

Researchers in India also found that *G. biloba* extract restored stress-induced increases in brain catecholamines (norepinephrine and dopamine), serotonin (5-HT), and plasma corticosterone to near normal levels (Shah, Sharma, Vohora 2003). In a recent study at Georgetown University Medical Center in Washington, D.C., ginkgolide B reduced glucocorticoid production by virtue of its direct suppression of the adrenal peripheral-type benzodiazepine receptor (Amri, Drieu, Papadopoulos 2003). This very specific effect has applications for emotional and medical disorders.

In a Chinese study of 82 patients with treatment-resistant chronic schizophrenia, patients receiving the classic antipsychotic haloperidol combined with *G. biloba* extract improved significantly compared to those treated with haloperidol plus placebo. Authors suggested that its antioxidant effect might have been part of the mechanism in the successful combination treatment protocol (Zhang, Zhou, Su et al. 2001). In a follow-up double-blind, placebo-controlled study of 109 schizophrenic patients, the same authors joined forces with Yale University's School of Medicine Neuropsychopharmacology Laboratory and reported that *G. biloba* EGb 761 treatment enhanced the effectiveness of haloperidol and also reduced extrapyramidal side effects that are so typical of this drug (Zhang, Zhou, Zhang et al. 2001).

G. biloba may also help to counteract sexual dysfunction as an adverse effect of SSRI antidepressants such as fluoxetine (Prozac) (Ashton, Ahrens, Gupta et al. 2000; Ellison, DeLuca 1998; Cohen, Bartlik 1998). In addition to fewer side effects compared to sildenafil (Viagra®), *G. biloba* could be of interest as a more cost-effective treatment of sexual dysfunction (Russo 2001).

G. biloba was not found to be any more effective than placebo in the prevention of winter depression. In an early German placebo-controlled, double-blind randomized study, *G. biloba* extract appeared to have an antidepressant effect on the treatment group of middle-aged to elderly patients (Halama 1990). In contrast, a 10-week, placebo-controlled, double-blind study of *G. biloba* extract PN246 in 27 Norwegian patients suffering from seasonal affective disorder showed no significant difference compared to placebo (Lingaerde, Foreland, Magnusson 1999). *G. biloba* extract EGb Li 1370 was shown to reverse the effects of sleep disturbance and cognitive impairment in depressed Swiss patients medicated with the tricyclic antidepressant trimipramine (Hemmeter, Annen, Bischof et al. 2001). It was suggested that *G. biloba* extract might have improved sleep by reducing corticotrophin-releasing hormone.

A Canadian study of 36 children between the ages of 3 and 17 years diagnosed with attention-deficit hyperactivity disorder (ADHD) determined that a commercial herbal remedy containing *Panax quinquefolium* (200 mg) and *G. biloba* extract (50 mg) was effective on symptoms of ADHD within two weeks of administration (Lyon, Cline, Totosy de Zepetnek et al. 2001). It is unfortunate that a combination herbal product was selected for this clinical trial although it may well be that the effect was in fact due to their synergy. These preliminary results should prompt other researchers to explore the contribution of individual herbs compared to simple herbal mixtures as alternative or adjunctive treatment to conventional amphetamine-based treatment of ADHD.

Cardiovascular Effects

Gingkolides have shown significant anticoagulant properties. Specifically, they inhibit platelet-activating factor, which is implicated in platelet aggregation, allergic inflammatory processes, and is also found in brain cells. This would help to explain the CNS neuroprotection linked to *G. biloba* extract and ginkgolides (Russo 2001; Smith, Maclennan, Darlington 1996). The mechanism of this action remains unclear although Ca^{++} (Zhu, Wu Gao et al. 1997) and Na^{+} and K^{-} ATPase activities are implicated (Pierre, Jamme, Droy-Lefaix et al. 1999). Ginkgolides appear to stabilize mast cells, which may be useful in the treatment of diseases involving mastocytes, and antagonize the response of eosinophils to platelet activating factor (Guinot, Summerhayes, Berdah et al. 1988; Barnes, Chung, Page 1988).

G. biloba has been shown to be more effective than dozens of other conventional drugs in improving cerebral blood flow in stroke victims (Heiss, Zeiler 1978). In a recent Brazilian study conducted over an eight-month period, *G. biloba* treatment was associated with reduced blood viscosity and improved cerebral perfusion and cognitive function (Santos, Galudorz, Barbieri et al. 2003).

G. biloba's anticoagulant effect could be of clinical benefit in pets with high risk of clot formation (e.g., cardiomyopathy or polycythemia, cerebrovascular or pulmonary thromboemboli). This effect may be of particular interest in cats as a less toxic alternative to aspirin. Concurrent administration of *G. biloba* with other antithrombolytic drugs is not advised; veterinary patients taking *G. biloba* extract should be closely monitored with tests of bleeding and clotting at regular intervals. Patients who are taking *G. biloba* products should be withdrawn from the herb in advance of elective surgery and should be evaluated for clotting problems prior to surgery.

G. biloba EGb 761 is now thought to decrease blood pressure in addition to its potent antithrombotic and antioxidant activity. These effects are of interest for the treatment of hypertension and, in particular, for the treatment or prevention of stroke (Sasaki, Noguchi, Yamamoto et al. 2002). A comparative *in vitro* study of *G. biloba* extract, bilobalide, ginkgolides A, B, and C, as well as flavonoid components proved that all constituents tested have an independent, concentration-dependent vasorelaxant property (Nishida, Satoh 2004). Despite its promise, a recent placebo-controlled double-blind study of healthy volunteers did not demonstrate any short-term effects on blood pressure, heart rate, or ECG parameters (Kalus JS, Piotrowski AA, Fortier CR et al. 2003). *G. biloba* is under current investigation for the treatment of cardiovascular diseases by the National Center for Complementary and Alternative Medicine, a special division of the National Institutes of Health in Bethesda, Maryland, created in 1998 (Wong, Nahin 2003).

The activation of T lymphocytes is an important part of the inflammatory process of vascular diseases of the heart and brain. *G. biloba* extract inhibits a number of cytokines including interleukins, tumor necrosis factor-alpha, and interferon-gamma (Cheng, Yang, Ho et al. 2003). These authors also demonstrated that *G. biloba* has a specific inhibitory action on activator protein-1 of T cells, implying *G. biloba's* potential use in the treatment of cardiovascular and cerebrovascular diseases as well as in activated T cell–mediated illnesses.

Miscellaneous Effects

In a small British study of postmenopausal women, modest but significant improvement in cognitive tests was demonstrated compared to placebo; other menopausal symptoms were unaffected (Hartley, Heinze, Elsabagh et al. 2003).

One study investigated the effectiveness of *G. biloba* as an aid to withdrawal treatment from chronic cocaine use with the hypothesis that an improvement in cognitive function might reduce relapse in addicts. *G. biloba* failed to provide any therapeutic benefit for the treatment of cocaine dependence (Kampman, Majewska, Tourian et al. 2003).

G. biloba compounds bilobetin, gingketin, and amentoflavone exhibited antifungal properties and were among *G. biloba* components identified in the needles of *Taxus baccata* (European yew tree) for the first time (Krauze-Baranowska, Wiwart 2003).

G. biloba extract has been shown to reduce acute gastric mucosal damage induced by indomethacin, and provided moderate analgesia at doses of 100 mg/kg administered subcutaneously. It also enhanced the anti-inflammatory effects of NSAIDs including indomethacin, rofecoxib, celecoxib, and dexamethasone (Abdel-Salam, Baliuomy, El-batran et al. 2004). In another study, *G. biloba* extract boosted the anti-inflammatory effects of cimetidine and also displayed protective effects of its own in the treatment of acute gastric mucosal injury (Wang, Zhao, Ma 2000). In Turkey, prophylactic treatment of rats with EGb 761 resulted in significant decreases in both serum amylase and lipase, and histopathology indicated its therapeutic benefit in the treatment of acute pancreatitis (Zeybek, Gorbulu, Yagci et al. 2003).

Its neuroprotective and immune-stimulating effects suggest the use of *G. biloba* in the treatment of multiple sclerosis; however, further research is needed (Bowling, Stewart 2003). *G. biloba* has also shown promise in animal models of Parkinson's disease, a finding that has been attributed to its antioxidant effect and protection of mitochondria (Beal 2003). *G. biloba* extract was shown to enhance the effects of levodopa in rat models of Parkinson's disease, and combined therapy may prove helpful to humans suffering from the disease (Cao, Sun, Tong 2003).

In addition to its neuroprotective and vascular antioxidant effects (Ponto, Schultz 2003), EGb 761 has now been shown to rejuvenate degenerated thymus, pointing to its benefits on the immune system as well as on cell proliferation

(Tian, Tian, Zhang et al. 2003). Researchers in Mexico have found that EGb 761 has immunostimulatory effects (Puebla-Prez, Lozoya, Villasenor-Garcia 2003). *G. biloba* extract (100 mg/kg/day) moderated corticosterone levels in stressed rats and improved the immune response (e.g., proliferation index of splenocytes, delayed-type hypersensitivity response to dinitrofluorobenzene) of test subjects.

Among the most exciting new findings are indications that *G. biloba* extract inhibits human breast cancer cells and also impacts human bladder cancer cells (Chao, Chu 2004; DeFeudis, Papadopoulos, Drieu 2003). The mechanism is attributed to the antioxidant, anti-angiogenic, and gene-regulatory actions involving flavonoid (e.g., kaempferol) and terpenoid (e.g., ginkgolide B) constituents of *G. biloba* (DeFeudis, Papadopoulos, Drieu 2003). EGb 761 and ginkgolide B inhibited cell proliferation in highly aggressive cell lines of a human breast cancer cell line that is rich in peripheral-type benzodiazepine receptors (PBR), but were ineffective against another human breast cancer cell line that is low in PBR (Papadopoulos, Kapsis, Li et al. 2000). Further analysis showed that EGb actually altered the expression of 36 gene products involved in cell proliferation. The cytostatic effect of *G. biloba* extract and its affinity for PBR are promising indicators of its use in oncology. In addition, *G. biloba* extract EGb 761 significantly inhibited the *in vitro* proliferation of specific human hepatocellular carcinoma cell lines (Chao, Chu 2004). EGb 761 is now known to function at the level of DNA, impacting gene transcription, cellular metabolism, and signaling pathways (Smith, Luo 2004). Future studies are anticipated with great interest.

Adverse Effects

Adverse effects of *G. biloba* include mild gastrointestinal complaints, allergic reaction (skin reaction, spasm, cramps) and a possible reduction of female fertility (PDR 2000). Italian cardiologists reported a case of ventricular arrhythmia induced by *G. biloba* extract that resolved with withdrawal of the herb (Cianfrocca, Pelliccia, Auriti et al. 2002), but the mechanism of this alleged reaction was not proven.

There have also been reports of hematologic effects including increased bleeding time, spontaneous bilateral subdural hematomas, and subarachnoid hemorrhage associated with the use of *G. biloba* (PDR 2000, Vale 1998; Rown, Lewish 1996). Cases of spontaneous hemorrhage in patients treated with *G. biloba* have been reported. However, a double-blind, placebo-controlled study of 32 healthy male volunteers did not reveal altered platelet function based on measures of hemostasis, coagulation, and fibrinolysis. These French researchers suggested that reports of bleeding problems associated with *G. biloba* extract might not be related to the herb (Bal Dit Sollier, Caplain, Drouet 2003). Nonetheless, sporadic cases of bleeding disorders have been published and associated with *G. biloba* consumption. Isolated cases of hemorrhage, however, cannot be conclusive evidence although they should prompt clinicians to monitor and forewarn patients who use

G. biloba products. One case of retrobulbar hemorrhage was reported in a patient following cataract surgery and was later attributed to self-treatment with *G. biloba* (Fong, Kinnear 2003). A case of post-surgical bleeding in a patient who underwent laparoscopic cholecystectomy was reported and also linked to *G. biloba* intake (Fessenden, Wittenborn, Clarke 2001). Finally, a patient suffered a spontaneous intracerebral hemorrhage that was ascribed to self-medication with *G. biloba* extract (Benjamin, Muir, Briggs et al. 2001).

G. biloba leaves contain a neurotoxin (4'-O-methylpyridoxine) with antivitamin B_6 effects. However, this ginkgotoxin is inactivated by modern commercial preparation of EGb 761 or LI 1370. Nonetheless, sporadic reports of fatalities and seizure (Ginnan-sito-toxism) have been reported in Asia when famine caused the consumption of higher volume of *G. biloba* nuts (Russo 2001). Generalized convulsions occurred in a Japanese patient with no known history of epilepsy. In the hours prior to the seizure, the patient had consumed between 70 and 80 *G. biloba* nuts (Miwa, Iijima, Tanaka et al. 2001). *G. biloba* treatment was suggested to have precipitated seizures in two British patients with well-controlled epilepsy who suffered recurrent seizure activity two weeks after taking *G. biloba* (Granger 2001). This finding was not challenged with repeat courses of *G. biloba* supplement.

Given the worldwide distribution and concentration of trees in Asia, the risk of allergic reaction to the tree's pollen is also a consideration. *G. biloba* pollen has high cross-reactivity with other pollens and accounted for 4.7% of skin prick reactions in a population of Korean subjects with respiratory allergy (Yun, Ko, Park et al. 2000). The potential for allergic reactions to medicinal plants is always possible, although none have been reported thus far for *G. biloba*.

Drug Interactions

Herb and drug interaction is a recognized risk, and *G. biloba* is no exception. For example, a coma associated with concomitant use of *G. biloba* extract and trazodone has been reported (Galluzzi, Zanetti, Binetti et al. 2000). In a recent Harvard University study of presurgical patients at Brigham and Women's Hospital in Boston, MA, 22% reported the use of herbal medicines; *G. biloba* was the second most popular herb (following *Echinacea purpura* and preceding *Hypericum perforatum*) used in this sample (Tsen, Segal, Pothier et al. 2000). One third of geriatric patients attending a memory clinic in Toronto, Canada, were at risk of an interaction between a conventional drug and herbal medicine; the most common one identified was concomitant use of *G. biloba* and aspirin (Dergal, Gold, Laxer et al. 2002).

G. biloba did not appear to have any significant effect on the pharmacokinesis of oral digoxin in eight healthy human volunteers (Mauro, Mauro, Kleshinski et al. 2003). In addition, *G. biloba* did not interact with warfarin treatment (Engelsen, Nielsen, Hansen 2003).

G. biloba extract was administered to 12 healthy volunteers, and metabolites of alprazolam (CYP3A4 activity) and dextromethorphan (CYP2D6 activity) were measured in blood and urine. Researchers determined that there was no significant difference in drug metabolism associated with *G. biloba* and concluded that drugs primarily dependent on cytochrome P450 2D6 and 3A4 pathways would be unaffected by concomitant use of *G. biloba* (Markowitz, Donovan, Lindsay DeVane et al. 2003). Nonetheless, it seems more prudent to conduct larger studies on a wider variety of drugs before this conclusion becomes certain.

In contrast, studies elsewhere have discovered significant impact of *G. biloba* extract on cytochrome P450 1A1, 1A2, and 2B1 isozymes and altered metabolism of drugs (Yang, Wang, Lu et al. 2003). In a rodent study, concomitant administration of *G. biloba* leaf extract and diltiazem, a common probe of cytochrome P450 3A, indicated that the combination increased the bioavailability of diltiazem. The mechanism was by *G. biloba's* suppression of the drug's metabolism in the intestine and liver as well as inhibition of CYP3A (Ohnishi, Kusuhara, Yoshioka et al. 2003).

Availability

G. biloba is widely available in many commercial preparations in combination with other compounds or alone. In general, it may be preferable to avoid the use of most polyherbal preparations to better isolate any clinical improvement benefit or undesired side effects.

The oral LD50 value of standardized *G. biloba* extract in mice was 7.7 g/kg. Doses as high as 500 mg/kg/day did not cause organ damage, and at 900 mg/kg/day to rabbits and 1600 mg/kg/day to rats did not affect reproduction (Mills, Bone 2000).

Although dosage has not yet been firmly established for veterinary patients, a daily dose of 40 to 80 mg BID to TID of standardized extracts corresponding to EGb 761 or LI 1370 is suggested for aging pets with signs of cognitive decline or at risk for thromboemboli caused by various illnesses. This dose range has been used extensively in clinical trials in geriatric people. However, doses of standardized *G. biloba* extract in animal studies have been as high as 10 times greater than the doses used in people (Smith, Maclennan, Darlington 1988). For example, a dosage of 120–240 mg/day for a human patient who weighs approximately 80 kg is between 1.5 to 3 mg/kg/day of standardized extract. In animal studies, doses as high as 100 mg/kg/day or higher have been used (Mills, Bone 2000).

The effective dose range in dogs and cats remains to be determined, but it is reasonable to start at a lower dose (50 mg for small dogs and cats; 100 mg for medium dogs; 150 mg for large dogs) and increase to effect (maximum dose 240 mg). At least six weeks of treatment has been recommended to determine a therapeutic benefit to the patient (Mills, Bone 2000), although results may be seen within days or weeks. To further complicate the question of dosage, there is also considerable variation in the quality of commercial preparations of *G. biloba*, which is known to impact the antioxidant activity of the herb (Mantle, Wilkins, Gok 2003). The biopharmaceutical quality of herbal OTC preparations is also subject to variation in different commercial products; this will impact the absorption rate and affect of their ingredients (Kressmann, Biber, Wonnemann et al. 2002).

Clinical Application in Veterinary Behavior Medicine

Geriatric patients with cognitive decline would likely benefit from standardized preparations of ginkgo extract. *G. biloba* might be a useful adjunct or an alternative to treatment with selegiline, which has become the conventional drug of choice for pets diagnosed with cognitive dysfunction syndrome.

The antidepressant and anxiolytic effects of *G. biloba* have not been extensively studied, despite occasional reports, and deserve focus. The effects of *G. biloba* on serotonergic, GABA-ergic and MAO systems, as well as its direct impact on adrenal glucocorticoid production, support the potential of its psychoactive properties. For example, young and older pets might be helped to adjust to new homes or new owners. This might be an important benefit, for example, to pets adopted from rescue shelters that have a higher risk of adjustment problems, including separation anxiety syndrome (Schwartz 2003). In addition, newly acquired puppies and kittens might be helped to better integrate into their new homes.

A study of ADHD in children and adolescents demonstrated the clinical benefit of *G. biloba* combined with *Panax quinquefolium*. These preliminary results suggest its clinical usefulness in controlling dogs with hyper-reactivity that does not respond to an increase in exercise and basic obedience training, pathological canine hyperkinesis, and feline hyperesthesia. Future investigation may confirm or refute this suggestion. Pets with psychomotor seizures and peripheral or central vestibular syndromes may also benefit from treatment with *G. biloba.*

G. biloba might benefit pets of breeding value with sexual dysfunction, and could have potential in treating extroverted or introverted (self-directed) forms of compulsive behaviors.

Preliminary results on MAO_A KO mice introduced earlier suggest that *G. biloba* might be an effective agent in the treatment of aggressive problems in pets. Based on the murine study findings, *G. biloba* could be useful in the treatment of aggressive conflicts between house pets such as dominance conflicts between dogs, territorial and dominance aggression between cats, and perhaps to facilitate the introduction of new pets to resident pets. It is also possible that other types of aggression, such as fear, maternal, and instrumental aggression might be impacted with *G. biloba* treatment, either as the primary therapy or as an adjunct to other conventional or herbal medication.

G. biloba is the focus of a tremendous amount of scientific interest; details of its pharmacological and clinical potential are rapidly accumulating. *G. biloba* (and its derivatives) presents as one of the most exciting herbal prospects of human and veterinary medicine.

References

Abdel-Salam OM, Baiuomy AR, El-batran S et al. Evaluation of the anti-inflammatory, anti-nociceptive and gastric effects of *Ginkgo biloba* in the rat. Pharmacol Res. 2004;49:133–142.

Ahlemeyer B, Krieglstein J. Pharmacological studies supporting the therapeutic use of *Ginkgo biloba* extract for Alzheimer's disease. Pharmacopsychiatry. 2003;36(Suppl 1):S8–14.

Amri H, Drieu K, Papadopoulos V. Transcriptional suppression of the adrenal cortical peripheral-type benzodiazepine receptor gene and inhibition of steroid synthesis by ginkgolide B. Biochem Pharmacol. 2003;65:717–729.

Ashton AK, Ahrens K, Gupta S et al. Antidepressant-induced sexual dysfunction and *Ginkgo biloba.* Am J Psychiatry. 2000;157:836–837.

Bal Dit Sollier C, Caplain H, Drouet L. No alteration in platelet function or coagulation induced by EGb 761 in a controlled study. Clin Lab Haematol. 2003;25:251–253.

Barnes PJ, Chung KF, Page CP. Inflammatory mediators and asthma. Pharmacol Rev. 1988;40:49–84.

Benjamin J, Muir T, Briggs K et al. A case of cerebral haemorrhage—can *Ginkgo biloba* be implicated? Postgrad Med J. 2001;77:112–113.

Beal MF. Bioenergetic approaches for neuroprotection in Parkinson's disease. Ann Neurol. 2003;53 (Suppl 3):S39–47.

Biber A. Pharmacokinetics of *Ginkgo biloba* extracts. Pharmacopsychiatry. 2003;36(Suppl 1):S32–37.

Bowling AC, Stewart TM. Current complementary and alternative therapies for multiple sclerosis. Curr Treat Options Neurol. 2003;5:55–68.

Calapai G, Crupi A, Firenzuoli F et al. Neuroprotective effects of *Ginkgo biloba* extract in brain ischemia are mediated by inhibition of nitric oxide synthesis. Life Sci. 2000;67:2673–2683.

Canter PH, Ernst E. Multiple n=1 trials in the identification of responders and non-responders to the cognitive effects of *Gingko biloba.* Int J Clin Pharmacol Ther. 2003;41:354–357.

Cao F, Sun S, Tong ET. Experimental study on inhibition of neuronal toxical effects of levodopa by *Ginkgo biloba* extract on Parkinson disease in rats. J Huazhong Univ Sci Technolog Med Sci. 2003; 23:151–153.

Chandrasekaran K, Mehrabian Z, Spinnewyn B et al. Neuroprotective effects of bilobalide, a component of *Ginkgo biloba* extract (EGb 761) in global brain ischemia and in excitotoxicity-induced neuronal death. Pharmacopsychiatry. 2003;36(Suppl 1):S89–94.

Chao JC, Chu CC. Effects of *Ginkgo biloba* extract on cell proliferation and cytotoxicity in human hepatocellular carcinoma cells. World J Gastroenterol. 2004;10:37–41.

Cheng SM, Yang SP, Ho LJ et al. Down-regulation of c-jun N-terminal kinase-activator protein-1 signaling pathway by *Ginkgo biloba* extract in human peripheral blood T cells. Biochem Pharmacol. 2003;66:679–689.

Cianfrocca C, Pelliccia F, Auriti A et al. *Ginkgo biloba*-induced frequent ventricular arrhythmia. Ital Heart J. 2002;3:689–691.

Cieza A, Maier P, Poppel E. Effects of *Gingko biloba* on mental functioning in healthy volunteers. Arch Med Res. 2003;34:373–381.

Cohen AJ, Bartlik B. *Ginkgo biloba* for antidepressant-induced sexual dysfunction. J Sex Marit Ther. 1998;24:139–143.

Cott J. Medicinal plants and dietary supplements: Sources for innovative treatment or adjuncts? Psychopharm Bull. 1994:31:131–137.

Das A, Shanker G, Nath C et al. A comparative study in rodents of standardized extracts of *Bacopa monniera* and *Ginkgo biloba*: anticholinesterase and cognitive enhancing activities. Pharmacol Biochem Behav. 2002;73:893–900.

Davies JA, Johns L, Hones FA. Effects of bilobalide on cerebral amino acid neurotransmission. Pharmacopsychiatry. 2003;36(Suppl 1):S84–88.

DeFeudis FV, Papdopoulos V, Drieu K. *Ginkgo biloba* extracts and cancer: a research area in its infancy. Fundam Clin Pharmacol. 2003;17:405–417.

DeLaGarza VW. Pharmacologic treatment of Alzheimer's disease: an update. Am Fam Physician. 2003;68:1365–1372.

Dergal JM, Gold JL, Laxer DA et al. Potential interactions between herbal medicines and conventional drug therapies used by older adults attending a memory clinic. Drugs Aging. 2002;19:879–886.

Duverger D, DeFeudis FV, Drieu K. Effects of repeated treatments with an extract of *Ginkgo biloba* (EGb 761) on cerebral glucose utilization in the rat: an autoradiographic study. Gen Pharmacol. 1995;26:1375–1383.

Eckert A, Keil U, Kressmann S et al. Effects of EGb 761 *Ginkgo biloba* extract on mitochondrial function and oxidative stress. Pharmacopsychiatry. 2003;36(Suppl 1):S15–23.

Ellison JM, DeLuca P. fluoxetine-induced genital anesthesia relieved by *Ginkgo biloba* extract. J Clin Psychiat. 1998;59:199–200.

Engelsen J, Nielsen JD, Hansen KF. Effect of Coenzyme Q10 and *Ginkgo biloba* on warfarin dosage in patients on long-term warfarin treatment. A randomized, double-blind, placebo-controlled crossover trial. Ugeskr Laeger. 2003;165:1868–1871.

Fessenden JM, Wittenborn W, Clarke L. *Ginkgo biloba*: a case report of herbal medicine and bleeding postoperatively from a laparoscopic cholecystectomy. Am Surg. 2001;67:33–35.

Fong KC, Kinnear PE. Retrobulbar haemorrhage associated with chronic *Ginkgo biloba* ingestion. Postgrad Med J. 2003;79:531–532.

Fowler JS, Wang GJ, Volkow ND et al. Evidence that *Gingko biloba* extract does not inhibit MAO A and B in living human brain. Life Sci. 2000;66:PL141–146.

Galluzzi S, Zanetti O, Binetti G et al. Coma in a patient with Alzheimer's disease taking low dose trazodone and *Gingko biloba*. J Neurol Neurosurg Psychiatry. 2000;68:679–680.

Granger AS. *Ginkgo biloba* precipitating epileptic seizures. Age Ageing. 2001;30:523–525.

Guinot P, Summerhayes C, Berdah L et al. Treatment of adult systemic mastocytosis with a PAF-acether antagonist BN52063. Lancet. 1988;2:114.

Haguenauer JP, Cantenot F, Koskas H et al. Treatment of equilibrium disorders with *Ginkgo biloba* extract. A multicenter double-blind drug vs. placebo study. Presse Med. 1986;15:1569–1572.

Halama P. Was leistet der Spezialextract EGB 761?: Ergebnisse einer placebokontrollierten, randomisierten doppelblinden Pilotstudie. Therapiewoche. 1990;40:3760–3765.

Hanrahan JR, Chebib M, Davucheron NL et al. Semisynthetic preparation of amentoflavone: A negative modulator at GABA(A) receptors. Bioorg Med Chem Lett. 2003;13:2281–2284.

Hartley DE, Heinze L, Elsabagh S et al. Effects on cognition and mood in postmenopausal women of 1-week treatment with *Ginkgo biloba*. Phrmacol Biochem Behav. 2003;75:711–720.

Heiss WD, Zeiler K. Medikamentöse Beeinflussung der Hirndurchblutung. Pharmakotherapie. 1978;1:137–144.

Hemmeter U, Annen B, Bischof R et al. Polysomnographic effects of adjuvant *Ginkgo biloba* therapy in patients with major depression medicated with trimipramine. Pharmacopsychiatry. 2001;34:50–59.

Hoerr R. Behavioural and psychological symptoms of dementia (BPSD): effects of EGb 761. Pharmacopsychiatry. 2003;36(Suppl 1):S56–61.

Hoyer S. Memory function and brain glucose metabolism. Pharmacopsychiatry. 2003;36(Suppl 1): S62–67.

Huang SH, Duke RK, Chebib M et al. Bilobalide, a sesquitepene trilactone from *Ginkgo biloba*, an antagonist at recombinant alpha1beta2gamma2L GABA(A) receptors. Eur J Pharmacol. 2003;464:1–8.

Ihl R. The impact of drugs against dementia on cognition in aging and mild cognitive impairment. Pharmacopsychiatry. 2003;36(Suppl 1):S38–43.

Itil TM, Eralp E, Tsambis E et al. Central nervous system effects of *Ginkgo biloba*, a plant extract. Am J Ther. 1996;3:63–73.

Itil T, Martorano D. Natural substances in psychiatry (*Ginkgo biloba* in dementia). Psychopharm Bull. 1995;31:147–158.

Ivic L, Sands TT, Fishkin N et al. Terpene trilactones from *Ginkgo biloba* are antagonists of cortical glycine and GABA(A) receptors. J Biol Chem. 2003;278:49279–49285.

Kalus JS, Piotrowski AA, Fortier CR et al. Hemodynamic and electrocardiographic effects of short-term *Ginkgo biloba*. Ann Pharmacother. 2003;37:345–349.

Kampman K, Majewski MD, Tourian K et al. A pilot trial of piracetam and *Ginkgo biloba* for the treatment of cocaine dependence. Addict Behav. 2003;28:437–448.

Kanowski S, Herrmann WM, Stephan K et al. Proof of efficacy of the *Ginkgo biloba* special extract EGb 761 in outpatients suffering from mild to moderate primary degenerative dementia of the Alzheimer type or multi-infarct dementia. Pharmacopsychiatry. 1996;29:47–56.

Kanowski S, Hoerr R. *Ginkgo biloba* extract EGb 761(R) in dementia: Intent to treat analyses of a 24-week, multi-center, double-blind, placebo-controlled, randomized trial. Pharmacopsychiatry. 2003; 36:297–303.

Kennedy DO, Scholey AB, Drewery L et al. Electroencephalograph effects of single doses of *Ginkgo biloba* and *Panax ginseng* in healthy young volunteers. Pharmacol Biochem Behav. 2003;75:701–709.

Klein J, Weichel O, Hilgert M et al. Excitotoxic hippocampal membrane breakdown and its inhibition by bilobalide: role of chloride fluxes. Pharmacopsychiatry. 2003;36 (Suppl 1):S78–83.

Krauze-Baranowska M, Wiwart M. Antifungal activity of biflavones from *Taxus baccata* and *Ginkgo biloba*. Z Naturforsch [C]. 2003;58:65–69.

Kressmann S, Biber A, Wonnemann M et al. Influence of pharmaceutical quality on the bioavailability of active components from *Ginkgo biloba* preparations. J Pharm Pharmacol. 2002;54:1507–1514.

Kuribara H, Weintraub ST, Yoshihama T et al. An anxiolytic-like effect of *Ginkgo biloba* extract and its constituent, ginkgolide A, in mice. J Nat Prod. 2003;66:1333–1337.

Le Bars PL, Kieser M, Itil KZ. A 26-week analysis of a double-blind, placebo-controlled trial of the *Ginkgo biloba* extract EGb 761 in dementia. Dement Geriatr Cogn Disord. 2000;11:230–237.

Li HL. A horticultural and botanical history of ginkgo. Morris Arboretum Bull. 1956;7:3–12.

Li W, Trovero F, Cordier J et al. Prenatal exposure of rats to *Ginkgo biloba* extract (EGb761) increases neuronal survival/growth and alters gene expression in the developing fetal hippocampus. 2003;144: 169–180.

Lingaerde O, Foreland AR, Magnusson A. Can winter depression be prevented by *Ginkgo biloba* extract? A placebo-controlled trial. Acta Psychiatr Scand. 1999;100:62–66.

Lyon MR, Cline JC, Totsy de Zepetnek J et al. Effect of the herbal extract combination *Panax quinquefolium* and *Ginkgo biloba* on attention-deficit hyperactivity disorder: a pilot study. J Psychiatry Neurosci. 2001;26:221–228.

Mantle D, Wilkins RM, Gok MA. Comparison of antioxidant activity in commercial *Ginkgo biloba* preparations. J Altern Complement Med. 2003;9:625–29.

Markowitz JS, Donovan JL, Lindsay DeVane C et al. Multiple-dose administration of *Ginkgo biloba* did not affect cytochrome P-450 2D6 or 3A4 activity in normal volunteers. J Clin Psychopharmacol. 2003;23:576–581.

Markus CR, Lammers JH. Effects of *Ginkgo biloba* on corticosterone stress responses after inescapable shock exposure in the rat. Pharmacol Biochem Behav. 2003;76:487–492.

Mauro VF, Mauro LS, Kleshinski JF et al. Impact of *Ginkgo biloba* on the pharmacokinetics of digoxin. Am J Ther. 2003;10:247–251.

Mills S, Bone K. Principles and Practice of Phytotherapy. Churchill Livingstone, Philadelphia, PA. 2000; 404–417.

Miwa H, Iijima M, Tanaka S et al. Generalized convulsions after consuming a large amount of ginkgo nuts. Epilepsia. 2001;42:280–281.

Morris CA, Avorn J. Internet marketing of herbal products. JAMA. 2003;29:1505–1509.

Muller WE, Chatterjee SS. Cognitive and other behavioral effects of EGb 761 in animal models. Pharmacopsychiatry. 2003;36(Suppl 1):S24–31.

Nishida S, Satoh H. comparative vasodilating actions among terpenoids and flavonoids contained in *Ginkgo biloba* extract. Clin Chim Acta. 2004;339:129–133.

Ohnishi N, Kusuhara M, Yoshioka M et al. Studies on interactions between functional foods or dietary supplements and medicines. I. Effects of *Ginkgo biloba* leaf extract on the pharmacokinetics of diltiazem in rats. Biol Pharm Bull. 2003;26:1315–1320.

Oken BS, Storzbach DM, Kaye JA. The efficacy of *Ginkgo biloba* on cognitive function in Alzheimer disease. Archives Neurol. 1998:55:1409–1415.

Oyama Y, Fuchs PA, Katayama N et al. Myricetin and quercetin, the flavonoid constituents of *Ginkgo biloba* extract, greatly reduce oxidative metabolism in both resting and Ca(2+)-loaded brain neurons. Brain Research. 1994;635:125–129.

Pang Z, Pan F, He S. *Ginkgo biloba*: History, current status, and future prospects. J Alt Compl Med. 1996;2:359–363.

Papadopoulos V, Kapsis A, Li H et al. Drug-induced inhibition of the peripheral-type benzodiazepine receptor expression and cell proliferation of human breast cancer cells. Anticancer Res. 2000;20; 2835–2847.

PDR for Herbal Medicines. (2nd ed) Medical Economics Company Inc., Montvale, NJ. 2000;342–346.

Persson J, Bringlov E, Nilsson LG et al. The memory-enhancing effects of Ginseng and *Ginkgo biloba* in healthy volunteers. Psychopharmacology (Berl). 2004;172:430–434.

Pierre S, Jamme I, Droy-Lefaix MT et al. *Ginkgo biloba* extract EGb 761 protects Na,K-ATPase activity during cerebral ischemia in mice. Neuroreport. 1999:10:47–51.

Ponto LL, Schultz SK. *Ginkgo biloba* extract: review of CNS effects. Ann Clin Psychiatry. 2003;15: 109–119.

Porsolt RD, Roux S, Drieu K. Evaluation of a *Gingko biloba* extract (EGb 761) in function tests for monoamine oxidase inhibition. Arzneimittelforschung. 2000;50:232–235.

Puebla-Perez AM, Lozoya X, Villasenor-Garcia MM. Effect of *Ginkgo biloba* extract, EGb 761, on the cellular immune response in a hypothalamic-pituitary-adrenal axis activation model in the rat. Int Immunopharmacol. 2003;3:75–80.

Rapin JR, Lamproglou I, Drieu K et al. Demonstration of the "anti-stress" activity of an extract of *Ginkgo biloba* (EGb 761) using a discrimination learning task. Gen Pharmacol. 1994;25:1009–1016.

Rowen J, Lewis S. Spontaneous bilateral subdural hematomas associated with chronic *Ginkgo biloba* ingestion. Neurology. 1995;46:1775–1776.

Russo E. Handbook of Psychotropic Herbs: A Scientific Analysis of Herbal Remedies for Psychiatric Conditions. The Haworth Press, Binghamton, NY. 2001;138–153.

Santos RF, Galduroz JC, Barbieri A et al. Cognitive performance, SPECT, and blood viscosity in elderly non-demented people using *Ginkgo biloba*. Pharmacopsychiatry. 2003;36:127–133.

Sasaki K, Hatta S, Haga M et al. Effects of bilobalide on gamma-aminobutyric acid levels and glutamic acid decarboxylase in mouse brain. European J Pharm. 1999;367:165–173.

Sasaki K, Hatta S, Wada K et al. Bilobalide prevents reduction of gamma-aminobutyric acid levels and glutamic acid decarboxylase activity induced by 4-0-methylpyridoxine in mouse hippocampus. Life Sci. 2000;67:709–715.

Schulz V, Hansel R, Tyler VE. Rational phytotherapy: A physicians' guide to herbal medicine. (3rd ed) New York, NY: Springer. 1998.

Schwartz S. Separation anxiety syndrome in dogs and cats. JAVMA. 2003;222:1526–1532.

Shah ZA, Sharma P, Vohora SB. *Ginkgo biloba* normalizes stress-elevated alterations in brain catecholamines, serotonin and plasma corticosterone levels. Eur Neuropsychopharmacol. 2003;13: 321–325.

Shih JC, Chen K, Ridd MJ et al. *Ginkgo biloba* abolishes aggression in mice lacing MAO. Antioxid Redox Signal. 2000;2:467–471.

Smith JV, Luo Y. Studies on molecular mechanisms of *Ginkgo biloba* extract. Appl Microbiol Biotechnol. 2004;64:465–472.

Smith JV, Luo Y. Elevation of oxidative free radicals in Alzheimer's disease models can be attenuated by *Ginkgo biloba* extract EGb 761. J Alzheimers Dis. 2003;5:287–300.

Smith PF, Maclennan K, Darlington CL. The neuroprotective properties of the *Ginkgo biloba* leaf: a review of the possible relationship to platelet-activating factor (PAF). J Ethnopharmacol. 1996;50: 131–139.

Tang Y, Lou F, Wang J et al. coumaroyl flavonol glycosides from the leaves of *Ginkgo biloba*. Phytochemistry. 2001;58:1251–1256.

Tian YM, Tian HJ, Zhang GY et al. Effects of *Ginkgo biloba* extract (EGb 761) on hydroxyl radical-induced thymocyte apoptosis and on age-related thymic atrophy and peripheral immune dysfunctions in mice. Mech Ageing Dev. 2003;124:977–983.

Tsen LC, Segal S, Pothier M et al. Alternative medicine use in presurgical patients. Anesthesiology. 2000;93:148–151.

Vale S. Subarachnoid hemorrhage associated with *Ginkgo biloba*. Lancet. 1998;352:36.

Wang FM, Yao TW, Zeng S. Disposition of quercetin and kaempferol in human following an oral administration of *Ginkgo biloba* extract tablets. Eur J Drug Metab Pharmacokinet. 2003;28:173–177.

Wang Q, Zhao WZ, Ma CG. Protective effects of *Ginkgo biloba* extract on gastric mucosa. Acta Pharmacol Sin. 2000;21:1153–1156.

White HL, Scates PW, Cooper BR. Extracts of *Ginkgo biloba* leaves inhibit monoamine oxidase. Life Sci. 1996;58:1315–1321.

Winter JC, Dimineri D. The discriminative stimulus properties of EGb 761, an extract of *Ginkgo biloba*. Pharm Biochem Behav. 1999;62:543–547.

Wong SS, Nahin RL. National Center for Complementary and Alternative medicine perspectives for complementary and alternative medicine research in cardiovascular diseases. Cardiol Rev. 2003;11: 94–98.

Yang XF, Wang NP, Lu WH et al. Effects of *Ginkgo biloba* extract and tanshinone on cytochrome P-450 isozymes and glutathione transferase in rats. Acta Pharmacol Sin. 2003;24:1033–1038.

Yun YY, Ko SH, Park JW et al. IgE immune response to *Ginkgo biloba* pollen. Ann Allergy Asthma Immunol. 2000;85:298–302.

Zeybek N, Gorgulu S, Yagci G et al. The effects of *Ginkgo biloba* extract (EGb 761) on experimental acute pancreatitis. J Surg Res. 2003;115:286–293.

Zhang XY, Zhou DF, Su JM et al. The effect of extract of *Ginkgo biloba* added to haloperidol on superoxide dismutase in inpatients with chronic schizophrenia. J Clin Psychopharmacol. 2001;21:85–88.

Zhu L, Wu J, Gao J et al. Antagonistic effects of extract from leaves of *Ginkgo biloba* on glutamate neurotoxicity. Chung Kuo Li Hsueh Pao (Acta Pharmacologica Sinica). 1997;14:344–347.

Huperzia serrata

Huperzia serrata (Huperzine, Qian Ceng Ta, Shuangyiping, She zu shi shan, Jin bu huan, Chinese Club Moss, Toothed Clubmoss, formerly known as *Lycopodium serrata*) is a native Chinese moss in the *Lycopodiaceae* family (Russo 2001). It is a prehistoric plant dating back to the Devonian period. *H. serrata* is traditionally used as an analgesic, antispasmodic, antipyretic, diuretic, and a detoxicant to reduce edema and stop bleeding (Zangara 2003; Leung 1990).

Ingredients

At some point during its clinical use, observations of cholinergic effects associated with *H. serrata* led to further investigation and identification of the sesquiterpene alkaloids huperzine A and B (Zangara 2003).

CNS Effects

Huperzine A, first isolated in China in 1980, is a potent and reversible inhibitor of AChE (Zangara 2003). Both compounds exhibit potent AChE inhibition. In fact, huperzine A is at least three times stronger than physostigmine and 30 times as potent as galanthamine, which is currently prescribed in the United Kingdom for the treatment of Alzheimer's disease, without the adverse effects (Leung 1990). Huperzine A may also increase levels of norepinephrine and dopamine (Zhu, Giacobini 1995). Recently, a research group in Israel identified alkylene-linked dimmers of hupyridone derivatives of huperzine A (Wong, Greenblatt, Dvir et al. 2003). These compounds were shown to be even more potent inhibitors of AchE than huperzine A and indicate that the search for improved AchE inhibitors is far from over.

Neurological and Behavioral Effects

H. serrata has become the focus of attention for the treatment of cognitive impairment. A relative, *Lycopodium clavatum*, has also traditionally been used to balance behavioral and mood disturbances (PDR 2000).

H. serrata has emerged as a significant herbal alternative in the treatment of Alzheimer's disease (Howes, Perry, Houghton 2003). At least part of the mechanism of action is due to antagonism of beta-amyloid protein (Wang, Zhang, Tang 2001) and the inhibition of nitric oxide-induced neurotoxicity (Zhao, Li 2002). In comparative tests against synthetic drugs such as donepezil and tacrine used in the treatment of Alzheimer's disease, it has no reported side effects at therapeutic dosage, easily crosses the blood-brain barrier, and has a prolonged half-life (Jiang, Luo, Bai 2003).

In an *in vitro* rat study, both huperzine A and donepezil showed significant neuroprotection against oxidative injury (Zhou, Fu, Tang 2001). In another study of different AChE forms in various parts of the rat brain, huperzine A, donepezil, and tacrine were consistently high in their inhibitory properties (Zhao, Tang 2002).

Huperzine A has shown nootropic effects in rats (Wang, Zhou, Shao et al. 2003; Wang, Zhou, Shao et al. 2002; Wang, Zhang, Tang 2001). Gerbils with ischemic injury showed significant improvement in memory impairment and neuronal degeneration with huperzine A treatment (0.1 mg/kg BID for 14 days) (Zhou, Zhang, Tang 2001). Huperzine is currently in the final stages of clinical investigation in China, and studies are under way in the United States for the treatment of Alzheimer's disease. In July 2003, Savient Pharmaceuticals acquired exclusive European and American marketing rights to huperzine A from Marco Hi-TechJoint Venture, which has exclusive worldwide marketing and distribution rights (Anonymous 2004).

H. serrata is of worldwide interest for the treatment of neurodegenerative illnesses such as perinatal hypoxia as well as senile degenerative changes (Wang, Zhou, Shao et al. 2003). It is also considered a primary candidate for pretreatment of organophosphate nerve agents, which is of serious importance given current terrorist threats around the world (Lallement, Baille, Baubichon et al. 2002; Lallement, Foquin, Dorandeu et al. 2001).

Adverse Effects

A study of the effect of huperzine A on liver cytochrome P-450 was conducted in order to predict possible drug interaction and ensure safe administration (Ma, Wang, Xin et al. 2003). At therapeutic doses of 0.1 mg/kg, liver CYP isoenzymes were unaffected; however, slight inductive response of CYP1A2 was observed at toxicological doses of 1 or 2 mg/kg.

The acute effects of huperzine A and tacrine on rat liver were compared (Ma, Xin, Wang et al. 2003). Although both resulted in increased serum aspartate aminotransferase and alanine aminotransferase, tacrine was associated with histopathologic changes whereas huperzine was not. Furthermore, the effect of huperzine A (but not tacrine) on liver values was reversed by atropine.

Drug interaction has not been reported to date although the potential may exist. Slight dizziness is the only side effect reported in an earlier human clinical trial and it did not affect the therapeutic effect (Zhang, Tang, Han et al. 1991).

Availability

As with many TCM preparations, herbs are often used in combination to potentiate their effects or to counteract potential toxicity. *H. serrata* is available in commercial preparations in combination with *Ginkgo biloba* (Russo 2001).

Clinical Application in Veterinary Behavior Medicine

H. serrata is primarily of interest in the treatment of canine and feline cognitive dysfunction syndromes. It may be effective used alone, in combination with other herbal neuroprotectors, or as an adjunct to conventional treatment with selegiline. Further research will determine how it will be best applied.

References

Anonymous. Huperzine A. Drugs R D. 2004;5:44–45.

Howes MJ, Perry NS, Houghton PJ. Plants with traditional uses and activities, relevant to the management of Alzheimer's disease and other cognitive disorders. Phytother Res. 2003;17:1–18.

Jiang H, Luo X, Bai D. Progress in clinical, pharmacological, chemical and structural biological studies of huperzine A: a drug of traditional Chinese medicine origin for the treatment of Alzheimer's disease. Curr Med Chem. 2003;10:2231–2252.

Lallement G, Baille V, Baubichon D et al. Review of the value of huperzine as pretreatment of organophosphate poisoning. Neurotoxicology. 2002;23:1–5.

Lallement G, Foquin A, Dorandeu F et al. Subchronic administration of various pretreatments of nerve agent poisoning. II. Compared efficacy against soman toxicity. Drug Chem Toxicol. 2001;24: 165–180.

Leung AY. Chinese medicinals. In: Janick J, Simon JE (eds). Advances in new crops. Timber Press, Portland, OR. 1990;499–510.

Ma XC, Wang HX, Xin J et al. Effects of huperzine A on liver cytochrome P-450 in rats. Acta Pharmacol Sin. 2003;24:831–835.

Ma XC, Xin J, Wang HX et al. Acute effects of huperzine A and tacrine on rat liver. Acta Pharmacol Sin. 2003;24:247–250.

PDR for Herbal Medicines. (2nd ed) Medical Economics Company Inc., Montvale, NJ 2000:196–197.

Russo E. Handbook of Psychotropic Herbs: A Scientific Analysis of Herbal Remedies for Psychiatric Conditions. The Haworth Press, Binghamton, NY 2001;157–158.
Wang LS, Zhou J, Shao XM et al. Huperzine A attenuates cognitive deficits and brain injury after hypoxia-ischemic brain damage in neonatal rats. Zhonghua Er Ke Za Zhi. 2003;41:42–45.
Wang LS, Zhou J, Shao XM et al. Huperzine A attenuates cognitive deficits and brain injury in neonatal rats after hypoxia-ischemia. Brain Res. 2002;949:162–170.
Wang R, Zhang HY, Tang XC. Huperzine A attenuates cognitive dysfunction and neuronal degeneration caused by beta-amyloid protein–(1-40) in rats. Eur J Pharmacol. 2001;421:149–156.
Wong DM, Greenblatt HM, Dvir H et al. Acetylcholinesterase complexed with bivalent ligands related to huperzine A: experimental evidence for species dependent protein-ligand complementarity. J Am Chem Soc. 2003;125:363–373.
Zhang RW, Tang SC, Han YY et al. Drug evaluation of huperzine A in the treatment of senile memory disorders. Zhongguo Yao Li Xue Bao. 1991;12:250–252.
Zhao HW, Li XY. Ginkgolide A, B, and huperzide A inhibit nitric oxide-induced neurotoxicity. Int Immunopharmacol. 2002;2:1551–1556.
Zhao Q, Tang XC. Effects of huperzine A on acetylcholinesterase isoforms in vitro: comparison with tacrine, donepezil, rivastigmine and physostigmine. Eur J Pharmacol. 2002;455:101–107.
Zhou J, Fu Y, Tang XC. Huperzine A and donepezil protect rat pheochromocytome cells against oxygen-glucose deprivation. Neurosci Lett. 2001;306:53–56.
Zhou J, Zhang HY, Tang XC. Huperzine A attenuates cognitive deficits and hippocampus neuronal damage after transient global ischemia in gerbils. Neurosci Lett. 2001;313:137–140.
Zhu XD, Giacobini E. Second generation cholinesterase inhibitors: Effect of (L)—huperzine-A on cortical biogenic amines. J Neurosci Res. 1995;41:828–835.

Panax ginseng

Panax ginseng (Jen-hsien, Ren shen, Kuei-kai, Ninjin, Insam, Chinese Ginseng, Korean Ginseng, Asian Ginseng, Oriental Ginseng, Red berry, Five-fingers, Man root, Racine de ginseng, Ginsengwurzel; family Araliaceae) is a perennial native to eastern China. It grows between 30 and 60 cm high and prefers the shade and, in cool climates, facing north. Terminal groups of palm-like leaves are born atop a smooth, round stem. *P. ginseng* produces small red berries. Plants are harvested between August and October, but not before three years of growth to allow for peak concentrations of the primary active compounds (Russo 2001; PDR 2000; Mills, Bone 2000).

The medicinal part of *P. ginseng* is the root, which produces offshoots that taper like a carrot at the ends and give it a characteristic anthropomorphic feature. *Panax* is the Greek word for panacea, or cure-all. Chinese "*seng*" is a group of herbs with fleshy roots. The term Ginseng, therefore, implies a human-shaped root or plant (Russo 2001; Mills, Bone 2000).

P. ginseng has been used traditionally for digestive symptoms, inappetance, neuralgia, anxiety, insomnia, fatigue, reduced concentration, impotence, sterility, arthritis, and debility (PDR 2000). In TCM, *P. ginseng* strengthens the qi and benefits the yin. From the Chinese perspective, the yin encompasses all bodily fluids, blood, and lymph, which lubricate, nourish, and fill the muscles, organs, and all physical aspects of the body. *P. ginseng* is also advised to fortify the spleen and tonify the stomach and lungs; it is used to treat respiratory symptoms, abdominal distension, and lethargy. *P. ginseng* is said to reduce fatigue, sharpen the mind, and slow aging. It is considered to be a life-saving treatment in patients suffering from traumatic injuries and shock. Herbs that calm the spirit are advised for anxiety, agitation, and insomnia (Mills, Bone 2000; Tillotson, Tillotson, Abel 2001).

Historical Perspective

P. ginseng is one of the most ancient medicinal herbs. According to Chinese legend, the Emperor Shennong of the late Han Dynasty, who lived around 2800 CE, introduced *P. ginseng*. In his famous materia medica *Shennong Bencao (Pen-ts'ao-ching)*, he described *P. ginseng* as useful for "quieting the spirit, curbing the emotion, stopping agitation, removing noxious influence, brightening the eye, enlightening the mind, and increasing the wisdom." He also believed that long-term use of *P. ginseng* would lead to long life (Russo 2001).

Ingredients

Components of *P. ginseng* include an essential oil (limonene, citral, terpineol, polyacetylenes), polysaccharides (sugars, starches), and flavonoids (e.g., panaxasenoide, trifolin, kaempferol). The most important compounds are the ginsenosides, a group of triterpene saponins with a chemical structure similar to steroids (Russo 2001; PDR 2000). As many as 28 ginsenosides have been identified and named according to their migration patterns on thin layer chromatography (Fig. 4-4). These are classified as either the protopanaxadiols or protopanaxatriols. The ginsenosides Rb1, Rb2, Rc, Rd, Re, and Rg1 have emerged as the most important components of *P. ginseng*. The pharmacology of the ginsenosides is complex. Compounds may share effects but can have specific properties as well.

CNS Effects

P. ginseng has a direct impact on cerebroelectrical activity. Single doses of 200 mg of *P. ginseng* extract G115 led to significant reductions in alpha, theta, and beta activity, as well as significant shortening of the latency of the P300 component of the evoked potential. In a double-blind, placebo-controlled balanced crossover study, ECG changes associated with *P. ginseng* intake were more pronounced compared to *Ginkgo biloba* (Kennedy, Scholey, Drewery et al. 2003).

P. ginseng saponins may directly impact the hypothalamo-pituitary-adrenal axis and inhibit a stress-induced increase in plasma corticosterone by blocking ACTH action on the adrenal gland (Kim, Moon, Jung et al. 2003). Protopanaxatriol saponins inhibit ACh-stimulated catecholamines secretion (Tachikawa, Kudo, Hasegawa et al. 2003). In addition, protopanaxadiol saponins may act as prodrugs; their metabolites show potent inhibitory activity of catecholamines secretion by direct action on nicotinic ACh receptors.

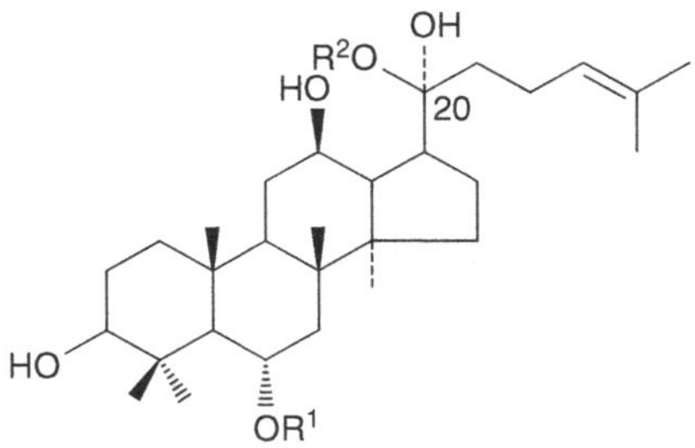

	R1	R2
20(S)-Protopanaxatriol	H	H
Ginsenoside Re	glc(2—1)rha	glc
Ginsenoside Rf	glc(2—1)glc	H
Ginsenoside Rg_1	glc	glc
Ginsenoside Rg_2	glc(2—1)rha	H

Protopanaxatriol Class

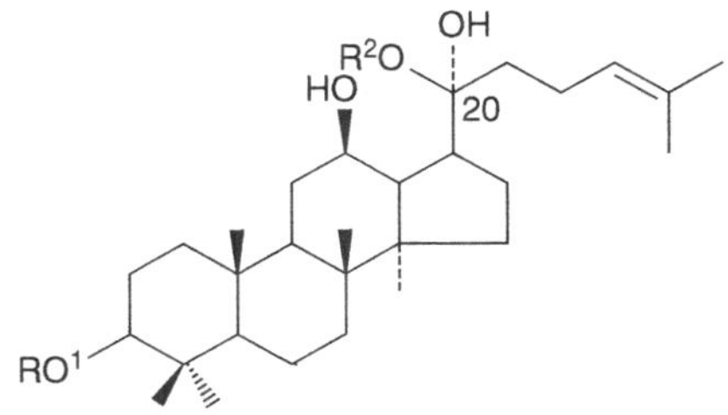

	R1	R2
20(S)-Protopanaxadiol	H	H
Ginsenoside Rb_1	glc(2—1)glc	glc(6—1)glc
Ginsenoside Rb_2	glc(2—1)glc	glc(6—1)ara *p*
Ginsenoside Rc	glc(2—1)glc	glc(6—1)ara *f*
Ginsenoside Rd	glc(2—1)glc	glc

Protopanaxadiol Class

glc = β-D-glucose
rha = α-L-rhamnose
ara = α-L-arabinose
p = pyranose
f = furanose

FIGURE 4-4. Active compounds of *Panax ginseng.* (Mills, Bone 2000)

Ginsenosides Rb1 and Rg1 have been suggested as the primary active agents of *P. ginseng* via stimulation of ACh, reduction in serotonin and free radicals, and enhanced metabolism of protein and nucleotide metabolism (Liu, Xiao 1992). In another study, ginsenosides Rg2,3 were shown to inhibit ACh-triggered catecholamines release by blockade of nicotinic ACh and GABA receptors. Another nonginsenoside compound has also shown nicotinic binding. Because senile cognitive changes have been improved by stimulation of nicotine receptors, these findings may help to explain the therapeutic benefit on age-related cognitive impairment (PDR 2000; Tachikawa, Kudo, Harada et al. 1999).

Cognitive and Psychological Effects

Recent double-blind, placebo-controlled studies found that a combination of *Ginkgo biloba* and *Panax ginseng* produced striking improvement on cognitive performance that was more impressive than the significant improvement demonstrated for either herb treatment group used alone (Kennedy, Scholey, Wesnes 2001a,b; Scholey, Kennedy 2002; Kennedy, Scholey, Wesnes 2002). *P. ginseng* appeared to improve self-rated mood and was associated with improved performance on memory and attentional tasks (Kennedy, Scholey, Wesnes 2002; Kennedy, Scholey, Wesnes 2001a). In early studies, ginsenoside Rb1 exerted a sedative effect and impaired cognitive performance, whereas ginsenoside Rg1 stimulated cognitive performance (Petkov 1978).

In cases of dementia, damage to neuronal networks may be compensated for and repaired by extensions of neuronal axons and dendrites (Tohda, Matsumoto, Zou et al. 2002). Interesting and potentially important neurotropic and neuroprotective properties have been attributed to ginsenoside Rb1 and Rg1 (Rudakewich, Ba, Benishin 2001). Both stimulated neurite outgrowth in the presence of a suboptimal dose of nerve growth factor, although neurite outgrowth was not significant in the absence of nerve growth factor. In addition, both Rb1 and Rg1 reversed cell death, although this effect was not reversed if cell death was induced by beta-amyloid. Deposition of beta amyloid is a consistent finding in the brains of aging pets with feline or canine cognitive dysfunction syndromes and in people with Alzheimer's disease (Cummings, Su, Cotman et al. 1993; Johnstone, Chaney, Norris et al. 1991).

Preliminary data on a new Panax species provides additional insight into the cognitive enhancement attributed to ginseng. *P. vietnamensis* was recently discovered in Vietnam. It has bamboo-like rhizomes and is closely related to *P. japonicus* and *P. pseudoginseng* (Komatsu, Zhu, Fushimi et al. 2001). In a recent Japanese study, protopanaxadiol-type saponins derived from *Panax ginseng, P. notoginseng,* and *P. vietnamensis* (Ye-Sanchi) all enhanced axonal and dendritic outgrowth (Tohda, Matsumoto, Zou et al. 2002).

P. ginseng may have greater clinical activity and, consequently, be of greater therapeutic benefit to the elderly (Sorensen, Sonne 1996). In a double-blind placebo-controlled study of standardized *P. ginseng* extract G115 in almost 400 healthy adults, psychological parameters were improved in both groups; however, the *P. ginseng* group showed significant improvement in alertness, relaxation, and overall well being compared to placebo (Wiklund, Karlberg, Lund 1994).

An anxiolytic effect has been confirmed in *P. ginseng* in rodent studies. An Indian study showed that anxiolytic activity for white (*Ren shen*) and red (*Hong shen*) varieties of *P. ginseng* root extract administered intraperitoneally was comparable to diazepam (Bhattacharya, Mitra 1991). In a more recent study (Bhattcharyya, Sur 1999), *P. ginseng* was again compared with diazepam in stressed rats. Both compounds exerted an antistress effect characterized by reduced levels of brain and hypothalamic 5-HT, possibly mediated by prostaglandins.

Antineoplastic Effects

Ginsenoside and nonginsenoside components of *P. ginseng* have been shown to possess potent antineoplastic effects via enzyme activation (Kim, Lee, Park et al. 1999a,b; Kim, Oh, Lee et al. 1999) as well as the inhibition of cancer cells (Lee, Sung, Lee et al. 1999). For example, red ginseng powder was shown to improve postoperative survival in patients with stage III gastric cancer (Suh, Kroh, Kim et al. 2002). *P. ginseng* extract also possesses a radioprotective effect that could become useful in patients undergoing radiation therapy (Kim, Jo, Kim 2003). Further clinical research is needed to confirm an antineoplastic application; however, cancer patients may feel invigorated by psychological and cognitive effects of the herb (Chang, Seo, Gyllenhaal et al. 2003).

Despite their antitumor activity, *P. ginseng* components may exert a carcinogenic effect. It has recently been demonstrated that ginsenosides Rb1 and Rh1 act as phytoestrogens and may promote activation of break cancer cells by binding to estrogen receptors (Lee, Jin, Lim et al. 2003a,b).

Antioxidant and Anti-inflammatory Effects

P. ginseng has shown antioxidant protection by free radical scavenging in hepatic and cardiac tissues, as well as at the level of a number of proteins and DNA (PDR 2000; Maffei, Carini, Aldini et al. 1999; Voces, Alvarez, Vila et al. 1999; Lee, Lee, Kim 1998). A traditional Chinese preparation called *Sheng mai san* (a mixture containing *Panax ginseng, Ophiopogon japonicus* and *Schisandra chinesis*) has been shown to possess antioxidant activity in the brain of rats (Ichikawa, Wang, Konishi 2003). *Sheng mai san* ("Generate the Pulse Powder") remains a popular treatment in Chinese hospitals, including for the treatment of emergency trauma cases (Tillotson, Tillotson, Abel 2001).

In recent studies of the antiallergic activities of ginsenosides, ginsenoside Rh2 and a *P. ginseng* extract called "compound K" displayed more potent cell membrane stabilizing activity than the antiallergenic drug disodium cromoglycate (Choo, Park Han et al. 2003; Park, Choo, Kim et al. 2003). Ginsenoside also exhibited anti-inflammatory properties by the inhibition of nitric oxide and prostaglandin E2 (Park, Choo, Kim et al. 2003). Ginsenosides and their metabolites may act as prodrugs with important antiallergic effects.

Cardiovascular and Pulmonary Effects

The ginsenosides exert important cardiac activity. Ginsenosides are antiarrhythmic, chronotrope negative, and inotrope positive and negative; they also elevate the ventricular fibrillation threshold (Rosado 2003; Wu, Zhang, Liu et al. 1995; Wu, Chen 1988). A recent electrocardiographic and hemodynamic study showed that *P. ginseng* increased the QT interval and decreased diastolic blood pressure within two hours of initial administration, although the clinical significance of these findings is uncertain (Caron, Hotsko, Robertson et al. 2002).

Platelet release reaction is suppressed by ginsenosides Ro, Rg1, and Rg2. Panaxynol blocks platelet aggregation, release, and thromboxane formation (Kuo, Teng, Lee et al. 1990).

Standardized *P. ginseng* extract G115 was recently shown to improve pulmonary function, including maximum inspiratory pressure and maximal oxygen consumption, in 92 patients with moderately severe chronic obstructive pulmonary disease (COPD). No side effects were reported at the treatment dose of 100 mg BID for three months (Gross, Shenkman, Bleiberg et al. 2002).

Hypoglycemic Effects

Ginsenosides produce a hypoglycemic effect by stimulation of insulin release as well as by adrenergic mechanisms (Guodong, Zhongqui 1987; PDR 2000). A dosage of 100–200 mg of oral standardize *P. ginseng* extract has been clinically effective in treating type 2 diabetes (non-insulin dependent) in people (Sotaniemi, Haapakoski, Rautio 1995). *P. ginseng* berry extract has also been shown to exert a hypoglycemic effect in mice (Attele, Zhou, Xie et al. 2002). Recently, a *P. ginseng* glycopeptide was shown to impact both blood glucose and liver glycogen. This hypoglycemic effect may be due to enhanced aerobic glycolysis by stimulation of beta-adrenergic receptors and enzymatic activity in the tricarboxylic acid cycle (Wang, Zhou, Yang et al. 2003).

Sexual Effects

P. ginseng has been shown to be an effective treatment for male erectile dysfunction (Hong, Ji, Hong et al. 2002). Erectile function is enhanced by peripheral and local neurophysiological mechanisms (Choi, Rha, Choi 1999; Choi, Seong, Rha 1995). Recently, ginsenoside Rb1 was associated with increased luteinizing hormone (LH) secretion by a direct effect on the anterior pituitary gland (Tsai, Chiao Lu et al. 2003). In addition, relaxation of the corpus cavernosum by *P. ginseng* may be associated with its apparent effect on sexual performance (Gillis 1997). *P. ginseng* has been shown to enhance sexual mounting in male rats and to increase sperm production in the rabbit (Tsai, Chiao Lu et al. 2003). The erectile properties of *P. ginseng* have led to its recommendation as an effective, safe, and less costly alternative to sildenafil (Viagra®) (Price, Gazewood 2003).

Miscellaneous Effects

Immunomodulatory effects induced by *P. ginseng* extract including the enhancement of killer T cell- and antibody-triggered cytotoxic activities, as well as stimulation of interferon production, also promote antiviral effects (Singh, Agarwal, Gupta 1984; Singh, George, Singh et al. 1983). Antiviral effects have been demonstrated against influenza and the common cold (Scaglione, Cattaneo, Alessandria et al. 1996).

P. ginseng has been shown to boost the clearance of blood alcohol by several mechanisms, including enzyme induction and delayed gastric emptying (PDR 2000).

Enzyme activation by *P. ginseng* saponins results in the reduction of serum triglycerides and cholesterol levels, and elevation of HDL-cholesterol (Kim, Park 2003; Inoue, Wu, Doue 1999). *P. ginseng* berry extract has also been shown to reduce plasma cholesterol levels (Attele, Zhou, Xie et al. 2002).

Availability

Statistics show that *P. ginseng* constitutes as much as 20% of the total botanical herbs market in the Unites States (Gillis 1997). Commercial over-the-counter *P. ginseng* products are very plentiful. Capsules are available between 100 mg to 1250 mg strengths. It is also supplied as a liquid (300 mg/ml), chewable lozenge, and tablet (350 mg, 500 mg) (Russo 2001; PDR 2000). It is also popular as a tea infusion. In TCM, red *P. ginseng* (*Hong shen, Hung seng*) refers to the root that has been steamed; sugared *P. ginseng* is called *Tang shen (T'ang seng*). It may be prepared sun-dried, boiled, and thinly sliced (Russo 2001).

Dosage depends on the condition to be treated as well as the preparation to be used. For example, erectile dysfunction in men has been shown to respond to red *P. ginseng* at a dose of 600 mg PO TID (Choi, Seong, Rha 1995). In general, between 0.5 to 3.0 g per day of the dried root or 100 to 200 mg of a quality standardized extract containing between 4 and 7 percent ginsenosides have been advised for people (Russo 2001; Mills, Bone 2000). Physical and psychological performance indices have been improved on 100 mg twice daily (Forgo, Schimert 1985). It is of note that the International Olympic Committee does not prohibit athletes from taking *P. ginseng* (Bahrke, Morgan 1994).

Many herbal products on the U.S. market contain trace to low amounts of the active ingredient (Anonymous 1995). The issue of quality control and product standardization is not exclusive to *P. ginseng*. However, the popularity of this product highlights the need for updating the current measures and regulations of commercial OTC herbal preparations.

Adverse Effects

Important side effects associated with *P. ginseng* use and abuse have been reported. General side effects include headache, nervousness, insomnia, epistaxis, and vomiting. These effects may result from hypertension. Other adverse effects include neonatal androgenization, vaginal bleeding, mastalgia, and mammary nodules (PDR 2000; Awang 1991). The anticoagulant effect could become of primary concern in patients undergoing surgical procedure, or those taking concomitant anticoagulants (e.g., warfarin) for other medical conditions (Rosado 2003; Janetzky, Morreale 1997). Patients taking *P. ginseng* products should withdraw from medication at least two weeks prior to scheduled surgery (Hodges, Kam 2002). If it is carefully monitored, however, the antithrombotic effect could be valuable in the prevention of clot formation in cats suffering from feline cardiomyopathy or post-trauma dogs at risk of pulmonary thromboembolism, for example.

The Ginseng Abuse Syndrome has been used to describe persistent heterogeneous complaints such as anxiety, insomnia, and diarrhea allegedly caused by prolonged high does of the herb (Siegel 1979). However, this was not a placebo-controlled study, and enormous quantities (as much as 15 g) of an unspecified quality of *P. ginseng* were administered (Russo 2001; Gillis 1997).

In mice, the LD50 of *P. ginseng* was between 10–30 gm/kg of whole root but was attributed to abdominal distension rather than actual pharmacological toxicity (Bahrke, Morgan 1994). In dogs, long-term supplementation of *P. ginseng* G115 had no clinically significant effects (Hess, Parent, Stevens et al. 1983). The risk of side effects increases with dosage and prolonged intake (Bisset, Wichtl 1994); the German Commission E advises that *P. ginseng* intake not exceed 90 consecutive days although repeat courses are an option (Russo 2001).

Drug Interaction

Drug interaction with insulin and other antidiabetic agents are also a potential risk given evidence of *P. ginseng's* hypoglycemic property. Patients taking antiplatelet or nonsteroidal anti-inflammatory drugs (NSAIDs) should avoid taking *P. ginseng* products due to its recognized antiplatelet properties. Concomitant use of *P. ginseng* with loop diuretics is inadvisable; there have been rare reports of nephrotoxicity in the same part of the kidney in which diuretics exert their effect (Becker, Greene, Evanson et al. 1996). However, these cases were not associated with a high-quality, standardized extract taken within therapeutic doses (Russo 2001).

Phenelzine (a monoamine oxidase inhibitor) and *P. ginseng* used in combination may lead to headache, tremor, and mania, and therefore concomitant use should be avoided (PDR 2000; Mills, Bone 2000).

Both *P. ginseng* and *Eleutherococcus senticosus* ("Siberian ginseng") contain glycosides that chemically resemble digoxin. Patients receiving digoxin and then supplemented with either of these herbs showed falsely elevated digoxin levels with one test and falsely decreased levels with another, although three other digoxin assays showed no interference (Dasgupta, Wu, Actor et al. 2003).

Clinical Application in Veterinary Behavior Medicine

Panax ginseng may facilitate recuperation from illness, although it should not be used in the immediate presurgical or postsurgical interval, to avoid increase risk of hemorrhage. Moreover, *P. ginseng* may be helpful in the treatment of blood clots, such as saddle thrombi related to feline cardiomyopathy and other clinical pathologies.

P. ginseng may also be valuable to treat cases of sexual dysfunction in pets, and its phytoestrogens affinity for estrogen receptors suggests its application in treating urinary incontinence for brief courses of administration.

In particular, cognitive impairment associated with senile changes may be particularly responsive to *P. ginseng* (Youdim, Joseph 2001). *P. ginseng* may be a useful alternative or adjunct to conventional medication with selegiline in cases of canine and feline cognitive dysfunction syndromes (Ruehl, Bruyette, DePaoli et al. 1995).

Evidence of its anxiolytic effect is eclipsed by proof of its cognitive-enhancing properties; additional research is needed to better evaluate its effect on mood, although it could be beneficial in treating mild forms of anxiety.

P. ginseng may enhance sexual performance in pets of particular breeding value; underlying physical causes must always be investigated. In these cases, *P. ginseng* may benefit sexual dysfunction by alleviating anxiety and supporting physiological mechanisms of sexual arousal. Due to its antithrombotic potential, however, *P. ginseng* administration requires very close monitoring in pets at higher risk for traumatic injury by fighting with other animals (e.g., outdoor cats and indoor pet experiencing conflicts with housemates) or in athletic dogs (e.g., dogs competing in agility, lure-coursing, field, herding trials).

In general, polyherbal preparations containing *P. ginseng* should be avoided in order to isolate the therapeutic effects of *P. ginseng* and to minimize the risk of side effects (Chang, Seo, Gyllenhaal et al. 2003). A dosage of 100 mg once to twice daily of a quality, dried-root preparation containing approximately 5% ginsenoside content is suggested for debilitated pets or those suffering from cognitive impairment. Although prolonged therapy may be accompanied by greater risk of adverse effects, continuous use may be worthwhile in chronic and debilitating conditions affecting aging pets.

Comparative studies between *P. ginseng* and conventional psychoactive medication deserve further attention. Its effect on mood remains unclear and difficult to interpret. Comparative or basic clinical studies of the behavioral and psychological effects of *P. ginseng* will provide additional direction and clarity.

References

Anonymous 1995. Herbal roulette. Consumer Reports (November):698–705.

Attele AS, Zhou YP, Xie JT et al. Antidiabetic effects of *Panax ginseng* berry extract and the identification of an effective component. Diabetes. 2002;51:1851–1858.

Awang DV. Maternal use of ginseng and neonatal androgenization. JAMA 1991;266:363.

Bahrke MS, Morgan WP. Evaluation of the ergogenic properties of ginseng. Sports Medicine 1994;18:229–248.

Becker BN, Greene J, Evanson J et al. Ginseng-induced diuretic resistance. JAMA 1996;276:606–607.

Bhattcharyya D, Sur TK. Effect of *Panax ginseng* and diazepam on brain 5-hydroxytryptamine and its modification by diclofenac in rats. Indian J Physiol Pharmacol. 1999;43:505–509.

Bhattacharya SK, Mitra SK. Anxiolytic activity of *Panax ginseng* roots: an experimental study. J Ethnopharmacol. 1991;34:87–92.

Bisset NG, Wichtl M. Herbal drugs and phytopharmaceuticals: A handbook for practice on a scientific basis. Med-Pharm Scientific Publishers, CRC Press: Boca Raton, FL 1994.

Chang YS, Seo EK, Gyllenhaal C et al. *Panax ginseng*: a role in cancer therapy? Integr Cancer Ther. 2003;2:13–33.

Choi H, Seong D, Rha K. Clinical efficacy of Korean red ginseng for erectile dysfunction. Int J Impot Res 1995;7:181–186.

Choo MK, Park EK, Han MJ et al. antiallergic activity of ginseng and its ginsenosides. Planta Med. 2003;69:518–522.

Choi Y, Rha K, Choi H. In vitro and in vivo experimental effect of Korean red ginseng on erection. J Urol 1999;162:1508–1511.

Caron MF, Hotsko AL, Robertson S et al. Electrocardiographic and hemodynamic effects of *Panax ginseng*. Ann Pharmacother. 2002;36:758–763.

Cummings BJ, Su JH, Cotman CW et al. Beta-amyloid accumulation in aged canine brain: a model of early plaque formation in Alzheimer's disease. Neurobiol Aging. 1993:14;547–560.

Dasgupta A, Wu S, Actor J et al. Effect of Asian and Siberian ginseng on serum digoxin measurement by five digoxin immunoassays. Significant variation in digoxin-like immunoreactivity among commercial ginsengs. Am J Clin Pathol. 2003;119:298–303.

Forgo I, Schimert G. Zur Frage der Wirkungsdauer des standarisierten Ginseng-Extraktes G 115 bei gesunden Leistungssportiern. Notabene medici 1985;9:636–649.

Gillis, CN. *Panax ginseng* pharmacology: a nitric oxide ink? Biochem Pharmacol. 1997;54:1–8.

Gross D, Shenkman Z, Bleiberg B et al. Ginseng improves pulmonary functions and exercise capacity in patients with COPD. Monaldi Arch Chest Dis. 2002;57:242–246.

Guodong L, Zhongqui L. Effects of ginseng saponins on insulin release from isolated pancreatic islets of rats. Chin J Integr Trad Western Med. 1987;7:326.

Hess FG, Parent RA, Stevens KR et al. Effects of subchronic feeding of ginseng extract G115 in beagle dogs. Food Chem Toxicol 1983;21:95–97.

Hodges PJ, Kam PC. The peri-operative implications of herbal medicines. Anaesthesia. 2002;57: 889–899.

Hong B, Ji YH, Hong JH et al. A double-blind crossover study evaluating the efficacy of Korean red ginseng in patients with erectile dysfunction: a preliminary report. J Urol. 2002;168:2070–2073.

Inoue, Wu, Dou et al. Lipoprotein lipase activation by red ginseng saponins in hyperlipidemia model animals. Phytomedicine 1999;6:257–265.

Janetzky K, Morreale AP. Probable interaction between warfarin and ginseng. Am J Health-System Pharm. 1997;54:692–693.

Johnstone E, Chaney M, Norris F et al. Conservation of the sequence of the Alzheimer's disease amyloid peptide in dog, polar bear and five other mammals by cross-species polymerase chain reaction analysis. Brain Res. 1991;10:299–305.

Kennedy DO, Scholey AB, Drewery L et al. Electroencephalograph effects of single doses of *Ginkgo biloba* and *Panax ginseng* in healthy young volunteers. Pharmacol Biochem Behav. 2003;75:701–709.

Kennedy DO, Scholey AB, Wesnes KA. Modulation of cognition and mood following administration of single doses of *Ginkgo biloba*, ginseng, and a ginkgo/ginseng combination to healthy young adults. Physiol Behav. 2002;75:739–751.

Kennedy DO, Scholey AB, Wesnes KA. Dose dependent changes in cognitive performance and mood following acute administration of Ginseng to healthy young volunteers. Nutr Neurosci. 2001a;4: 295–310.

——. Differential, dose dependent changes in cognitive performance following acute administration of a *Ginkgo biloba/Panax ginseng* combination to healthy young volunteers. Nutr Neurosci. 2001b;4: 399–412.

Kim DH, Moon YS, Jung JS et al. Effects of ginseng saponin administered intraperitoneally on the hypothalamo-pituitary-adrenal axis in mice. Neurosci Lett. 2003;343:62–66.

Kim SE, Lee YH, Park JH et al. Ginsenoside Rs4, a new type of ginseng saponin concurrently induces apoptosis and selectively elevates protein levels of p53 and p21WAF1 in human hepatoma SK-HEP-1 cells. Eur J Cancer. 1999a;35:507–511.

——. Ginsenoside Rs3, a new diol-type ginseng saponins, selectively elevates protein levels of p53 and p21WAF1 leading to induction of apoptosis in SK-HEP-1 cells. Anticancer Res 1999b;19:487–491.

Kim SE, Oh JH, Lee SK et al. Ginsenoside RH-2 induces apoptotic cell death in rat C6 glioma via a reactive oxygen and caspase dependent but Bcl-X(L)-independent pathway. Life Sci 1999;65:PL33–40.

Kim SH, Park KS. Effects of *Panax ginseng* extract on lipid metabolism in humans. Pharmacol Res. 2003;48:511–513.

Kim SR, Jo SK, Kim SH. Modification of radiation response in mice by ginsenosides, active components of *Panax ginseng*. In Vivo. 2003;17:77–81.

Komatsu K, Zhu S, Fushimi H et al. Phylogenetic analysis based on 18S rRNA gene and matK gene sequences of *Panax vietnamensis* and five related species. Planta Med. 2001;67:461–465.

Kuo SC, Teng CM, Lee JC et al. Antiplatelet components in *Panax ginseng*. Planta Med 1990;56: 164–167.

Lee BM, Lee SK, Kim HS. Inhibition of oxidative DNA damage, 8-OhdG, and carbonyl contents in smokers treated with antioxidants (vitamin E, vitamin C, beta-carotene and red ginseng). Cancer Lett. 1998;132:219–227.

Lee SJ, Sung JH, Lee SJ et al. Antitumor activity of a novel ginseng saponins metabolite in human pulmonary adenocarcinoma cells resistant to cisplatin. Cancer Lett. 1999;144:39–43.

Lee YJ, Jin YR, Lim WC et al. Ginsenoside Rb1 acts as a weak phytoestrogens in MCF-7 human breast cancer cells. Arch Pharm Res. 2003a;26:58–63.

—. A ginsenoside Rh1, a component of ginseng saponin, activates estrogen receptor in human breast carcinoma MCF-7 cells. J Steroid Biochem Mol Biol. 2003b;84:463–468.

Liu CX, Xiao PG. Recent advances on ginseng research in China. J Ethnopharmacol 1992;36:27–38.

Maffei F, Carini M, Aldini G et al. *Panax ginseng* administration in the rat prevents myocardial ischemia—reperfusion damage induced by hyperbaric oxygen: evidence for an antioxidant intervention. Planta Med. 1999;65:614–619.

Mills S, Bone K. Principles and Practice of Phytotherapy. Churchill Livingstone, Philadelphia, PA. 2000; 418–432.

Park EK, Choo MK, Kim EJ et al. Antiallergic activity of ginsenoside Rh2. Biol Pharm Bull. 2003; 26:1581–1584.

PDR for Herbal Medicines. (2nd ed) Medical Economics Company Inc., Montvale, NJ. 2000;346–351.

Petkov V. Effect of ginseng on the brain biogenic monoamines and 3',5'-AMP system. Experiments on rats. Arzneimittelforschung. 1978;28:388–393.

Price A, Gazewood J. Korean red ginseng effective for treatment of erectile dysfunction. J Fam Pract. 2003;52:20–21.

Rosado MF. Thrombosis of a prosthetic aortic valve disclosing a hazardous interaction between warfarin and a commercial ginseng product. Cardiology. 2003;99:111.

Rudakewich M, Ba F, Benishin CG. Neurotrophic and neuroprotective actions of ginsenosides Rb1 and Rg1. Planta Med. 2001;533–537.

Ruehl WW, Bruyette DS, DePaoli A et al. Canine cognitive dysfunction as a model for human age-related cognitive decline, dementia and Alzheimer's disease: clinical presentation, cognitive testing, pathology and response to 1-deprenyl therapy. Prog Brain Res. 1995;106:217–225.

Russo E. Handbook of Psychotropic Herbs: A Scientific Analysis of Herbal Remedies for Psychiatric Conditions. The Haworth Press, Binghamton, NY. 2001;182–191.

Scaglione F, Cattaneo G, Alessandria M et al. Efficacy and safety of the standardized Ginseng extract G115 for potentiating vaccination against the influenza syndrome and protection against the common cold. Drugs Exp Clin Res. 1996;22:65–72.

Scholey AB, Kennedy DO. Acute, dose-dependent cognitive effects of *Ginkgo biloba, Panax ginseng* and their combination in healthy young volunteers: differential interactions with cognitive demand. Hum Psychopharmacol. 2002;17:35–44.

Siegel RK. Ginseng abuse syndrome. Problems with the panacea. JAMA. 1976;241:1614–1615.

Singh VK, George CS, Singh N et al. Combined treatment of mice with *Panax ginseng* extract and interferon inducer; Amplification of host resistance to Semliki forest virus. Planta Med. 1983;47; 234–236.

Singh VK, Agarwal SS, Gupta BM. Immunomodulatory activity of *Panax ginseng* extract. Planta Med. 1984;50:462–465.

Sorensen H, Sonne J. A double-masked study of the effects of ginseng on cognitive functions. Curr Therapeut Res. 1996;57:959–968.

Sotaniemi E, Haapakoski E, Rautio A. Ginseng therapy in non-insulin dependent diabetic patients. Diabetes Care. 1995;18:1373–1375.

Suh SO, Kroh M, Kim NR et al. Effects of red ginseng upon posteroperative immunity and survival in patients with stage III gastric cancer. Am J Chin Med. 2003130:483–494.

Tachikawa E, Kudo K, Hasegawa H et al. In vitro inhibition of adrenal catecholamine secretion by steroidal metabolites of ginseng saponins. Biochem Pharmacol. 2003;66:2213–2221.

Tachikawa W, Kudo K, Harada K et al. Effects of ginseng saponins on responses induced by various receptor stimuli. Eur J Pharmacol. 1999;369:23–32.

Tillotson AK, Tillotson HSH, Abel R. The One Earth Herbal Sourcebook. Kensington Publishing, New York, NY 2001;141–143.

Tierra M. The Way of Chinese Herbs. Pocket Books, New York, NY 1998;259–262.

Tohda C, Matsumoto N, Zou K et al. Axonal and dendritic extension by protopanaxadiol-type saponins from ginseng drugs in SK-N-SH cells. Jpn J Pharmacol. 2002;90:254–22.

Tsai SC, Chai YC, Lu CC et al. Stimulation of the secretion of luteinizing hormone by ginsenoside Rb1 in male rats. Chin J Physiol. 2003;46:1–7.

Voces J, Alvarez A, Vila L et al. Effects of administration of the standardized *Panax ginseng* extract G115 on hepatic antioxidant function after exhaustive exercise. Comp Biochem Physiol C Pharmacol Toxicol Endocrinol. 1999;123:175–184.

Wang BX, Zhou QL, Yang M et al. Hypoglycemic mechanism of ginseng glycopeptide. Acta Pharmacol Sin. 2003;24:61–66.

Wiklund I, Karlberg J, Lund B. A double-blind comparison of the effect on quality of life of a combination of vital substances including standardized ginseng G115 and placebo. Curr Terapeut Res. 1994;55:32–42.

Wu JX, Chen JX. Negative chronotropic and inotropic effects of *Panax notoginseng* saponins. Chung Kuo Yao Li Hseuh Pao 1988;9:409–412.

Wu W, Zhang XM, Liu PM et al. Effects of *Panax notoginseng* saponins Rg1 on cardiac eletrophysiological properties and ventricular fibrillation threshold in dogs. Chung Kuo Yao Li Hsueh Pao 1995; 16:459–463.

Youdim KA, Joseph JA. A possible emerging role of phytochemicals in improving age-related neurological dysfunctions: a multiplicity of effects. Free Radic Biol Med. 2001;30:583–594.

Salvia miltiorrhiza

Native to China and Japan, *Salvia miltiorrhiza* (Dan shen, Red-Rooted Sage, Red-Rooted Salvia, Asian Red Sage, Salvia Root, Red Ginseng; family *Labiatae* or *Lamiacaea*) is a flowering perennial with violet purple blowers. It grows as high as 80 cm; upper leaves are crenate and lower leaves are ovate. The thick, stubby rhizome is the medicinal part of the plant. It is collected in spring or fall and dried. The plant must be distinguished from *S. trijuga* and *S. przelwalskii.* In addition, it should not be confused with *Dang sheng (Codonopsis pilulosa)*, which also differs in its activity as a qi tonic (PDR 2000). *Salvia officinalis,* a Mediterranean species naturalized in North America, was used by Native Americans and is discussed elsewhere in this book.

S. miltiorrhiza enters the Heart and Liver channels and is considered a Heart Blood mover (Heart Xue) with bitter and slightly cold traits (Zhong, Wiseman, Ellis 1996). It is traditionally used for the treatment of obstetric and gynecological complaints including menstrual pain and irregularity. *S. miltiorrhiza* is believed to expel pus and relieve pain. Combined with *Scutellaria baicalensis (Huang qin*) and *Stemona (Bai bu*) to prepare the Elixir known as *Qin bu dan*, it was used to treat pulmonary tuberculosis. It was one of many herbs used for the Fit-Settling Pill (*Ding xian wan*) to treat seizures. It is also used for angina pectoris, painful swelling of the skin and joints, and liver and spleen ailments (Tillotson, Tillotson, Abel 2001; PDR 2000; Zhong, Wiseman, Ellis 1996).

S. miltiorrhiza is used to restore calm to a troubled spirit and irritable mood by clearing heat and relieving blood stasis and a "heavy heart." Combined with Dilong (earthworm), it is a treatment for mania and insanity in conditions of excessive Heat and Xue stasis. Mixed with other Clear Heat and Calm Shen herbs, it is used to control restlessness, fright, and insomnia in conditions of Heart Heat, Heart Xue Xu with disturbed Shen. *S. miltiorrhiza* is mixed with *Shui niu jiao* (Water Buffalo Horn), *Xuan shen* (Scrophularia Root), and *Huang lian* (Coptis Root) in conditions of impaired yin with insomnia, delirium, and vexation. When mixed in liquor at bedtime, it is used to treat neurasthenia (PDR 2000; Zhong, Wiseman, Ellis 1996).

Ingredients

Compounds include diterpenes (e.g., tanshinones, isotanshinones, salviol) and caffeic acid derivatives (e.g., rosmarinic acid, salvianolic acids) (PDR 2000).

CNS Effects

Unfortunately, the calmative and sedative action of *S. miltiorrhiza* recognized by traditional Chinese herbalists has not been the focus of intense study. Nonetheless, there is some evidence to support its use for patients with emotional disruptions and cognitive impairment. In a study of a rat model of focal cerebral infarct, pretreatment (15 and 30 mg/kg IP) with Salvia extract resulted in reduced ischemic injury (Lo, Lin, Kuo et al. 2003). The neuroprotective effect was also reported in a study of cerebral ischemia in mice treated with Salvia tanshinones, which are lipid soluble and readily cross the blood-brain barrier (Lam, Lo, Sun et al. 2003). In a one-week study comparing the cognitive effects of Chinese herbs, *S. miltiorrhiza* did not produce significant enhancement compared to other herbs such as Chinese Ginseng (Hsieh, Pen, Wu et al. 2000).

In an earlier study in mice, a diterpene quinone isolated from *S. miltiorrhiza* called miltirone behaved as a partial central benzodiazepine agonist that was not accompanied by muscle relaxation, drug dependence, or withdrawal reactions following chronic administration (Lee, Wong, Chui et al. 1991). Miltirone has also been isolated in *Salvia officinalis* and other herbs (Miura K, Kikuzaki H, Nakatani N et al. 2002). A miltirone analog has been synthesized that is six times more potent than miltirone at the central benzodiazepine receptor (Chang, Chui, Tan et al. 1991). Regrettably, research into the psychoactive potential of *S. miltiorrhiza* has apparently stalled.

Miscellaneous Effects

S. miltiorrhiza has been shown to possess antimicrobial (including anti-HIV; Abd-Elazem, Chen, Bates et al. 2002; Lee, Lee, Noh et al. 1999), antihypertensive (Kang, Yun, Ryoo et al. 2002), anti-inflammatory (Kim, Moon, Chang et al. 2002; Kang, Chung, Kim et al. 2000), anticancer (Chang, Chang, Kuo et al. 2004; Yuan, Wang, Wei 2003), antioxidant (Lo, Lin, Kuo et al. 2003), and antithrombotic (Chan 2001) properties. It also boosts the immune system (Wong, Tse, Wong et al. 2004). *S. miltiorrhiza* prevents the formation of adhesions following abdominal surgery.

S. miltiorrhiza helps to improve hemodynamics of the heart muscle by improving coronary blood flow (Xia, Gu, Ansley et al. 2003; Ji, Tan, Zhu 2000; PDR 2000; Liu, Lu 1999). However, *S. miltiorrhiza* did not perform as well as *Valeriana officinalis* in the control of angina pectoris (Yang, Wang 1994).

The plant appears to impact alcohol addiction behaviorally and physiologically. *S. miltiorrhiza* displayed the ability to reduce voluntary alcohol intake; this suggests its use in the treatment of alcohol dependence and perhaps other addictions (Vacca, Colombo, Brunetti et al. 2003; Carai, Agabio, Bombardelli et al. 2000); (PDR 2000; Zhong, Wiseman, Ellis 1996). A hepatoprotective action (Liu, Hu, Liu et al. 2001) and anticirrhotic effect (Huang YT, Lee TY, Lin HC et al. 2001) have also been found.

Adverse Effects

S. miltiorrhiza is contraindicated in patients with bleeding disorders (e.g., hemophilia in dogs, warfarin poisoning) or those taking antithrombotic drugs, due to its antiplatelet action (e.g., aspirin therapy for feline cardiomyopathy) (Tillotson, Tillotson, Abel 2001; Chan 2001; Fugh-Berman 2000; PDR 2000). An aqueous extract of *S. miltiorrhiza* (100 mg/kg PO) markedly decreased plasma concentration and doubled the total body clearance of diazepam in rats, suggesting an impact on cytochrome P450 that is relevant to many other pharmaceutical drugs (Jinping, Peiling, Yawei et al. 2003).

Availability

One of the traditional methods of preparation of *S. miltiorrhiza* calls for root slices to be roasted and dried with wine (*Jiu dan shen*; daily dosage is 9 to 15 g). It may also be stir fried. It is also available in powders or pills. Infused in tea, the recommended dose is 3 to 15 g of dried *S. miltiorrhiza*. It may also be topically applied as a paste (prepared by boiling), for example, to treat skin infection. Prepared as a decoction, daily dosage is 1 to 4 g (Tillotson, Tillotson, Abel 2001; PDR 2000; Zhong, Wiseman, Ellis 1996).

Consumers should be aware that the content of active ingredients and the quality of the contents can vary widely in commercial preparations of *S. miltiorrhiza*

(Zhang, Yu, Jia et al. 2002). This has been reported in an increasing number of OTC herbal preparations.

Clinical Application in Veterinary Behavior Medicine

According to traditional application, *S. miltiorrhiza* may be useful for the treatment of pets suffering from conditions characterized by restlessness, anxiety, mild irritability, or depression (e.g., mild to moderate forms of separation anxiety syndrome or compulsive behavior, irritable aggression). At present, there is insufficient clinical or laboratory data to substantiate these uses.

Based upon current scientific evidence, *S. miltiorrhiza* may be helpful by virtue of its neuroprotective and antioxidant effects as an adjunct to the treatment of pets with behavioral disorders characterized by CNS hyperactivity (e.g., psychomotor seizure, feline hyperesthesia syndrome). Although *S. miltiorrhiza* does not appear to benefit cognitive impairment at this time, it may complement the effect of other herbal or conventional remedies in the treatment of canine and feline cognitive dysfunction syndrome or patients with normal senile decline.

References

Abd-Elazem IS, Chen HS, Bates RB et al. Isolation of two highly potent and non-toxic inhibitors of human immunodeficiency virus type 1 (HIV-1) integrase from *Salvia miltiorrhiza*. Antiviral Res. 2002;55:91–106.

Carai MA, Agabio R, Bombardelli E et al. Potential use of medicinal plants in the treatment of alcoholism. Fitoterapia. 2000;71(Suppl 1):S38–42.

Chan TY. Interaction between warfarin and danshen (*Salvia miltiorrhiza*). Ann Pharmacother. 2001;35: 501–504.

Chang JY, Chang CY, Kuo CC et al. Salvinal, a novel microtubule inhibitor isolated from *Salvia miltiorrhiza* Bunge (Danshen), with antimitotic activity in multidrug-sensitive and -resistant human tumor cells. Mol Pharmacol. 2004;65:77–84.

Chang HM, Chui KY, Tan FW et al. Structure-activity relationship of miltirone, an active central benzodiazepine receptor ligand isolated from *Salvia miltiorrhiza* Bunge (Danshen). J Med Chem. 1991; 34:1675–1692.

Fugh-Berman A. Herb-drug interactions. Lancet. 2000;355:1020.

Hsieh MT, Peng WH, Wu CR et al. The ameliorating effects of the cognitive-enhancing Chinese herbs on scopolamine-induced amnesia in rats. Phytother Res. 2000;14:375–377.

Huang YT, Lee TY, Lin HC et al. Hemodynamic effects of *Salvia miltiorrhiza* on cirrhotic rats. Can J Physiol Pharmacol. 2001;79:566–572.

Ji XY, Tan BK, Zhu YZ. *Salvia miltiorrhiza* and ischemic diseases. Acta Pharmacol Sin. 2000 Dec.; 21(12):1089–1094.

Jinping Q, Peiling H, Yawei L et al. Effects of the aqueous extract from *Salvia miltiorrhiza* Bge on the pharmacokinetics of diazepam and on liver microsomal cytochrome P450 enzyme activity in rats. J Pharm Pharmacol. 2003;55:1163–1167.

Kang BY, Chung SW, Kim SH et al. Inhibition of interleukin-12 and interferon-gamma production in immune cells by tanshinones from *Salvia miltiorrhiza*. Immunopharmacology. 2000;49:355–361.

Kang DG, Yun YG, Ryoo JH et al. Anti-hypertensive effect of water extract of danshen on renovascular hypertension through inhibition of the renin angiotensin system. Am J Chin Med. 2002;30:87–93.

Kim SY, Moon TC, Chang HW et al. Effects of tanshinone I isolated from *Salvia miltiorrhiza* bunge on arachidonic acid metabolism and in vivo inflammatory responses. Phytother Res. 2002;16:616–620.

Lee CM, Wong HN, Chui KY et al. Miltirone, a central benzodiazepine receptor partial agonist from a Chinese medicinal herb *Salvia miltiorrhiza*. Neurosci Lett. 1991;127:237–241.

Lee DS, Lee SH, Noh JG et al. Antibacterial activities of cryptotanshinone and dihydrotanshinone I from a medicinal herb, *Salvia miltiorrhiza* Bunge. Biosci Biotechnol Biochem. 1999;63:2236–2239.

Liu Q, Lu Z. Effect of *Salvia miltiorrhiza* on coronary collateral circulation in dogs with experimental acute myocardial infarction. J Tongji Med Univ. 1999;19:40–41, 69.

Liu P, Hu Y, Liu C et al. Effects of salviainolic acid A (SA-A) on liver injury: SA-A action on hepatic peroxidation. Liver. 2001;21:384–390.

Lo CJ, Lin JG, Kuo JS et al. Effect of *Salvia miltiorrhiza* Bunge on cerebral infarct in ischemia-reperfusion–injured rats. Am J Chin Med. 2003;31:191–200.

Miura K, Kikuzaki H, Nakatani N et al. Antioxidant activity of chemical components from sage (*Salvia officinalis* L.) and thyme (*Thymus vulgaris* L.) measured by the oil stability index method. J Agric Food Chem. 2002;50:1845–1851.

PDR for Herbal Medicines. (2nd ed) Medical Economics Company Inc., Montvale, NJ. 2000:636–639.

Tillotson AK, Tillotson HSH, Abel R. The One Earth Herbal Sourcebook. Kensington Publishing, New York, NY 2001;193–194.

Vacca G, Colombo G, Brunetti G et al. Reducing effect of *Salvia miltiorrhiza* extracts on alcohol intake: influence of vehicle. Phytother Res. 2003;17:537–541.

Wong CK, Tse PS, Wong EL et al. Immunomodulatory effects of Yun Zhi and Danshen capsules in health subjects—a randomized, double-blind, placebo-controlled, crossover study. Int Immunopharmacol. 2004;4:201–211.

Xia Z, Gu J, Ansley DM et al. Antioxidant therapy with *Salvia miltiorrhiza* decreases plasma endothelin-1 and thromboxane B2 after cardiopulmonary bypass in patients with congenital heart disease. J Thorac Cardiovasc Surg. 2003;126:1404–1410.

Yang GY, Wang W. Clinical studies on the treatment of coronary heart disease with *Valeriana officinalis* var latifolia. Zhongguo Zhong Xi Yi Jie He Za Zhi. 1994;14:540–542.

Yuan SL, Wang XJ, Wei YQ. Anticancer effect of tanshinone and its mechanisms. Ai Zheng. 2003;22: 1363–1366.

Zhang H, Yu C, Jia JY et al. Contents of four active components in different commercial crude drugs and preparations of danshen (*Salvia miltiorrhiza*). Acta Pharmacol Sin. 2002;23:1163–1168.

Zhong YX, Wiseman N, Ellis A. Fundamentals of Chinese medicine. Paradigm Publications: Brookline, MA. 1996;324, 394, 396.

Schisandra chinensis

Schisandra chinensis (Wu wei zi, Schisandra berries, Five-flavored fruit; family *Magnoliaceae*) is native to Korea and northeastern China. The plant may be dioecious or monoecious. Clustered flowers are followed by the medicinal berries, which have a reddish mahogany color and may appear to be dusted with powder (PDR 2000; Tierra 1998; Chen, Tian 1992). The fruit is harvested in autumn and is first steamed and then sun dried.

In TCM, *S. chinensis* affects the Lung, Heart, and Kidney meridians. It is considered to be astringent, warm in energy and predominantly sour in flavor. Its Chinese name *Wu wei zi* (five-flavored fruit) refers to the fact that it is thought to contain all five tastes described in fundamental Chinese philosophy; this helps to make this herb particularly important (Tillotson, Tillotson, Abel 2001).

S. chinensis is considered to have revitalizing, adaptogenic, tonic, antitussive, and expectorant properties. It is a remedy for digestive, urinary, hepatic, and sleep disorders. In particular, it is considered to be calming in cases of heart and kidney deficiencies with symptoms of palpitations, irritability, lack of focus, restless dreams, and insomnia. It has been used for the treatment of anxiety, depression, and neurasthenia (chronic fatigue) and enhances the yin (Tillotson, Tillotson, Abel 2001; Tierra 1998; Zhong, Wiseman, Ellis 1996a).

Ingredients

Components of *S. chinensis* berry include: vitamin C (ascorbic acid); fatty acids (e.g., linoleic acid); lignans (e.g. gomisins, schizandrines, schizandrols, schizantherines, wuweizisus); and volatile oil (e.g., chamigrenes, chamigrenals, ylangene) (PDR 2000; Yasukawa, Ikeya, Mitsuhashi et al. 1992; Wang, Tong, Song 1990).

CNS Effects

Combined with *Panax ginseng, S. chinensis* has been shown to improve memory (Tillotson, Tillotson, Abel 2001; Tierra 1998; Zhong, Wiseman, Ellis 1996a). *S. chinensis* berries are traditionally combined with *Panax ginseng* and *Ophiopogon japonicus* roots in the preparation of "Generate the Pulse" (Pulse-engendering) powder (Sheng mai san).

Treatment with *Sheng mai san* has been effective in protecting against induced brain ischemia and has improved oxidative damage; however, independently administered ingredients did not have the same activity (Xuejiang, Magara, Konishi 1999). This phenomenon was the subject of additional study, which suggested specific synergy of the polyherbal formula on ischemic cerebral injury and oxidative damage (Ichikawa, Wang, Konishi 2003). A novel formula composed of *S. chinensis, Panax ginseng,* and *Biota orientalis* was found to enhance cognitive function, particularly for memory consolidation, in mice (Nishiyama, Wang, Saito 1995).

Miscellaneous Effects

Schisadrin B protected against oxidative hepatotoxicity in mice that was induced by menadione (Ip, Yiu, Ko 2000) as well as tacrine, a pharmaceutical drug used in the treatment of Alzheimer's disease with recognized hepatotoxic effects (Pan, Han, Carlier et al. 2002).

In a Japanese study of mice, gomisin A, gomisin J, and wuweizisu C displayed anti-inflammatory and antitumor effects (Yasukawa, Ikeya, Mitsuhashi et al. 1992).

Sheng mai san is of particular focus in research. *Sheng mai san,* a documented treatment of coronary artery disease, showed significant cardioprotective properties against isoproterenol-induced myocardial injury in rats; the lignan-enriched extract of *Schisandra chinensis* was found to be the primary responsible component (Li, Poon, Ko 1996). The effects of *Sheng mai ye* (*Panax ginseng, Ophiopogon japonicus, Schisandra chinensis*) and Dan shen (*Salvia miltiorrhiza*) on adriamycin-induced glomerulosclerosis in rats were studied (Peng, Liu, Luo et al. 1999). Results showed lower BUN, cholesterol, and protein in the herbal treatment groups and less renal injury compared to control groups; this confirmed its traditional application and suggested its clinical potential in the treatment of glomerulosclerosis.

A novel polyherbal dietary supplement (Equiguard®), containing nine herbs including *S. chinensis* and *Astragalus membranaceus* and consistent with TCM principles, significantly reduced the growth of androgen-responsive and androgen-refractory prostate carcinoma cells *in vitro* (Hsieh, Lu, Guo et al. 2002).

Adverse Effects and Dosage

Recommended daily doses of *S. chinensis* in people are 1 to 6 g of dried powder; 1 to 3 g of dried decoction; and 25 to 35 drops of tincture every eight hours. The dried powder may be taken in a beverage or applied topically as needed (Tillotson, Tillotson, Abel 2001; Zhong, Wiseman, Ellis 1996). *Sheng mai san* is prepared with 9–15 g of *Panax ginseng* (Dang shen or Ren shen), 9 to 12 g of *Ophiopogon japonicus* (Ophiopogon, Mai men dong) and 3 to 6 g of *S. chinensis* (Wu wei zi) (Zhong, Wiseman, Ellis 1996b).

Clinical Application in Veterinary Behavior Medicine

The mechanism of action and therapeutic benefit of *S. chinensis* is unclear at this time; however, there is accumulating evidence of the effectiveness of its polyherbal preparations. In veterinary behavior medicine, *Sheng mai san* may be useful in the treatment of psychomotor seizures and cognitive dysfunction syndromes for its neuroprotective and antioxidant properties. It may also be helpful in the prevention of renal and hepatic toxicity of conventional anticonvulsant medication. Based on its traditional and anti-inflammatory properties, *Sheng mai san* may also be helpful in the control of compulsive behaviors, such as excessive licking and forms of pica in pets.

References

Chen J, Tian G. Ecological investigation on *Schisandra chinensis* (Turcz.) Baill. of the Changbai Mountain. Zhongguo Zhong Yao Za Zhi. 1992;17:204–205, 255.

Chiu PY, Mak DH, Poon MK et al. In vivo antioxidant action of a lignan-enriched extract of Schisandra fruit and an anthraquinone-containing extract of Polygonum root in comparison with schisandrin B and emodin. Planta Med. 2002;68:951–956.

Hsieh TC, Lu X, Guo J et al. Effects of herbal preparation Equiguard on hormone-responsive and hormone-refractory prostate carcinoma cells: mechanistic studies. Int J Oncol. 2002;20:681–689.

Ichikawa H, Wang X, Konishi T. Role of component herbs in antioxidant activity of shengmai san—a traditional Chinese medicine formula preventing cerebral oxidative damage in rat. Am J Chin Med. 2003;31:509–521.

Ip SP, Yiu HY, Ko KM. Schisandrin B protects against menadione-induced hepatotoxicity by enhancing DT-diaphorase activity. Mol Cell Biochem. 2000;208:151–155.

Li PC, Poon KT, Ko KM. *Schisandra chinensis*-dependent myocardial protective action of sheng-mai-san in rats. Am J Chin Med. 1996;24:255–262.

Nishiyama N, Wang YL, Saito H. Beneficial effects of S-113m, a novel herbal prescription, on learning impairment model in mice. Biol Pharm Bull. 1995;18:1498–1503.

Pan SY, Han YF, Carlier PR et al. Schisandrin B protects against tacrine- and bis(7)-tacrine–induced hepatotoxicity and enhances cognitive function in mice. Planta Med. 2002;68:217–220.

PDR for Herbal Medicines. (2nd ed) Medical Economics Company Inc., Montvale, NJ. 2000;669–671.

Peng Y, Liu F, Luo J et al. Effects of danshen and shengmaiye on glomerulosclerosis by adriamycin in rats. Hunan Yi Ke Da Xue Xue Bao. 1999;24:332–334.

Tierra M. The Way of Chinese Herbs. Pocket Books, New York, NY. 1998;270.

Tillotson AK, Tillotson HSH, Abel R. The One Earth Herbal Sourcebook. Kensington Publishing, New York, NY. 2001;196–197.

Wang K, Tong YY, Song WZ. Determination of the active ingredients in Chinese drug wuweizi (*Schisandra chinensis*) by TLC-densitometry. Yao Xue Xue Bao. 1990;25:49–53.

Xuejiang W, Magara T, Konishi T. Prevention and repair of cerebral ischemia-reperfusion injury by Chinese herbal medicine, shengmai san, in rats. Free Radic Res. 1999;31:449–455.

Yasukawa K, Ikeya Y, Mitsuhashi H et al. Gomisin A inhibits tumor promotion by 12-O-tetradecanoylphorbol-13-acetate in two-stage carcinogenesis in mouse skin. Oncology. 1992;49:68–71.

Zhong YX, Wiseman N, Ellis A. Fundamentals of Chinese medicine. Paradigm Publications. Brookline, MA 1996;350–351a; 411–412b.

Zingiber officinale

Zingiber officinale (Sheng jiang, Gan jiang, Adrak, Ardrakam, Shoga, Shokyo, Ginger, Gingembre, Ingwer; family *Zingiberaceae*) is a creeping perennial that is indigenous to southwest Asia; it is thought to have originated in India. The long (15 to 30 cm) lanceolate leaves die each year (Fig. 4-5). A white or yellow flower grows from a spiked flower scape that grows directly from the rhizome. Although it grows wild in some regions, *Z. officinale* is widely cultivated in the tropics around the world, including the United States, as a condiment and for medicinal purposes. The medicinal part is the branched, tuberous rhizome (Ginger root), which is peeled and used fresh or dried (Fig. 4-6). The aromatic and pungent flavor is characteristic (Anjaria, Parabia, Dwivedi 2002; Mills, Bone 2002; PDR 2000).

In TCM, dried ginger (*Gan jiang*) is considered to be more appropriate for patients with "interior cold" as a heating or metabolic and circulatory booster; fresh ginger (*Sheng jiang*) is thought to disperse "exterior cold" by promoting sweating (Mills, Bone 2002). It enters the body via the spleen, stomach, and lung channels. Fresh or dried, ginger is considered pungent and hot and is often used for the common cold caused by "Wind Cold" (chills, fever, malaise, rhinitis, congestion) or "Cold" (inappetance, GI upset, pale tongue) (Mills, Bone 2002). *Z. officinale* is considered to enhance the yang and, for this reason, is not recommended for pregnant women.

In TCM, *Z. officinale* is used as an antiemetic and to treat asthma and respiratory conditions as well as vomiting (Mills, Bone 2002; Zhong, Wiseman, Ellis 1996).

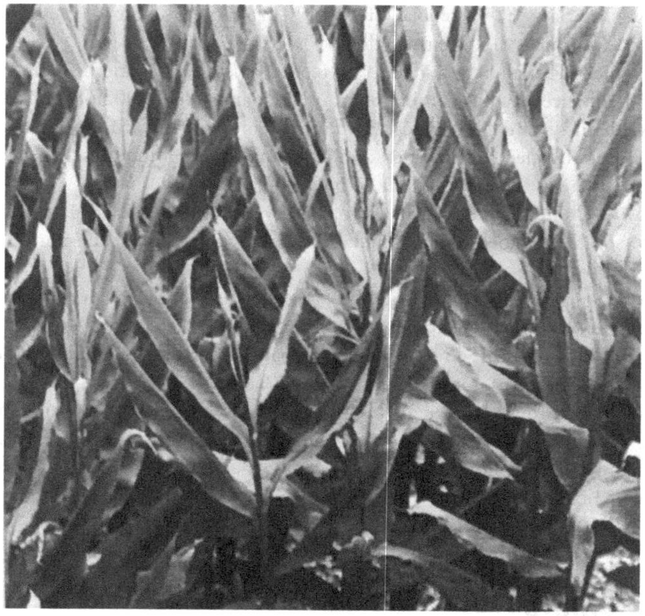

FIGURE 4-5. Commercial plantation of *Zingiber officinale* in India. (Photo courtesy of Dr. Jayvir Anjaria)

Z. officinale is used in Ayurvedic medicine as a laxative, antihelminthic, expectorant, aphrodisiac, and digestive (e.g., dyspepsia) agent. Ayurveda also considers *Z. officinale* to be useful in the treatment of restless and anxious symptoms (Anjaria, Parabia, Dwivedi 2002).

Ingredients

Compounds include: gingerdiols; starch (50%); aryl alkanes; gingerols; shogaols; diarylheptanoids (e.g., gingerenones A, B); and the volatile oil (2–3%). The components of the volatile oil vary according to the source but may contain zingiberol, zingiberene, ar-curcumene, and linalool, among others.

CNS Effects

An invertebrate study indicated that [6]-gingerol, a component of *Z. officinale*, had anticholinergic, antidopaminergic, and antiserotonergic effects (Singh, Singh, Singh 1999), although it is unclear whether the anticholinergic effect is central as well as peripheral (Mills, Bone 2002). *Z. officinale* also displayed an anticonvulsant property as one of the ingredients in a traditional Chinese formula (Minami, Shibata, Nomoto et al. 2000). Its antioxidant effect has been shown to be equivalent to that of vitamin C (Ahmed, Seth, Banerjee 2000).

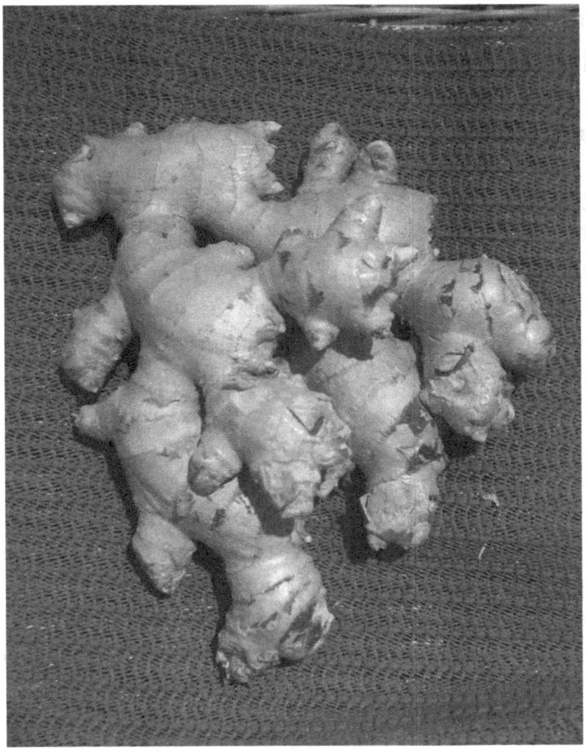

FIGURE 4-6. Rhizome of *Zingiber officinale.* (Photo courtesy of Dr. Stefanie Schwartz)

In a recent Indian investigation, *Z. officinale* root extract was found to possess anticonvulsant, anxiolytic, and antiemetic properties (Vishwakarma, Pal, Kasture et al. 2002). A commercial preparation containing a combination of *Z. officinale* and *Ginkgo biloba*, both known to possess antiserotonergic activity, was tested against diazepam in rats. The product showed anxiolytic properties comparable to diazepam; however, at higher dosage it also showed anxiogenic effects (Hasenohrl, Nichau, Frisch et al. 1996). In follow-up studies of this combination product (Zingicomb®), the German team concluded that unlike diazepam, the product did not produce lingering amnesic effect. This finding distinguishes the commercial preparation from other serotonin antagonists, which are typically associated with memory disruption (Topic, Hasenohrl, Hacker et al. 2002; Hasenohrl, Topic, Frisch et al. 1998). They also found that the *Z. officinale* and *Gingko biloba* mixture enhanced cognitive function and exhibited antioxidant effect after chronic administration (Topic, Tani, Tsiakitzis et al. 2002).

Behavioral and Psychological Effects

Chinese researchers investigated the antidepressant effects of the ancient Chinese formula *Banxia Houpu* that has been traditionally used for alleviating depression (Luo, Nong Wang, Kong et al. 2000). The decoction, which contains *Pinellia ternata, Poria cocos, Magnolia officinalis, Perilla frutescens,* and *Zingiber officinale,* was shown to possess an antidepressant property in mice that was comparable to fluoxetine (Prozac®).

The antiserotonergic effect of *Z. officinale* extract, in polyherbal combinations or alone, supports its potential as an anxiolytic agent. However, it may be best used in combination with other antioxidant herbs to enhance cognitive impairment, particularly in pets affected with age-related senility or cognitive dysfunction syndrome.

Miscellaneous Effects

Z. officinale has proven cholagogic, antiemetic, antithrombotic, antimicrobial, antidiabetic, anti-inflammatory, and antioxidant effects; it is also known to reduce cholesterol and plasma triglycerides, although this last effect is more pronounced when *Z. officinale* is given in combination with *Allium sativum* (Garlic) (Akhani, Vishwakarma, Goyal 2004; Konning, Agyare, Ennison 2004; Ficker, Smith, Akpagana et al. 2003; Nurtjahja-Tjendraputra, Ammit, Roufogalis et al. 2003; Penna, Medeiros, Aimbire et al. 2003; Sripramote, Lekhyananda 2003; Altman, Marcussen 2001; Fuhrman, Rosenblat, Hayek et al. 2000; Ahmed, Sharma 1997).

In a recent study on rats in Cameroon, the aqueous extract of *Z. officinale* root showed an androgenic activity including increased serum testosterone, testicular mass, and prostate (Kamtchouing, Mbongue Fandio, Dimo et al. 2002).

An antiplatelet effect is attributed to the gingerols and is of interest as an alternative to aspirin in cardiovascular illness (Koo, Ammit, Tran et al. 2001).

Z. officinale root has also been shown to inhibit the growth of *Helicobacter pylori,* which is associated not only with gastric ulcer formation but also gastric and colon cancer (Mahady, Pendland, Yun et al. 2003).

Z. officinale extract (25, 50, 100 and 200 mg/kg PO) in an ethanol and acetone but not aqueous extract showed significant antiemetic activity in dogs treated with the chemotherapy agent cisplatin (Sharma, Kochupillai, Gupta et al. 1997). Its antiemetic effect failed when tested against apomorphine-induced nausea. These findings suggest its potential use to control the side effects associated with cancer chemotherapy. The significance of this finding relates to the fact that 5-HT receptors are involved in the vomiting reflex and in anxiety, which is relevant to understanding the visceral effects of extreme emotional responses.

Z. officinale also appears to increase the absorption of synthetic drugs (Mills, Bone 2002); this may be an advantage in some patients but is considered to be problematic in others depending on their health status and the other drugs prescribed for their care.

Adverse Effects

The acute oral LD50 for *Z. officinale* oil in rats was greater than 5 g/kg; chronic administration of 100 mg/kg per day produced no adverse effects (Mills, Bone 2002). Side effects are rare except for the development of hypersensitivity (which is possible with any botanical preparation) and gastric ulceration in doses above 6 grams. Marked overdosage may be associated with cardiac arrhythmia and CNS depression (PDR 2000). It was recently found to be without side effects, including teratogenic effects, in a study conducted in Canada (Portnoi, Chng, Karimi-Tabesh et al. 2003).

Availability

The dried root may be used in powder form or its extract used in tea. *Z. officinale* is commercially available in capsules (100 to 1000 mg), chewable tablets, powder (1 to 4 g per diem depending on the condition treated), liquid, tincture, oil, and in tea bags (PDR 2000). It can also be applied directly to muscle spasm or inflamed joints (Zhong, Wiseman, Ellis 1996). The recommended human dosage is 500 mg two to four times a day, 0.7 to 2 ml per diem of liquid extract, and 1.7 to 5 ml per diem of tincture (Mills, Bone 2002).

Clinical Application in Veterinary Behavior Medicine

Used alone or as an important ingredient in the TCM antidepressant formula *Banxia Houpu, Z. officinale* deserves recognition for its psychoactive properties. The antidepressant effects of *Banxia Houpu* were comparable to fluoxetine (Luo, Nong Wang, Kong et al. 2000); this TCM formula would be of particular interest in clinical diagnoses known to respond to fluoxetine such as dominance behavior in dogs and house-soiling problems in cats.

Z. officinale appears to exert cognitive-enhancing and neuroprotective effects that would benefit patients with canine or feline cognitive dysfunction syndrome and psychomotor seizures. Combined with other herbal or conventional drugs, *Z. officinale* might also benefit cats with feline hyperesthesia syndrome. Its anxiolytic effect, which has been compared to diazepam, is applicable to a wide range of behavior problems in pets.

Preliminary indications of its androgenic effect in an African study (Kamtchouing, Mbongue Fandio, Dimo et al. 2002) support its traditionally attributed yang quality; *Z. officinale* could therefore be valuable in the treatment of low libido and infertility in breeding animals. However, this effect may limit its usefulness in single herb treatment of anxiety-related urine marking or dominance behavior, for instance, which could be exacerbated by this property. This effect might be useful in cases of hormone-deficient urinary incontinence in neutered male dogs. Used in combination with other herbs, this reported effect might be inconsequential. The results of ongoing research, and their relevance to veterinary behavior practice, are anticipated with great interest.

References

Ahmed RS, Seth V, Banerjee BD. Influence of dietary ginger (*Zingiber officinales* Rosc) on antioxidant defense system in rat: comparison with ascorbic acid. Indian J Exp Biol. 2000;38:604–606.

Ahmed RS, Sharma SB. Biochemical studies on combined effects of garlic (*Allium sativum* Linn) and ginger (*Zingiber officinale* Rosc) in albino rats. Indian J Exp Biol. 1997;35:841–843.

Akhani SP, Vishwakarma SL, Goyal RK. Anti-diabetic activity of *Zingiber officinale* in streptozotocin-induced type I diabetic rats. J Pharm Pharmacol. 2004;56:101–105.

Altman RD, Marcussen KC. Effects of a ginger extract on knee pain in patients with osteoarthritis. Arthritis Rheum. 2001;44:2531–2538.

Anjaria J, Parabia M, Dwivedi S. Ethnovet Heritage: Indian Ethnoveterinary Medicine, An Overview. Pathik Enterprise Publishers: Ahmedabad, India. 2002;546.

Ficker C, Smith ML, Akpagana K et al. Bioassay-guided isolation and identification of antifungal compounds from ginger. Phytother Res. 2003;17:897–902.

Fuhrman B, Rosenblat M, Hayek et al. Ginger extract consumption reduces plasma cholesterol, inhibits LDL oxidation and attenuates development of atherosclerosis in atherosclerotic, apolipoprotein E-deficient mice. J Nutr. 2000;130:1124–1131.

Hasenohrl RU, Nichau CH, Frisch CH et al. Anxiolytic-like effect of combined extracts of *Zingiber officinale* and *Ginkgo biloba* in the elevated plus-maze. Pharmacol Biochem Behav. 1996;53:271–275.

Hasenohrl RU, Topic B, Frisch C et al. Dissociation between anxiolytic and hypomnestic effects for combined extracts of *Zingiber officinale* and *Ginkgo biloba*, as opposed to diazepam. Pharmacol Biochem Behav. 1998;59:527–535.

Kamtchouing P, Mbongue Fandio GY, Dimo T et al. Evaluation of androgenic activity of *Zingiber officinale* and *Pentadiplandra brazzeana* in male rats. Asian J Androl. 2002;4:299–301.

Konning GH, Agyare C, Ennison B. Antimicrobial activity of some medicinal plants from Ghana. Fitoterapia. 2004;75:65–67.

Koo KL, Ammit AJ, Tran VH et al. Gingerols and related analogues inhibit arachidonic acid-induced human platelet serotonin release and aggregation. Thromb Res. 2001;103:387–397.

Luo L, Nong Wang J, Kong LD et al. Antidepressant effects of Banxia Houpu decoction, a traditional Chinese medicinal empirical formula. J Ethnopharmacol. 2000;73:277–281.

Mahady GB, Pendland SL, Yun GS et al. Ginger (*Zingiber officinale*) and the gingerols inhibit the growth of Cag A+ strains of *Helicobacter pylori*. Anticancer Res. 2003;23:3699–3702.

Mills S, Bone K. Principles and Practice of Phytotherapy. Churchill Livingstone: Philadelphia, PA. 2000:394–403.

Minami E, Shibata H, Nomoto M et al. Effect of shitei-to, a traditional Chinese medicine formulation, on pentylenetetrazol-induced kindling in mice. Phytomedicine. 2000;7:69–72.

Nurtjahja-Tjendraputra E, Ammit AJ, Roufogalis BD et al. Effective anti-platelet and COX-1 enzyme inhibitors from pungent constituents of ginger. Thromb Res. 2003;111:259–265.

PDR for Herbal Medicines. (2nd ed) Medical Economics Company Inc., Montvale, NJ. 2000:339-342.

Penna SC, Medeiros MV, Aimbire FS et al. Anti-inflammatory effect of the hydralcoholic extract of *Zingiber officinale* rhizomes on rat paw and skin edema. Phytomedicine. 2003;10:381–385.

Portnoi G, Chng LA, Karimi-Tabesh L et al. Prospective comparative study of the safety and effectiveness of ginger for the treatment of nausea and vomiting in pregnancy. Am J Obstet Gynecol. 2003;189:1374–1377.

Sharma SS, Kochupillai V, Gupta SK et al. Antiemetic efficacy of ginger (*Zingiber officinale*) against cisplatin-induced emesis in dogs. J Ethnopharmacol. 1997;57:93–96.

Singh VK, Singh S, Singh DK. Effect of active molluscicidal component of spices on different enzyme activities and biogenic amine levels in the nervous tissue of *Lymnaea acuminata*. Phytother Res. 1999;13:649–654.

Sripramote M, Lekhyananda N. A randomized comparison of ginger and vitamin B6 in the treatment of nausea and vomiting of pregnancy. J Med Assoc Thai. 2003;86:846–853.

Topic B, Hasenohrl RU, Hacker R et al. Enhanced conditioned inhibitory avoidance by a combined extract of *Zingiber officinale* and *Ginkgo biloba*. Phytother Res. 2002;16:313–315.
Topic B, Tani E, Tsiakitzis K et al. Enhanced maze performance and reduced oxidative stress by combined extracts of *Zingiber officinale* and *Ginkgo biloba* in the aged rat. Neurobiol Aging. 2002;23: 135–143.
Vishwakarma SL, Pal SC, Kasture VS et al. Anxiolytic and antiemetic activity of *Zingiber officinale*. Phytother Res. 2002;16:621–626.
Zhong Y, Wiserman N, Ellis A. Fundamentals of Chinese Medicine. Paradigm Publications: Brookline, MA. 1996;317.

Miscellaneous Chinese Herbs

Aconitum spp.

Aconitum spp. (*Bhugara, Vachnag*) are employed for medicinal purposes in Ayurveda and are said to possess narcotic, sedative, diuretic, antidiabetic, and antiarthritic properties (Anjaria, Parabia, Dwivedi 2002) (color plate 4-2; Fig. 4-7). Aconitum is also a common ingredient in a variety of TCM formulas. The tuberous

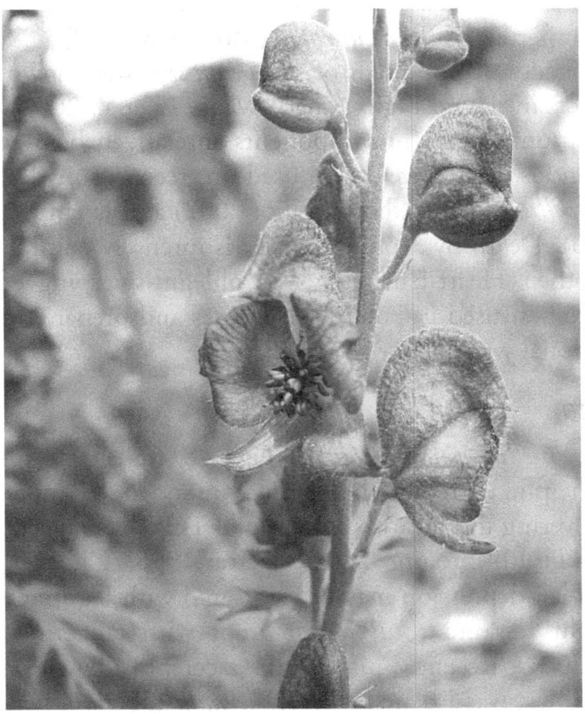

FIGURE 4-7. Close-up of *Aconitum spp.* flower. (Photo courtesy of Prof. George Ellmore)

root is prepared in a variety of ways and used distinctly. For example, the main aconite tuber (*Chuan wu tou*) is thought to enter the Spleen, Liver, Kidney, and Life Gate channels and is used to treat Damp and Wind conditions. The accessory aconite tuber enters the Heart, Spleen, and Kidney channels to balance yang. Both preparations are considered to be Hot and Bitter, although the accessory aconite (*Fu zi*) is also considered to have Sweet. The tuber may be salted (*Xian fu zi*), cooked (*Shou fu zi*), boiled and sliced (*Hei shun pian*), boiled, sliced, steamed, and smoked (*Bai fu pian*), or used as a powder (*Cao wu tou*) (Zhong, Wiseman, Abel 1996).

There are three groups of aconite alkaloids. One is considered extremely toxic. Another has little toxicity and has been shown to possess antiarrhythmic activity. A third group possesses potent antinociceptive, antiarrhythmic, and anticonvulsant effects due to sodium channel blockade (Ameri 1998). For example, aconitine is a potent neurotoxin derived from *Aconitum spp.* (Ameri, Simmet 1999; Chan, Tomlinson, Critchley et al. 1994). Adverse effects of *Aconitum spp.* also include cardiac arrhythmias (Chan, Tomlinson, Tse et al. 1994). In fact, *A. ferox* is used by the hill people of India and the Himalayas to poison arrowheads, in addition to its having applications in healing (Anjaria, Parabia, Dwivedi 2002). Native American tribes such as the Eskimo, Cree, Blackfoot, and Aleut recognized the poisonous properties of *Aconitum spp.* (Moerman 2002).

Recently, an alkaloid component of *Aconitum spp.* was shown to have GABA-antagonistic effects in the rat brain (Zhao, Wang, Li et al. 2003). Clinical studies are lacking. Aconitum species, or components of relatively benign varieties, can be extremely poisonous and have been used in recent suicides in the United Kingdom (*A. napellus* or Monskhood; Elliot 2002) and Japan (Ito, Tanaka, Funayama et al. 2000). Death by aconite toxicity is intensely painful and slow (PDR 2000). Despite their Heart-balancing and phlegm-sweeping effects, medicinal *Aconitum spp.* are best used in polyherbal recipes and prepared strictly according to ancient traditional wisdom, or not at all.

Pinellia ternata

In TCM theory, *Pinellia ternata* (*Ban xia;* Fig. 4-8) transforms phlegm and therefore would be a helpful ingredient in formulas intended to treat emotional disruptions; phlegm covering the Heart is intrinsic to TCM's perspective on mental illness (http://tcm.health-info.org 2004; Tierra 1998; Zhong, Wiseman, Ellis 1996). In particular, depression may be associated with dampness and phlegm or mucus and might respond to *P. ternata* root with tangerine peel (Tillotson, Tillotson, Abel 2001). Recently, pinelloside, a cerebroside with antibacterial and antifungal properties, was isolated from *P. ternata* tubers (Chen, Ciu, Liu et al. 2003). Four distinct fractions derived from an extract of *Banxia Houpu Tang* (Pinellia and Magnolia Bark Decoction), a TCM formula prescribed to relieve Liver qi stagnation and transform phlegm. The formula, which contains *Ban xia*

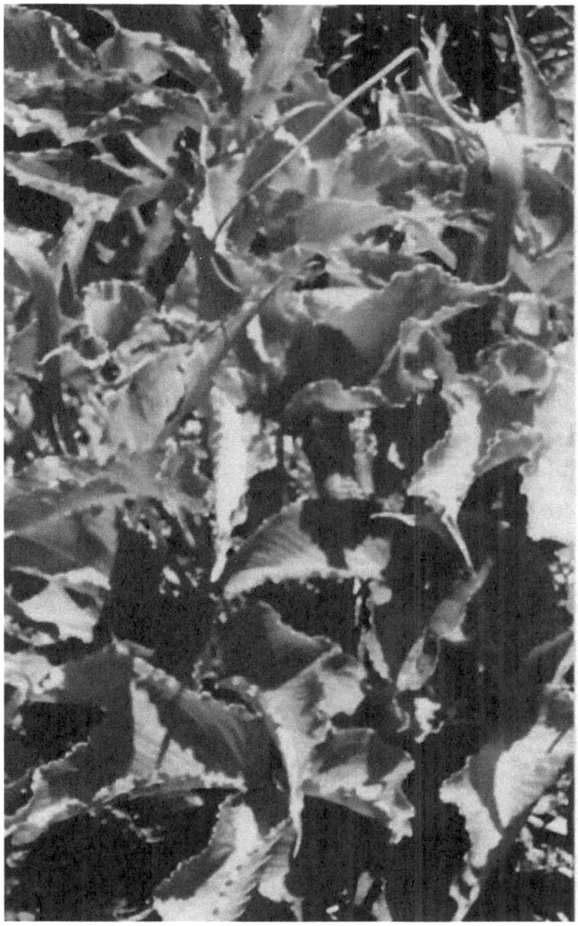

FIGURE 4-8. *Pinellia ternata* (*Ban xia*). (Photo courtesy of Dr. Susan Wynn)

and *Zingiber officinale* among its other ingredients, demonstrated antidepressant effects in mice (Huang, Kong, Wang 2002). Significant increases in brain serotonin (5-HT), norepinephrine, and dopamine were reported. It was concluded that this traditional herbal formula has an antidepressant effect that is likely mediated by monoamine neurotransmitters.

Regrettably, the FDA has now banned *P. ternata* due to trace amounts of ephedrine alkaloids. Ephedra was used as the primary ingredient in commercially prepared and widely marketed over-the-counter (OTC) weight-loss remedies. Although this application was inconsistent with TCM wisdom and practice, serious side effects and fatalities from public misuse of the herb forced the government to take decisive action against compounds and products containing ephedra (e.g.,

Ephedra sinica, Ma huang). Although the FDA is warranted in banning OTC sale of potentially toxic herbs, this action prevents qualified TCM practitioners and herbalists from accessing valuable ingredients for use in age-old remedies.

Poria cocos

Poria cocos (*Fu ling*) is an Oriental fungus that is commonly used in TCM formulas. It is considered Sweet in taste and enters the heart, spleen, and small intestine channels. It is used to calm the heart and spirit, and promotes the circulation of water and phlegm. It enhances Spleen qi and harmonizes the stomach.

A polysaccharide fraction isolated from *P. cocos* has shown potential as a biological response modifier, rather than as a cytotoxin, for the treatment of human leukemia (Chen, Chang 2004). It has also shown anti-inflammatory and antioxidant properties (Lee, Jeon 2003; Schinella, Tournier, Prieto et al. 2002). In an earlier study, a formula containing *Poria cocos*, *Codonopsis pilosula*, *Astragalus membranaceus*, and *Glycyrrhiza uralensis* improved cognitive function in a murine model of senile dementia (Liu, Yang, Zheng 1997). *Ban xia Hou pu Decoction*, an ancient TCM formula for the treatment of depressive illness and schizophrenia, is composed of *Poria cocos, Pinellia ternata*, *Magnolia officinalis*, *Perilla frutescens*, and *Zingiber officinale*. An ethanol extract of this mixture was shown to possess significant antidepressant effects in mice that were comparable to those of fluoxetine (Li, Kong, Wang et al. 2003; Luo, Nong Wang, Kong et al. 2000). Due to their Pinellia content, the availability of such interesting formulas will be impacted by the FDA's ban of ephedrine alkaloids. More research is required to determine the beneficial and adverse affects of TCM herbal formulas. It is hoped that these new regulations may be revised to allow skilled medical and veterinary professionals to study and use such formulas and ingredients for the benefit of their patients.

Scutellaria baicalensis

Scutellaria baicalensis (*Huang qin*, Chinese Scullcap), a traditional Chinese herb used to treat respiratory symptoms, has demonstrated psychoactive properties. It is discussed in conjunction with *Scutellaria lateriflora*, a Native American herb that also has interesting clinical potential.

Zyzyphus jujube

Zyzyphus jujube (Jujube, *Da zao*) is a berry-producing plant that grows in Asia, the Middle East, Africa, and southern Europe. The sweet, shiny, red fruit may be eaten raw or dried and follows small, pale-yellow flowers. Compounds include triterpenes saponins, tannins, hydroxycoumarins, sugars, triterpenes, flavonoids, and peptide and isoquinoline alkaloids. The medicinal berries are traditionally used as a tonic to prevent stress ulcers and protect the liver and for a variety of abdominal and respiratory complaints (PDR 2000; Zhong, Wiseman, Abel 1996).

It is considered Warm and Sweet and enters the spleen, stomach, and lung channels. *Z. jujube* is used to resolve qi insufficiency, palpitations, insomnia, fear, and visceral agitation, particularly in women. It nourishes Heart yin, enhances liver blood, and calms the spirit. It is a frequent ingredient in several Harmonizing formulas (e.g., Minor Bupleurum Decoction, Bupleurum and Cinnamon Twig Decoction, Pinellia Heart-Draining Decoction) (Zhong, Wiseman, Abel 1996).

In China, *Z. jujube* has been used as a sedative, anxiolytic, and hypnotic drug. A study of jujuboside A, a derivative of jujubogenin, on the hippocampal dentate gyrus formation showed inhibitory effects on neuronal firing (Shou, Feng, Wang et al. 2003). In a follow-up study, the same Chinese team observed that jujuboside A exerted an inhibitory effect on glutamate-mediated pathways of the hippocampus (Zhang, Ning, Shou et al. 2003). There is still no scientific confirmation of any clinical psychological effect attributed to *Z. jujube*.

Kampo

Historical Perspective

Kampo is the ancient practice of traditional Japanese medicine. Buddhist priest-physicians traveling through Asia prior to the sixth century AD, and during a second wave during the Tang dynasty between the seventh and tenth centuries AD, influenced Kampo. *Jian Zhen* (*Chien Chen*; 683–763 AD) was one of the most revered and loved of the Buddhist monks who brought TCM to Japan (Anonymous 2004). The Japanese government recently authorized more than 140 traditional Kampo formulas for mainstream use in Japan.

Japanese healing includes many of the same categories recognized in TCM. In addition, the Japanese scholar Mikao Usui rediscovered and reinterpreted the practice of *Reiki* (universal life energy) in the 1800s. It is based on a reference in ancient Sanskrit writings by a student of the Buddha's and incorporates meditation, knowledge of the *chakras* and the flow of qi or prana, and healing touch (Muller, Gunther1995). Although this healing practice is not strictly Kampo, it borrows from the philosophies of Ayurvedic and Oriental medicine. Reiki is not an herbal practice but bears mention because it can be used in conjunction with both Western and Eastern techniques of medicine.

Kampo Herbs in Veterinary Behavior Medicine

Saiboku-to is a polyherbal formula of Kampo that contains 10 herbs including *Magnolia officinalis* (Magnoliae Cortex), *Perilla frutescens* (Perillae Herba), and *Bupleurum chinense* root (Ikarashi, Yuzurihara, Sakakibara et al. 2001). An anxiolytic effect was associated with CNS histaminergic systems (Yuzurihara, Ikarashi, Ishige et al. 2000). The effects of *Saiboku-to* were later investigated in the striatum and hippocampus and compared with the effects of diazepam on ACh concentrations. Both *Saiboku-to* and diazepam were found to decrease ACh in both regions; however, *Saiboku-to* was shown to further potentiate diazepam-induced inhibition of ACh release (Ikarashi, Yuzurihara 2002), confirming earlier results that the anxiolytic effect of *Saiboku-to* is not due to an inhibition of diazepam metabolism (Yuzurihara, Ikarashi, Ishihara et al. 2000). Further investigation is warranted.

The Kampo medicines *Kami-shoyo-san* and *Hange-koboku-to* were shown to relieve panic attacks, anticipatory anxiety, and agoraphobia in four patients (Mantani, Hisanaga, Kogure et al. 2002). In particular, *Hange-koboku-to* and other Kampo herbal formulas traditionally used to regulate gastrointestinal function were investigated for their modulatory effects on human plasma adrenocorticotropic hormone and cortisol levels and were found to suppress plasma cortisol levels under stressful conditions (Naito, Itoh, Takeyama 2003). The active compound for the anxiolytic effect of *Hange-koboku-to* and *Saiboku-to* appears to be honokiol, derived from *Magnolia officinalis*, which is an ingredient in both formulas (Kuribara, Kishi, Hattori et al. 2000, 1999).

References

Ameri A. The effects of Aconitum alkaloids on the central nervous system. Prog Neurobiol. 1998;56: 211–235.

Ameri A, Simmet T. Interaction of the structurally related aconitum alkaloids, aconitine and 6-benzyolheteratisine, in the rat hippocampus. Eur J Pharmacol. 1999;386:187–194.

Anjaria J, Parabia M, Dwivedi S. Ethnovet Heritage: Indian Ethnoveterinary Medicine, An Overview. Pathik Enterprise Publishers, Ahmedabad, India. 2002;2, 181–182.

Anonymous. Chinese Medicine History. http://www.taijichinesemedicine.com/TCMhistory.htm, 2004.

Anonymous. Classics of Traditional Chinese Medicine. National Library of Medicine Online, History of Medicine Division. http://www.nlm.nih.gov/hmd/chinese/emperors.html, 2000.

Bensky D, Gamble A. Chinese Herbal Medicine Formulas and Strategies. Seattle, Washington, Eastland Press Inc. 1993.

Chan TY, Tomlinson B, Tse LK et al. Aconitine poisoning due to Chinese herbal medicines: a review. Vet Hum Toxicol. 1994;36:452–455.

Chan TY, Tomlinson B, Critchley JA et al. Herb-induced aconitine poisoning presenting as tetraplegia. Vet Hum Toxicol. 1994;36:133–134.

Chen JH, Cui GY, Liu JY et al. Pinelloside, an antimicrobial cerebroside from *Pinellia ternata.* Phytochemistry. 2003;64:903–906.

Chen YY, Chang HM. Antiproliferative and differentiating effects of polysaccharide fraction from fu-ling (*Poria cocos*) on human leukemic U937 and HL-60 cells. Food Chem Toxicol. 2004;42:759–769.

Elliott SP. A case of fatal poisoning with the aconite plant: quantitative analysis in biological fluid. Sci Justice. 2002;42:111–1115.

Ikarashi Y, Yuzurihara M. Potentiation by saiboku-to of diazepam-induced decreases in hippocampal and striatal acetylcholine release in rats. Phytomedicine. 2002;9:700–708.

Ikarashi Y, Yuzurihara M, Sakakibara I et al. Effects of an oriental herbal medicine, “Saiboku-to,” and its constituent herbs on Compound 48/80-induced histamine release from peritoneal mast cells in rats. Phytomedicine. 2001;8:8–15.

Ito K, Tanaka S, Funayama M et al. Distribution of Aconitum alkaloids in body fluids and tissues in a suicidal case of aconite ingestion. J Anal Toxicol. 2000;24:348–353.

Kuribara H, Kishi E, Hattori N et al. The anxiolytic effect of two oriental herbal drugs in Japan attributed to honokiol from magnolia bark. J Pharm Pharmacol. 2000;52:1425–1429.

Kuribara H, Kishi E, Hattori N et al. Application of the elevated plus-maze test in mice for evaluation of the content of honokiol in water extracts of magnolia. Phytother Res. 1999;13:593–596.

Lee KY, Jeon YJ. Polysaccharide isolated from *Poria cocos sclerotium* induces NF-kappaB/Rel activation and iNOS expression in murine macrophages. Int Immunopharmacol. 2003;3:1353–1362.

Li JM, Kong LD, Wang YM et al. Behavioral and biochemical studies on chronic mild stress models in rats treated with a Chinese traditional prescription *Banxia-houpu* decoction. Life Sci. 2003;74: 55–73.

Liu ZY, Yang YG, Zheng B. Effect of improving memory and inhibiting acetylcholinesterase activity by invigorating-qi and warming-yang recipe. Zhongguo Zhong Xi Yi Jie He Za Zhi. 1993;13:675–676, 646.

Luo L, Nong Wang J, Kong LD et al. Antidepressant effects of *Banxia Houpu* decoction, a traditional Chinese medicinal empirical formula. J Ethnopharmacol. 2000;73:277–281.

Mantani N, Hisanaga A, Kogure T et al. Four cases of panic disorder successfully treated with Kampo (Japanese herbal) medicines: Kami-shoyo-san and Hange-koboku-to. Psychiatry Clin Neurosci. 2002;56:617–620.

Mills S, Bone K. Principles and Practice of Phytotherapy. Churchill Livingstone, Philadelphia, PA. 2000;5–10.

Moerman DE. Native American Ethnobotany. Timber Press, Portland, OR. 2002;46.

Muller B, Gunther HH. A complete book of Reiki healing. LifeRhythm, Mendocino, CA. 1995;9–20.

Naito T, Itoh H, Takeyama M. Some gastrointestinal function regulatory Kampo medicines have modulatory effects on human plasma adrenocorticotropic hormone and cortisol levels with continual stress exposure. Biol Pharm Bull. 2003;26:101–104.

PDR for Herbal Medicines (2nd ed) Medical Economics Company Inc., Montvale, NJ. 2000;439–440.

Schinella GR, Tournier HA, Prieto JM et al. Antioxidant activity of anti-inflammatory plant extracts. Life Sci. 2002;70:1023–1033.

Shou C, Feng Z, Wang J et al. The inhibitory effects of jujuboside A on rat hippocampus in vivo and in vitro. Planta Med. 2002;68:799–803.

Tierra M. The Way of Chinese Herbs. Pocket Books, New York, NY. 1998;1–79;204-205, 357.

Tillotson AK, Tillotson HSH, Abel R. The One Earth Herbal Sourcebook. Kensington Publishing, New York, NY 2001;102–104,338.

Wang YM, Kong LD, Huang ZQ. Screening of antidepressant fractions of banxia houpu decoction. Zhongguo Zhong Yao Za Zhi. 2002;27:932–936.

Yuzurihara M, Ikarashi Y, Ishihara K et al. Effects of subacutely administered saiboku-to, an oriental herbal medicine, on pharmacodynamics and pharmacokinetics of diazepam in rodents. Eur J Drug Metab Pharmacokinet. 2000;25:127–136.

Yuzurihara M, Ikarashi Y, Ishige A et al. Anxiolytic-like effect of saiboku-to, an oriental herbal medicine, on histaminergics-induced anxiety in mice. Pharmacol Biochem Behav. 2000;67:489–495.

Zhang M, Ning G, Shou C et al. Inhibitory effect of jujuboside A on glutamate-mediated excitatory signal pathway in hippocampus. Planta Med. 2003;69:692–695.

Zhao XY, Wang Y, Li Y et al. Songorine, a diterpenoid alkaloid of the genus Aconitum, is a novel GABA(A) receptor antagonist in rat brain. Neurosci Lett. 2003;337:33–36.

Zhong YX, Wiseman N, Ellis A. Fundamentals of Chinese medicine. Paradigm Publications; Brookline, MA. 1996;316–317, 331, 343, 374–376, 399.

CHAPTER

5

Miscellaneous Psychoactive Herbs

"What is a weed?
A plant whose virtues have not yet been discovered."
—*Ralph Waldo Emerson* (1803–1882)

Introduction

This section discusses psychoactive herbs of interest that could not be easily categorized elsewhere in this book. For example, *Acorus calamus* has been used medicinally by Native Americans and is known in both TCM and Ayurveda. The commercial floral essence preparations known as Bach's Flower Essences™ are included here as well.

Cannabis sativa is an ancient herb that has been used in Ayurveda, TCM, and in the Western world for medicinal purposes. Although it is an illicit substance in many places because of its widespread use as a recreational drug, it is of increasing interest for the treatment of physical and psychological illness. Although it cannot be recommended for medicinal application in pets, its derivatives may some day find their way into mainstream use.

Theobroma cacao, the source of cocoa and chocolate, has well-known toxicity in dogs and cats that precludes its use as a psychoactive substance. However, its potential psychoactive properties are sure to be of interest to the reader.

Acorus calamus

Acorus calamus (Calamus, Sweet Flag, Grass Myrtle, Sweet Grass, Sweet Myrtle, Sweet Root, Sweet Cane, Myrtle Sedge, Cinnamon Sedge, *Shi chang pu*, Acori rhizoma; family *Araceae*) is a medicinal plant known to many ethnic groups. It was indigenous to India and North America but is found around the world. The plant grows one-half to 1 m tall. The triangular stem bears sword-shaped leaves arranged in pairs (Fig. 5-1). The medicinal rhizome has a characteristic aromatic

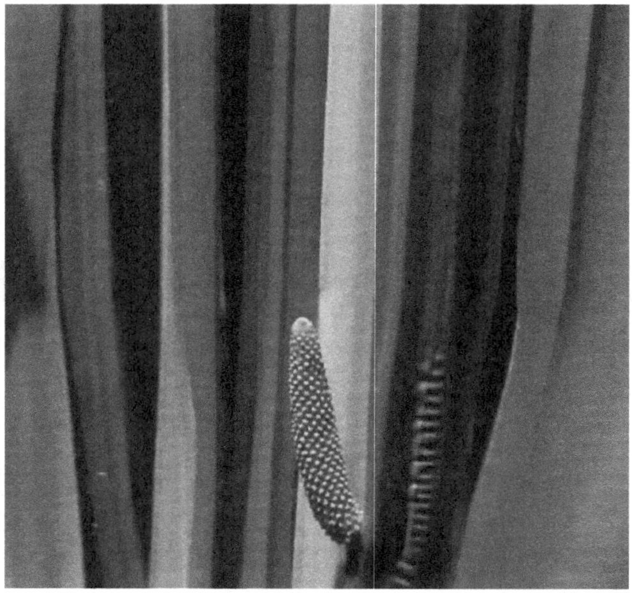

FIGURE 5-1. Sword-like leaves of *Acorus calamus.* (Photo courtesy of Dr. Jayvir Anjaria)

fragrance but is bitter in taste (Fig. 5-2). Compounds include the volatile oil (e.g., α,β-asarones) (PDR 2000).

In Ayurveda, *A. calamus* is used as an analgesic, antihelminthic, calmative, and to treat digestive complaints (PDR 2000). The dried rhizome is taken as a tea to treat dyspepsia or as an additive for medicinal baths. The powdered form should be discarded after 24 hours, although the root can be stored for up to 18 months (PDR 2000).

A. calamus was well-known to many Native American tribes (Moerman 2002). It was used as an analgesic (e.g., by the Cree, Blackfoot, Cheyenne, Mohegan), cough and cold remedy (e.g., by the Algonquin, Chippewa, Blackfoot, Cheyenne, Cree, Delwaware, Iroquois, Ojibwa, Meskwaki). It was used by various tribes to treat heart disease, digestive ailments, and gynecologic complaints in addition to toothache, earache, fever, and more. The Cree chewed the root as a stimulant; Dakota Indians rubbed a paste of the root of the face of warriors to keep them fearless and calm.

In TCM, *A. calamus* is known as *Shi chang pu* and is considered to be a slightly Warm and Bitter substance that frees yang. It enters the Heart, Spleen, and Liver channels to eliminate Dampness and Wind and enhance qi. It is said to open the orifices and is used whenever Phlegm is excessive or stagnant. This might occur in conditions characterized by abdominal discomfort, digestive disorders, poor

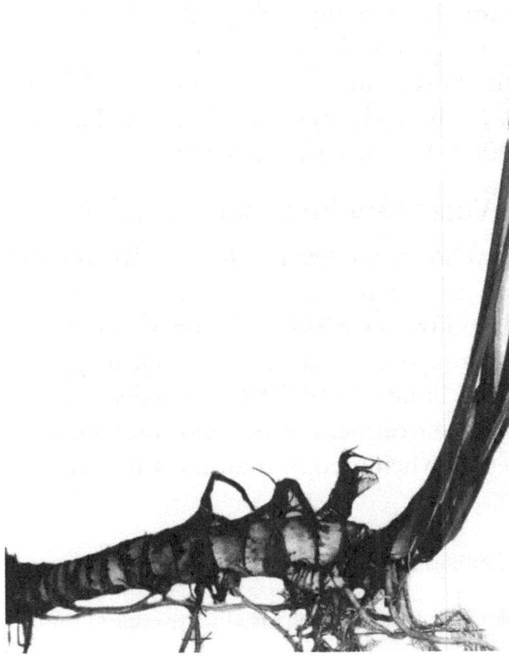

FIGURE 5-2. *Acorus calamus* showing plant rhizome. (Photo courtesy of Dr. Jayvir Anjaria)

memory, withdrawal, mania, vexation, and other symptoms (PDR 2000; Zhong, Wiseman, Ellis 1996).

CNS and Neuroprotective Effects

A Korean investigation of the central effects of the essential oil from *Acorus gramineus* in mice showed that inhalation of the oil produced significant inhibition of the degrading enzyme GABA-transaminase. This resulted in a significant increase in GABA and glutamate. An anticonvulsive and sedative effect was reported (Koo, Park, Ha et al. 2003).

A central dopaminergic and GABAergic***Q2*** mechanism was suggested to explain the effects of *A. gramineus* in mice (Liao, Huang, Jan et al. 1998). In this study, *Shi chang pu* showed weak anticonvulsant effects, competitive affinity for $GABA_A$ receptors, GABA agonistic action, prolonged barbiturate anesthesia, and inhibited apomorphine-induced stereotypic behavior. An anticonvulsant property was not confirmed for *A. calamus* root extract in a study of frogs (Panchal, Venkatakrishna-

Bhatt, Doctor et al. 1989); however, it counteracted amphetamine-triggered hyperactivity. In addition, a sedative and tranquilizing effect was weaker than chlorpromazine.

An early study demonstrated a tranquilizing effect for *A. calamus* (Menon, Dandiya 1967). Indian researchers described a neuroprotective effect in rats (Shukla, Khanna, Ali et al. 2002). An *in vitro* antiproliferative and immunosuppressive effect (Mehrotra, Mishra, Maurya et al. 2003) and antioxidant property (Acuna, Atha, Ma et al. 2002) have been demonstrated.

Clinical Application in Veterinary Behavior Medicine

Laboratory evidence of a psychoactive effect for *Acorus calamus* is unconvincing, although its GABAergic and modest sedative properties may be promising. There have been no clinical trials to investigate isolated properties of this herb. Although no adverse effects have been reported, calamus oils rich in β-asarone have been linked with malignant tumors in rats (PDR 2000). This does not appear to be a reliable psychoactive herb for the treatment of behavior problems in pets, although it may have a synergistic effect when used in traditional polyherbal formulas.

References

Acuna UM, Atha DE, Ma J et al. Antioxidant capacities of ten edible North American plants. Phytother Res. 2002;16:63–65.

Liao JF, Huang SY, Jan YM et al. Central inhibitory effects of water extract of Acori graminei rhizoma in mice. J Ethnopharmacol. 1998;61:185–193.

Mehrotra S, Mishra KP, Maurya R et al. Anticellular and immunosuppressive properties of ethanolic extract of *Acorus calamus* rhizome. Int Immunopharmacol. 2003;3:53–61.

Menon MK, Dandiya PC.The mechanism of the tranquillizing action of asarone from *Acorus calamus* Linn. J Pharm Pharmacol. 1967;19:170–175.

Moerman DE. Native American Ethnobotany. Timber Press, Portland, OR. 2002;46–48.

Panchal GM, Venkatakrishna-Bhatt H, Doctor RB et al. Pharmacology of *Acorus calamus* L. Indian J Exp Biol. 1989;27:561–567.

PDR for Herbal Medicines. (2nd ed) Medical Economics Company Inc., Montvale, NJ. 2000;138–139.

Shukla PK, Khanna VK, Ali MM et al. Protective effect of *Acorus calamus* against acrylamide induced neurotoxicity. Phytother Res. 2002;16:256–260.

Zhong YX, Wiseman N, Ellis A. Fundamentals of Chinese medicine. Paradigm Publications; Brookline, MA. 1996;331,343, 374–376,399.

Bach's Flower Essences

Edward Bach was a British physician of the twentieth century. During the 1930s he developed a series of flower extractions that he believed had medicinal value. He called these 37 flower extractions "flower essences." A thirty-eighth essence was spring water that he claimed had a healing property (Howard 1998; Mantle 1997). These collectively became known as The Bach Flower Essences™ or the Bach Flower Remedies®. The flower extracts are divided into seven groups accord-

Table 5-1: The Bach Flower Essences™ Categorized by Edward Bach in the 1930s According to the Emotional State They Are Supposed to Target[1]

Despondency and Despair	Larch (*Latrix deciduas*)
	Pine (*Pinus sylvestris*)
	Elm (*Ulmus procera*)
	Sweet Chestnut (*Castanea sativa*)
	Star of Bethlehem (*Ornithogalum umbellatum*)[2]
	Willow Oak (*Salix vitellina*)
	Crab Apple (*Malis pumila*)
Fear	Rock Rose (*Helianthemum nummularium*) [2]
	Mimulus (*Mimulus guttatus*)
	Cherry Plum (*Prunus cerasifera*) [2]
	Aspen (*Populus tremula*)
	Red Chestnut (*Aesculus carnea*)
Lack of Interest in Present Circumstances	Clematis (*Clematis vitalba*) [2]
	Honeysuckle (*Lonicera caprifolium*)
	Wild Rose (*Rosa canina*)
	Olive (*Olea europaea*)
	White Chestnut (*Aesculus hippocastanum*)
	Mustard (*Sinapis arvensis*)
	Chestnut Bud (*Aesculus hippocastanum*)
Loneliness	Water Violet (*Hottonia palustris*)
	Impatiens (*Impatiens glandulifera*)[2]
	Heather (*Calluna vulagris*)
Overcare for Others' Welfare	Chicory (*Cichorium intybus*)
	Vervain (*Verbena officinalis*)
	Vine (*Vitis vinifera*)
	Beech (*Fagus sylvatica*)
	Rock Water (*Water from a well or source with recognized healing power*)
Oversensitivity	Agrimony (*Agrimonia eupatoria*)
	Centaury (*Centaurium umbellatum*)
	Walnut (*Juglans regia*)
	Holly (*Ilex aquifolium*)
Uncertainty	Cerato (*Ceratostigma willmottiana*)
	Scleranthus (*Scleranthus annuus*)
	Gentian (*Gentiana amarelle*)
	Gorse (*Ulex europaeus*)
	Hornbeam (*Carpinus betulus*)
	Wild Oat (*Bromus ramosus*)

[1] *The Bach Centre, Mount Vernon, Sotwell, Wallingford, Oxfordshire, OX10 0PZ, United Kingdom*
[2] *The five components of Bach's Rescue Remedy®*

ing to the emotion they are intended to treat (Table 5-1). Approximately one third of the "flower essences" are from trees. Bach also prepared a cocktail of five of these flower extracts (rock rose, impatiens, star of Bethlehem, cherry plum, clematis) and called it Rescue Remedy® (Fig. 5-3).

These substances have been incorporated into homeopathic practice and are supposed to be able to "liberate the vital force from an alien disease process" (Richardson-Boedler 2000). Although there are differences between homeopathy and the Bach system of flower remedies, there is some common ground (van

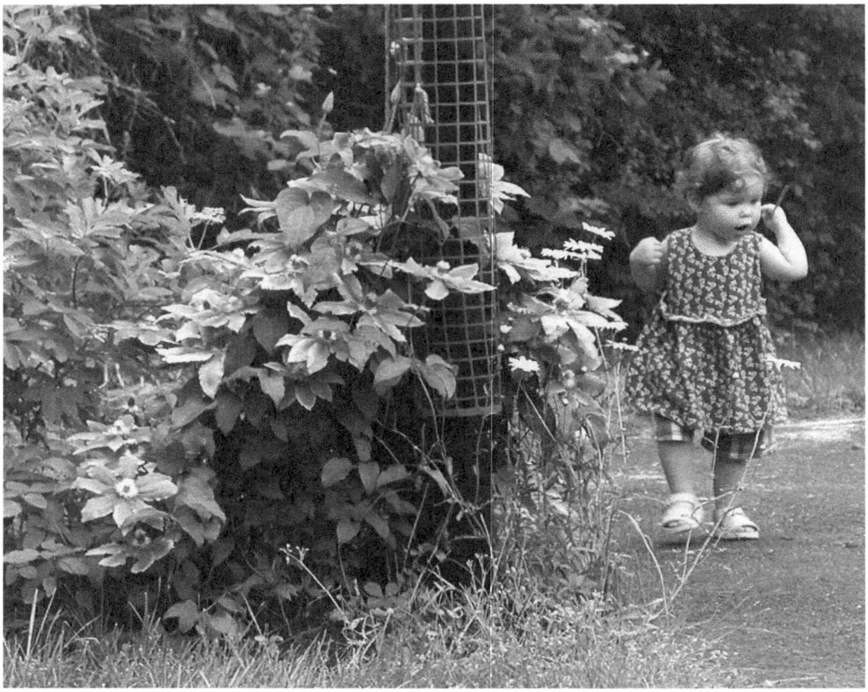

FIGURE 5-3. Clematis "Star of India" and Julia (18 mos.), both growing in the author's garden. (Photo courtesy of Dr. Stefanie Schwartz)

Haselen 1999). This book does not address homeopathic treatments, but because the Bach flower extracts are largely botanical and not exclusively homeopathic, they bear mention here.

The product brochure of Rescue Remedy® states that it is a "natural reliever of everyday stress . . . proven to be as helpful with animals as with people." It is supposed to be used in "emergencies and accidents." The Bach Centre, based in Oxfordshire, England, claims that it is "very powerful." In fact, these statements are unfounded by data.

In a randomized, placebo-controlled, blinded parallel study with crossover of the placebo group to the flower remedies after the first phase, anxiety was measured with a standardized anxiety test. There was no significant difference between the two groups. Authors concluded that Bach floral preparations had no specific effect (Walach, Rilling, Engelke 2001). In a doctoral dissertation, Weisglas (1979) conducted a double-blind experiment in 31 healthy subjects. His results suggested an interference effect between the essences of some of the groups and a significantly positive effect on measures of self-acceptance, humor, creativity, and libido.

Further research is urged. In a recent British review of research on Bach's extract (Ernst 2002), two studies suggested a clinical benefit, which was not deemed to be valid because of design flaws. Two other studies that controlled for placebo effects and minimized selection bias by randomization found no demonstrable effects beyond a placebo response.

Clinical Application in Veterinary Behavior Medicine

To date, there are no consistent or reliable data to support any effect from the flower remedies beyond a placebo effect. In its product inserts, The Bach Centre claims that Rescue Remedy® has an immediate calming effect and can be used for pets to help overcome emotional or behavioral problems such as veterinary visits, fear of loud noises, excessive barking or hissing, stress due to being left alone, adapting to the loss of owner or companion, anxiety in new surroundings, shock, trauma or mistreatment, and more. Although there are no reports of drug interaction or side effects (Mantle 1997), Bach extracts cannot be recommended for the treatment of behavior problems in pets without further research of their efficacy or potential adverse reactions (Table 5-1).

References

Ernst E. "Flower remedies": a systematic review of the clinical evidence. Wien Klin Wochenschr. 2002;114:963–966.

Howard J. Bach Flower Remedies: a personal commentary on the work of Dr. Edward Bach. Complement Ther Nurs Midwifery. 1998;4:148–149.

Mantle F. Bach flower remedies. Complement Ther Nurs Midwifery. 1997;3:142–144.

Richardson-Boedler C. The Doctrine of Signatures: a historical, philosophical, scientific view (II). Br Homeopath J. 2000;89:26–28.

van Haselen RA. The relationship between homeopathy and the Dr. Bach system of flower remedies: a critical appraisal. Br Homeopath J. 1999:88:121–127.

Walach H, Rilling C, Engelke U. Efficacy of Bach-flower remedies in test anxiety: a double blind, placebo-controlled, randomized trial with partial crossover. J Anxiety Disord. 2001;15:359–366.

Weisglas MS. Personal growth and conscious evolution through Bach flower essences. PhD Thesis, California Institute of Asian Studies, 1979; Dissertation Abstracts International 1981;41:9.

Cannabis sativa

Cannabis sativa, the hemp plant, is a dioecious annual or biennial plant that grows as high as 5 m (Fig. 5-4). Indigenous to the Middle East, it is now cultivated around the world. The medicinal parts of the plant are the twig tips of the female plant with either flowers or fruit attached. *C. sativa* is well known as the source of marijuana (also referred to as pot, grass, weed, ganja, reefer, and kif), which is in widespread use as an illegal substance. A resinous exudate that accumulates on the leaves of the plant is also psychoactive and known as hash, hashish, or charas (PDR 2000; Russo 2000).

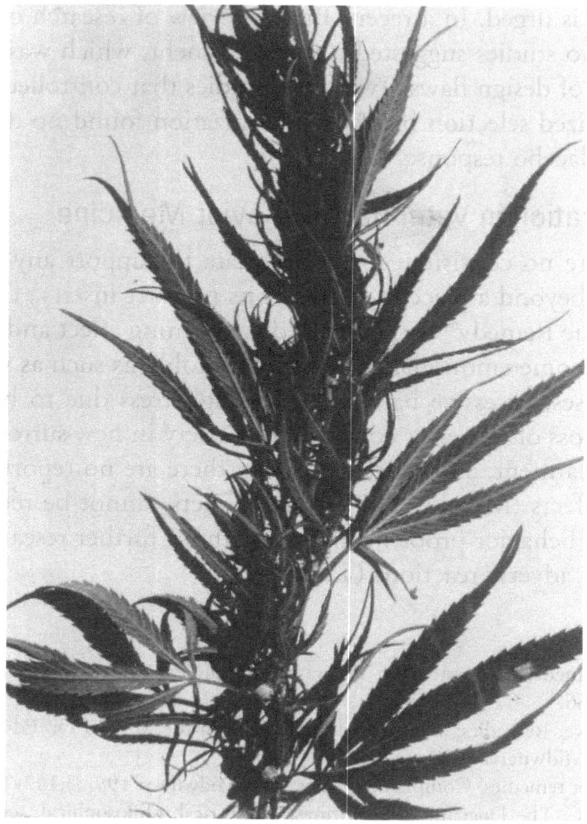

FIGURE 5-4. *Cannabis sativa.* (Photo courtesy of Dr. Jayvir Anjaria)

Recreational drug users either smoke or ingest it to induce psychoactive reactions. Dried marijuana leaves, seeds, and stems are rolled into marijuana cigarettes. When the pungent smoke is inhaled, the psychotropic effects of marijuana take minutes to occur and last several hours. When taken by mouth, the effect appears 30 to 60 minutes later and lasts up to eight hours (PDR 2000; Russo 2000). It is commonly used in conjunction with other drugs such as morphine, methadone, and methamphetamine and may potentiate the effects of these drugs (Reid, Bornheim 2001).

Historical Perspective

The first record of the euphoric effect of marijuana appeared in India in ancient texts dated between 2000 and 1400 BCE, where it was first referred to as "bhanga." The extract of Indian hemp was used as a sedative and sleep inducer. It was also used for pain associated with arthritis and gastrointestinal disease; epilepsy; respiratory ailments such as asthma, bronchitis, and whooping cough; and dystocia. Medical texts from ancient Assyria note its psychogenic effect. The Scythians used it in funeral rituals.

In China, *C. sativa* was used to treat malaria, arthritis, gout, constipation, gynecological disorders, and "absentmindedness." Preparations of *C. sativa* were described in medical texts through the Middle Ages and into the eighteenth and nineteenth centuries, in both Europe and the Middle East (Russo 2000). It was often advocated for the treatment of opium addiction and delirium tremens associated with alcohol withdrawal. By the late 1800s (Indian Hemp Drugs Commission) and early 1900s (League of Nations' Second Opium Conference), stricter commercial control impacted the legal use of *C. sativa*, although it continued to be used more freely in the East (Kendell 2003).

Ingredients

Chief among the active agents is delta 9-tetrahydrocannabinol (THC), one of 60 cannabinoids. THC was identified and isolated in the 1960s and is concentrated in the flowering parts of female plants. However, within the last decade, selection has pushed the usual THC content from 1–3% to as much as 6–13% or more (Baker, Pryce, Giovannoni et al. 2003). Other active compounds include the volatile oil complex (e.g., pinenes, humules) and the flavonoids (e.g., canniflavone1 and 2) (PDR 2000).

Cannabidiol (CBD) is another cannabinoid compound derived from *C. sativa.* Compared with THC, it is more sedative and anxiolytic. It has been noted that THC may be anxiogenic despite its euphoric effect (Russo 2000). In fact, cannabidiol alleviates anxiety caused by THC and possesses anti-inflammatory and analgesic activity (Williamson, Evans 2000). It is also of interest in the treatment of chemotherapy-induced nausea (Parker, Mechoulam, Schlievert 2002). Another nonpsychoactive cannabinoid, ajulemic acid, has been the focus of study for its promising anti-inflammatory and immune-mediating properties (Zurier 2003).

Industrial preparations of hemp contain little THC and are used to make a number of products, such as textiles and cosmetics (Stadtmauer, Beyer, Bardina 2003). Hempseed and hempseed oil are free of THC and are used in the food industry (Stadtmauer, Beyer, Bardina 2003).

CNS and Physiological Effects

Marijuana's effect is due to a coincidental mimicry of one of its cannabinoids with an endogenous cannabinoid called anandamide (N-arachidonoylethanolamine), a lipid-derived compound that has pharmacological effects that resemble THC (Martin, Mechoulam, Razdan 1999; Adams, Martin 1996). Activity of this compound is highest in the hippocampus, parahippocampal cortex, cerebellum, thalamus, and striatum, which may explain many of THC's effects (Devane, Hanus, Breuer et al. 1992).

THC has recently been found to be primarily responsible for the psychotropic effects of whole plant marijuana (Wachtel, ElSohly, Ross et al. 2002). The psychotropic action includes cognitive impairment, difficulty concentrating, impaired short-term memory and time perception, reduced drive, mood swings, and heightened or altered sensory perception. Anxiety, panic, and psychotic episodes are also reported (PDR 2000; Iversen 2003). In people, marijuana also causes reduced body temperature and intraocular pressure, bronchodilation, peripheral vasodilatation, and increased systolic blood pressure and heart rate (PDR 2000; Hillard 2000). In animals, bradycardia and hypotension are more characteristic but is rapidly normalized (Jones 2002). Antiemetic, anticonvulsive, analgesic, antimicrobial and antitumor effects are also recognized. Immune suppression and appetite stimulation are also associated with THC administration (PDR 2000).

Surprisingly few long-term studies on the cognitive, behavioral, or physical effects of *C. sativa* are available. Furthermore, few studies have examined the effects of *in utero* exposure despite the fact that cannabis preparations are the most commonly used recreational drugs during pregnancy. One study in rats showed significant behavioral differences in adults exposed *in utero* to *C. sativa*. In addition, there were sexually dimorphic changes of the endocrine system in exposed rats (Navarro, Rubio, de Fonseca 1995). Withdrawal from chronic *C. sativa* use may reduce dopaminergic transmission in the limbic system much like the effect of other addictive drugs (Ameri 1999; Diana, Melis, Muntoni et al. 1998; Tanda, Goldberg 2003).

Adverse Effects

It is now known that THC exerts its central effects via the CB1 cannabinoid receptors (Iversen 2003; Ameri 1999). These involve dopaminergic (Valjent, Pages, Rogard et al. 2001) and glutamate mechanisms (Ferraro, Tomasini, Gessa et al. 2001), and are concentrated primarily in the basal ganglia, globus pallidus, and substantia nigra and moderately so in the amygdala, hypothalamus, hippocampus, cerebellum, and caudate nucleus (Baker, Pryce, Giovannoni et al. 2003). Long-term administration of THC reduces sensitivity of GABAergic and glutamatergic pathways to cannabinoids as well as opioids; it also supports the addictive effect of marijuana (Hoffman, Oz, Caulder et al. 2003). Spatial memory impairment may be caused by inhibition of cholinergic transmission by acetylcholine suppression (Mishima, Egashira, Matsumoto et al. 2002). Repeated administration of THC to rats produced cognitive dysfunction attributed to changes in frontal cortex dysfunction, and specifically attributed to a reduction of dopamine turnover (Verrico, Jentsch, Roth 2003).

The CB2 receptors are found primarily in leukocytes and in the spleen and may provide an explanation for the immunosuppressive effects associated with marijuana (Baker, Pryce, Giovannoni et al. 2003; Gross, Terraza, Marchant et al.

2000; Ameri 1999). Many neurons with high density of CB1 receptors are also GABAergic interneurons in the hippocampus, amygdala, and cerebral cortex. The endocannabinoids anandamide and arachidonylglycerol may act as retrograde synaptic mediators (Iversen 2003). The psychoactive effects produced via CB1 receptors may be due to an increase of prostaglandin E2 in the brain (Yamaguchi, Shoyama, Watnabe et al. 2001). Research into CB1 and CB2 receptor antagonists may point to antimicrobial properties against intramacrophagic gram-negative bacteria (Gross, Terraza, Marchant 2000). Recently, additional cannabinoid receptors in the CNS and periphery (non-CB1-2) have been suggested (Wiley, Martin 2002).

Although fatal reactions are rare, chronic abusers are at higher risk for inflammation of the upper airways, cognitive and emotional decline, and sexual dysfunction (PDR 2000). *C. sativa*'s cardiovascular effects are benign in most recreational users; however, there have been reports of stroke, heart attacks, and other adverse reactions that are attributed to increased catecholamines, cardiac output, and other physiological effects (Jones 2002). In animal models, cannabinoids suppress the hypothalamic-pituitary-adrenal axis, gonadal steroids, growth hormone, prolactin, and thyroid hormone. Endocrine effects are due to binding with endocannabinoid receptors associated with the hypothalamus (Brown, Dobs 2002). Allergic and anaphylactic responses to hemp products have also been reported (Stadtmauer, Beyer, Bardina 2003).

There is evidence suggesting that the use of *C. sativa* may exacerbate or even cause psychosis and the risk of developing schizophrenia; however, this evidence is not yet conclusive (Dean, Sundram Bradbury et al. 2001; Iversen 2003; Dean, Bradbury, Copolov 2003). Recently, chronic administration of THC to rats elicited stereotypic oral behavior, suggesting that *C. sativa* use may cause effects similar to "hard" drugs (Rubino, Vigano, Massi et al. 2001).

Recently, marijuana smoke and THC have been implicated as cancer risk factors (Roth, Marques-Magallanes, Yuan et al. 2001). There have been reports of possible drug interaction with tricyclic antidepressants that include delirium, cognitive impairment, and tachycardia (Wilens, Biederman, Spencer 1997).

C. sativa has significant impact on safe driving when used alone, and there is also important interaction with alcohol on operating motor vehicles (Williamson, Evans 2000; O'Kane, Tutt, Bauer 2002; White House News Release 2003).

Medicinal Marijuana

Many traditional medicinal uses of marijuana have been substantiated by modern research. Moreover, new applications of its effects have emerged. For example, the appetite stimulant effect of "medicinal marijuana" is used to benefit patients suffering from anorexia associated with AIDS. This has led to research into the role of endocannabinoids in obesity (Cota, Marsicano, Lutz et al. 2003). Its antiemetic effect has helped cancer patients with nausea caused by chemotherapeutic agents

(PDR 2000; Williamson, Evans 2000; Soderpalm, Schuster, de Wit 2001). Considerable antioxidant and neuroprotective effects have been discovered (Hampson, Grimaldi, Lolic et al. 2000), suggesting that cannabinoids possess antioxidant effects superior to both alpha-tocopherol (vitamin E) and ascorbic acid (vitamin C). Its alleviation of painful muscle spasm and capacity for neuroprotection has found application in the treatment of multiple sclerosis (Iversen 2003; Baker, Pryce, Giovannoni et al. 2003; Smith 2002). A synthetic THC (dronabinol) has also been shown to reduce behavioral disturbance among Alzheimer's patients (Volicer, Stelly, Morris et al. 1997). Synthetic analogues of cannabinoids that may have fewer systemic side effects are being developed for the topical treatment of glaucoma (Buchwald, Derendorf, Ji et al. 2002; Jarvinen, Pate, Laine 2002; Green 1998).

C. sativa may also be effective in cases of Tourette's syndrome (Muller-Vahl, Schneider, Koblenz et al. 2002; Muller-Vahl, Koblenz, Jobges et al. 2001), although further research is warranted. Cannabinoid receptors are found in high concentration in the basal ganglia, which are implicated in Tourette's pathology. It is also suggested as a possible treatment of obsessive-compulsive disorder (OCD). Cannabinoids might interfere with repetitive thoughts and intense preoccupation by virtue of its cognitive and mood altering effects (Russo 2000).

Legal preparations of *C. sativa* are available in capsules of 2.5 mg, 5 mg, and 10 mg for the treatment of nausea and anorexia. Medicinal use of marijuana has been legalized in eleven of the United States since 1996 (Alaska, Arizona, California, Colorado, Hawaii, Maine, Montana, Nevada, Oregon, Vermont and Washington), although only a few have incorporated provisions that adequately protect the patient. In some other states, medicinal marijuana laws have been repealed or have been allowed to expire without further revision or consideration (http://www.mpp.org 2004).

In a recent and controversial move, the Canadian government has allowed patients with specific medical conditions to use legally prescribed *C. sativa* (Hall, Degenhardt 2003). With strict guidelines for its prescription and distribution, Canadian patients must meet requirements to purchase and grow 30 marijuana seeds, or dried marijuana for medical use (Sibbald 2003).

In 2002, the Center for Medicinal Cannabis Research initiated clinical studies on the potential use of medicinal marijuana in California (Vastag 2003). There have been few trials examining the therapeutic potential of marijuana compared to it physiological effects. Efforts to reclassify marijuana from Schedule I (controlled drugs such as heroine and morphine) to Schedule III (drugs with less potential for abuse) are under way, despite much opposition. It is likely that the development of synthetic cannabinoid analogs will eventually bypass legal complications and any undesirable side effects of medicinal marijuana in Canada and elsewhere.

Clinical Application in Veterinary Behavior Medicine

Marijuana is an illicit substance in the United States and elsewhere unless its medicinal use is specifically provided for by law. *C. sativa* preparations are not recommended for use in veterinary behavior medicine at this time.

References

Adams IB, Martin BR. Cannabis: pharmacology and toxicology in animals and humans. Addiction. 1996;91:1585–1614.

Ameri A. The effects of cannabinoids on the brain. Prog Neurobiol. 1999;58:315–348.

Baker D, Pryce G, Giovannoni G et al. The therapeutic potential of cannabis. Lancet Neurol. 2003;2: 291–298.

Brown TT, Dobs AS. Endocrine effects of marijuana. J Clin Pharmacol. 2002;42(Suppl 11):90S–96S.

Buchwald A, Derendorf H, Ji F et al. Soft cannabinoid analogues as potential anti-glaucoma agents. Pharmazie. 2002;57:108–114.

Cota D, Marsicano G, Lutz B et al. Endogenous cannabinoid system as a modulator of food intake. Int J Obes Relat Metab Disord. 2003;27:289–301.

Diana M, Melis M, Muntoni AL, Gessa GL. Mesolimbic dopaminergic decline after cannabinoid withdrawal. Proc Natl Acad Sci USA. 1998;95:10269–10273.

di Tomaso E, Beltramo M, Piomelli D. Brain cannabinoids in chocolate. Nature. 1996;382:677–678.

Dean B, Bradbury R, Copolov DL. Cannabis-sensitive dopaminergic markers in postmortem central nervous system: changes in schizophrenia. Biol Psychiatry. 2003;53:585–592.

Dean B, Sundram S, Bradbury R et al. Studies on [3H]CP-55940 binding in the human central nervous system: regional specific changes in density of cannabinoid-1 receptors associated with schizophrenia and cannabis use. Neuroscience. 2001;103:9–15.

Devane WA, Hanus L, Breuer A, et al. Isolation and structure of a brain constituent that binds to the cannabinoids receptor. Science. 1992;258:1946–1949.

Ferraro L, Tomasini MC, Gessa GL et al. The cannabinoid receptor agonist WIN 55,212-2 regulates glutamate transmission in rat cerebral cortex: an in vivo and in vitro study. Cereb Cortex. 2001;11: 728–733.

Green K. Marijuana smoking vs cannabinoids for glaucoma therapy. Arch Ophthalmol. 1998;116: 1433–1437.

Gross A, Terraza A, Marchant J et al. A beneficial aspect of a CB1 cannabinoid receptor antagonist: SR141716A is a potent inhibitor of macrophage infection by the intracellular pathogen Brucella suis. J Leukoc Biol. 2000;67:335–344.

Hall W, Degenhardt L. Medical marijuana initiatives : are they justified? How successful are they likely to be? CNS Drugs. 2003;17:689–697.

Hampson AJ, Grimaldi M, Lolic M et al. Neuroprotective antioxidants from marijuana. Ann N Y Acad Sci. 2000;899:274–282.

Hillard CJ. Endocannabinoids and vascular function. J Pharmacol Exp Ther. 2000;294:27–32.

Hoffman AF, Oz M, Caulder T et al. Functional tolerance and blockade of long-term depression at synapses in the nucleus accumbens after chronic cannabinoid exposure. J Neurosci. 2003;23:4815–4820.

Iversen L. Cannabis and the brain. Brain. 2003;126(Pt 6):1252–1270.

James JS. Marijuana and chocolate. AIDS Treat News. 1996;257:3–4.

Jarvinen T, Pate DW, Laine K. Cannabinoids in the treatment of glaucoma. Pharmacol Ther. 2002;95:203–220.

Jones RT. Cardiovascular system effects of marijuana. J Clin Pharmacol. 2002;42(Suppl 11):58S–63S.

Kendell R. Cannabis condemned: the proscription of Indian hemp. Addiction. 2003;98:143–151.

Martin BR, Mechoulam R, Razdan RK. Discovery and characterization of endogenous cannabinoids. Life Sci. 1999;65:573–595.

Mishima K, Egashira N, Matsumoto Y et al. Involvement of reduced acetylcholine release in Delta9-tetrahydrocannabinol-induced impairment of spatial memory in the 8-arm radial maze. Life Sci. 2002;72:397–407.

Muller-Vahl KR, Koblenz A, Jobges M et al. Influence of treatment of Tourette syndrome with delta9-tetrahydrocannabinol (delta9-THC) on neuropsychological performance. Pharmacopsychiatry. 2001;34:19–24.

Muller-Vahl KR, Schneider U, Koblenz A, Jobges M, Kolbe H, Daldrup T, Emrich HM. Treatment of Tourette's syndrome with Delta 9-tetrahydrocannabinol (THC): a randomized crossover trial. Pharmacopsychiatry. 2002;35:57–61.

Navarro M, Rubio P, de Fonseca FR. Behavioural consequences of maternal exposure to natural cannabinoids in rats. Psychopharmacology (Berl). 1995;122:1–14.

O'Kane CJ, Tutt DC, Bauer LA. Cannabis and driving: a new perspective. Emerg Med (Fremantle). 2002;14:296–303.

Parker LA, Mechoulam R, Schlievert C. Cannabidiol, a non-psychoactive component of cannabis and its synthetic dimethylheptyl homolog suppress nausea in an experimental model with rats. Neuroreport. 2002;13:567–570.

PDR for Herbal Medicines. (2nd ed) Medical Economics Company Inc., Montvale, NJ. 2000;500–503.

Reid MJ, Bornheim LM. Cannabinoid-induced alterations in brain disposition of drugs of abuse. Biochem Pharmacol. 2001;61:1357–1367.

Roth MD, Marques-Magallanes JA, Yuan M et al. Induction and regulation of the carcinogen-metabolizing enzyme CYP1A1 by marijuana smoke and delta (9)-tetrahydrocannabinol. Am J Respir Cell Mol Biol. 2001;24:339–344.

Rubino T, Vigano D, Massi P et al. The psychoactive ingredient of marijuana induces behavioural sensitization. Eur J Neurosci. 2001;14:884–886.

Russo E. Handbook of Psychotropic Herbs: A Scientific Analysis of Herbal Remedies for Psychiatric Conditions. The Haworth Press, Binghamton, NY. 2001.

Sibbald B. Medical marijuana to sell for $5 per gram. CMAJ. 2003;169:222.

Smith PF. Cannabinoids in the treatment of pain and spasticity in multiple sclerosis. Curr Opin Investig Drugs. 2002;3:859–864.

Soderpalm AH, Schuster A, de Wit H. Antiemetic efficacy of smoked marijuana: subjective and behavioral effects on nausea induced by syrup of ipecac. Pharmacol Biochem Behav. 2001;69:343–350.

Stadtmauer, G, Beyer K, Bardina L et al. Anaphylaxis to ingestion of hempseed (*Cannibis sativa*). J Allerg Clin Immun. 2003;112:216–217.

State by State Medicinal Marijuana Laws, Marijuana Policy Project, State Policies Department, Washington DC, July 2004. Available online at http://www.mpp.org.

Tanda G, Goldberg SR. Cannabinoids: reward, dependence, and underlying neurochemical mechanisms—a review of recent preclinical data. Psychopharmacology (Berl). 2003;169:115–134.

Trudeau DL, Thuras P, Stockley H. Quantitative EEG findings associated with chronic stimulant and cannabis abuse and ADHD in an adult male substance use disorder population. Clin Electroencephalogr. 1999;30:165–174.

Valjent E, Pages C, Rogard M et al. Delta 9-tetrahydrocannabinol-induced MAPK/ERK and Elk-1 activation in vivo depends on dopaminergic transmission. Eur J Neurosci. 2001;14:342–352.

Vastag B. Medical Marijana Center Opens Doors. JAMA. 2003;290:877–879.

Verrico CD, Jentsch JD, Roth RH. Persistent and anatomically selective reduction in prefrontal cortical dopamine metabolism after repeated, intermittent cannabinoid administration to rats. Synapse. 2003;49:61–66.

Volicer L, Stelly M, Morris J et al. Effects of dronabinol on anorexia and disturbed behavior in patients with Alzheimer's disease. Int J Ger Psychiat. 1997;12:913–919.

Wachtel SR, ElSohly MA, Ross SA et al. Comparison of the subjective effects of Delta(9)-tetrahydrocannabinol and marijuana in humans. Psychopharmacology (Berl). 2002;161:331–339.

White House News Release: Recent Analysis Shows that One in Six High School Seniors Admitted Driving While High; Sept. 16, 2003. http://www.whitehousedrugpolicy.gov/news/press03/091603.html

Wilens TE, Biederman J, Spencer TJ. Case study: adverse effects of smoking marijuana while receiving tricyclic antidepressants. J Am Acad Child Adolesc Psychiatry. 1997;36:45–48.
Wiley JL, Martin BR. Cannabinoid pharmacology: implications for additional cannabinoid receptor subtypes. Chem Phys Lipids. 2002;121:57–63.
Williamson EM, Evans FJ. Cannabinoids in clinical practice. Drugs. 2000;60:1303–1314.
Yamaguchi T, Shoyama Y, Watanabe S et al. Behavioral suppression induced by cannabinoids is due to activation of the arachidonic acid cascade in rats. Brain Res. 2001;889:149–154.
Zurier RB. Prospects for cannabinoids as anti-inflammatory agents. J Cell Biochem. 2003;88:462–426.

Griffonia simplicifolia

Griffonia simplicifolia (Bandeiraea simplicifolia, family *Leguminosae*) is a perennial, climbing shrub that is native to Africa and found primarily in the west central nations of Ghana, Gabon, Liberia, Ivory Coast, Nigeria, and Togo. The shrub reaches 3 m tall and bears greenish flowers that are followed by black seedpods. It grows in thickets and is often associated with termite mounds. It is traditionally used as a chewing stick.

G. simplicifolia seeds are rich in 5-hydroxytryptophan (5-HTP), the immediate precursor of the neurotransmitter serotonin (5-HT) that derives from the essential amino acid L-tryptophan(Das, Bagchi, Bagchi et al. 2004). Levels of 5-HTP were highest in *G. simplicifolia* seeds from Ghana (Lemaire, Adosraku 2002).

Current research of *G. simplicifolia* is focused on its usefulness as a glial marker in neurological research (Sandelin, Zabihi, Liu et al. 2004; Garcia-Ovejero, Veiga, Garcia-Segura et al. 2002). It is also of particular interest as a xenograft immunodiagnostic reagent due to its high specificity for the xenoreactive antigens at the source of organ transplant rejection in humans (Tempel, Tschampel, Woods 2002). Another of its lectin components has interesting insecticidal properties (Zhu-Salzman, Shade, Koiwa et al. 1998).

Tryptophan was popular as a dietary supplement until its use was linked with the potentially fatal eosinophilia-myalgia syndrome. Although this was subsequently traced to contamination from a single manufacturer, the supplement was removed from the market. Since then, 5-HTP has risen in popularity as a mood-enhancer for the treatment of insomnia, depression, obesity, and symptoms attributed to serotonin deficiency. 5-Hydroxytryptophan (5-HTP) and tryptophan have been used as alternatives to pharmaceutical antidepressants in treating unipolar depression and dysthymia; however, at least one meta-analysis of 108 trials revealed only two studies that could be considered reliable. It was therefore concluded that 5-HTP and 5-HT should be considered of limited clinical usefulness, particularly in view of the absence of controlled study of potential toxicity in both compounds (Shaw, Turner, Del Mar 2001).

Toxic reactions to 5-HTP in dogs have been reported, and drug interactions with conventional psychiatric drugs (e.g., MAOIs, antidepressants) as well as other psychoactive herbs (e.g., *Hypericum perforatum*) have been identified (Gwaltney-Brant, Albretson, Khan 2000). Overdosage or synergistic effects with other drugs can result in the serotonin syndrome, which includes signs of gastrointestinal upset, lethargy, hyperesthesia, ataxia, tremors, and seizure.

5-HTP is rapidly absorbed and readily crosses the blood-brain barrier, after which it is converted to serotonin. In dogs, signs of intoxication can occur at doses of 23.6 mg/kg or higher and may be lethal at 128 mg/kg (Means 2002).

There is no direct clinical evidence that *G. simplicifolia* is of therapeutic benefit at this time. Given the evidence of its potential adverse effects, and the existence of other safer, proven compounds, *G. simplicifolia* is not considered to be of clinical importance. Further study will clarify its safety and therapeutic application, if any.

References

Das YT, Bagchi M, Bagchi D et al. Safety of 5-hydroxy-L-tryptophan. Toxicol Lett. 2004;150:111–122.

Garcia-Ovejero D, Veiga S, Garcia-Segura LM et al. Glial expression of estrogen and androgen receptors after rat brain injury. J Comp Neurol. 2002;450:256–271.

Gwaltney-Brant SM, Albretson JC, Khan SA. 5-Hydroxytryptophan toxicosis in dogs: 21 cases (1989–1999). JAVMA. 2000;216:1937–1940.

Lemaire PA, Adosraku RK. An HPLC method for the direct assay of the serotonin precursor, 5-hydroxytrophan, in seeds of *Griffonia simplicifolia*. Phytochem Anal. 2002;13:333–337.

Means C. Selected herbal hazards. Vet Clin Small Anim Pract. 2002;32:367–382.

Sandelin M, Zabihi S, Liu L et al. Metastasis-associated S100A4 (Mts1) protein is expressed in subpopulations of sensory and autonomic neurons and in Schwann cells of the adult rat. J Comp Neurol. 2004;473:233–243.

Shaw K, Turner J, Del Mar C. Tryptophan and 5-hydroxytryptophan for depression. Cochrane Database Syst Rev. 2001;1:CD003198.

Tempel W, Tschampel S, Woods RJ. The xenograft antigen bound to *Griffonia simplicifolia* lectin 1-B(4). X-ray crystal structure of the complex and molecular dynamics characterization of the binding site. J Biol Chem. 2002;277:6615–6621.

Zhu-Salzman K, Shade RE, Koiwa H et al. Carbohydrate binding and resistance to proteolysis control insecticidal activity of *Griffonia simplicifolia* lectin II. Proc Natl Acad Sci USA. 1998;95: 15123–15128.

Theobroma cacao

Theobroma cacao (Cocoa, Chocolate) is a small tree between 4 and 8 m in height. Native to the South American Andes, the tree is now cultivated in tropical regions around the world, and principally in West Africa (Nigeria, Ghana, Ivory Coast), Brazil, and the Dominican Republic. Surface roots form a mass at the tree's base; the taproot extends 2 m deep but is shorter in compact soil. The fruits of the plant are commonly referred to as pods. Pods vary in shape and size and can be oblong, spherical, or blunted (Fig. 5-5). Each pod contains five rows of between 20 to 60 beans (large seeds), which also vary in size. At harvest, pods are cut from the trees

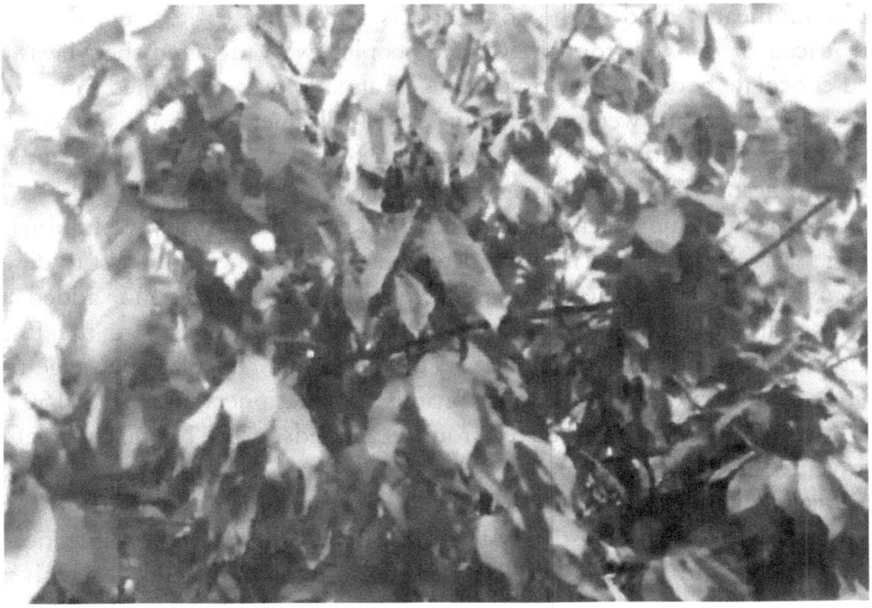

FIGURE 5-5. *Theobroma cocoa* tree showing leaves and fruit pods. (Photo courtesy of Dr. Jayvir Anjaria)

and allowed to rest on the ground before they are cracked open. Beans are then briefly fermented before drying in the sun (New Crop Resource Online, Purdue University 2003).

Theobroma cacao is the source of a number of commercially important products, containing several hundred volatile compounds alone. A well-known example of a medicinal compound derived from this plant is the CNS and cardiovascular stimulant theophylline. Now largely replaced by other pharmaceutical compounds, it also possessed diuretic and bronchial smooth muscle relaxant properties (PDR 2000; Graziano 1998). Perhaps the best recognized product that comes from this tree is chocolate; milk chocolate, for example, is prepared by the addition of sugar, milk, and flavoring to dry, crushed cocoa beans. Theobroma is also the source of cocoa butter used by both pharmaceutical and cosmetic industries (New Crop Resource Online, Purdue University 2003; PDR 2000).

Historical Perspective

The earliest evidence of the consumption of chocolate has been attributed to the Preclassic Maya in 600 BC in what is now northern Belize in Central America (Hurst, Tarka, Powis et al. 2002), although the Mayan and Aztecs may have cultivated cocoa trees as early as 1500 BC. They considered it to be a sacred plant.

Theobroma means "food of the gods" and is a reference to its original use. The word "cacao" is derived from the Olmec peoples, who predated the Mayas. The sacred chocolate beverage they prepared ("cacahuatl") was consumed from golden cups, and cocoa beans were used as currency. (Dillinger, Barriga, Escarcega et al. 2000). Indigenous people of Mexico continue to use chocolate as a sacred part of rituals and fiestas (Dillinger, Barriga, Escarcega et al. 2000).

Europeans first enjoyed chocolate in the mid sixteenth century. Columbus may have been the first to report it, but Cortes seems to have been the first to describe the recipe for preparing the chocolate beverage. Spanish aristocracy added sugar to it to counteract the bitter brew. Sir Hans Soane, physician to the English throne, created milk chocolate in 1727; his medicinal chocolate beverage recipe continued to be used by the Cadbury brothers confectioners more than 150 years later. Theobromine was first isolated from cacao seeds in 1841. The chocolate bar was invented in 1848 (Graziano 1998).

In folk medicine, cocoa beans have been advocated for the treatment of intestinal parasites and other digestive system ailments, burns and topical infection, diabetes, malaria, and listlessness (New Crop Resource Online, Purdue University 2003; PDR 2000).

Ingredients

Cocoa contains theobromine (0.5 to 2.7%), caffeine (0.25% in cocoa), tyramine, tryptamine, dopamine, nicotinic acid, free amino acids, and tannins. Chocolate is high in phenylethylamine, which may explain some of its medicinal properties (New Crop Resource Online, Purdue University 2003; PDR 2000). Cocoa and chocolate contain flavonoids that have antioxidant effects and modulate cholesterol levels and vascular homeostasis (Steinberg, Bearden, Keen 2003; Schramm, Karim, Schrader et al. 2003; Zhu, Holt, Lazarus et al. 2002; Wan, Vinson, Etherton et al. 2001). The cocoa flavanols (−)−epicatechin and (+)−catechin are particularly effective antioxidants (Zhu, Holt, Lazarus et al. 2002; Rein, Lotito, Holt et al. 2000). Their uptake may be augmented by concurrent carbohydrate ingestion (Schramm, Karim, Schrader et al. 2003). Cocoa flavonoids may also modulate platelet function, although this effect is not as marked as that of aspirin (Pearson, Paglieroni, Rein et al. 2002).

Clinical Effects

The caffeine content of chocolate may explain part of the effect of chocolate consumption on mood (Bastia, Schwarzschild 2003). Caffeine is the most widely consumed psychomotor stimulant and psychoactive substance. Its catabolic products theobromine and xanthine are found in tea, coffee, and chocolate. These compounds have significant antioxidant and pro-oxidant action (Azam, Hadi, Khan et al. 2003). The psychoactive effect of chocolate may emanate from a synergistic effect between caffeine, theobromine, and elevated central anandamide levels (di Tomaso, Beltramo, Piomelli 1996). Cocoa amines may cause migraines in susceptible individuals. Some people are allergic to chocolate products (New Crop Resource Online, Purdue University 2003; PDR 2000).

The ingestion of carbohydrates increases tryptophan and, therefore, central serotonergic activity. It is thought that depression and changes in food cravings reflect a self-medication. Several types of cyclical depressive states have been associated with cravings for sweets, chocolate in particular (Moller SE 1992). Craving sweets is increased by induced depressive moods in both animals and people (Willner, Benton, Brown et al. 1998). One study documented that 49% of all food cravings in a healthy group of women was for chocolate (Hill, Heaton-Brown 1994). This study confirmed a premenstrual increase in food cravings and noted that consumption of highly palatable foods reduced hunger and improved mood. Eating chocolate did not improve mood in a group of self-identified female chocolate "addicts." In these women, eating chocolate provoked feelings of guilt (Macdiarmid, Hetherington 1995). In another study of self-labeled chocoholics, eating chocolate resulted in feeling less anxious and more energetic and able to concentrate (Dallard, Cathebras, Sauron et al. 2001).

Because even small quantities of protein in a meal will block the bioavailability of tryptophan, it is unlikely that carbohydrate ingestion can explain the impact by chocolate on mood (Benton, Donohoe 1999). Chocolate components such as caffeine, phenylethylamine, anandamines, and magnesium are in such low levels that they are also unlikely to contribute to the mood-altering effects of chocolate. Although chocolate cravings have also been attributed to a hedonistic attraction for palatable but "forbidden" foods (Rogers, Smit 2000), it is plausible that all palatable foods stimulate central endorphin release (Benton, Donohoe 1999; Dum, Herz 1984).

Chocolate contains a number of bioactive compounds that may regulate neurotransmitter levels such as serotonin and dopamine. It also contains components that parallel other addictive substances (Bruinsma, Tern 1999). Cocoa powder and chocolate have been shown to contain compounds that may mimic cannabinoids. The mechanism may be direct by activation of endogenous cannabinoid receptors, or indirect by raising anandamide levels. Anandamide is a brain lipid with high affinity for cannabinoid receptors and psychoactive effects resembling plant cannabinoids. This may also explain cravings for chocolate. It is also possible that elevations in anandamide levels may combine with other chocolate components such as caffeine and theobromine to contribute to a short-lived euphoric effect (di Tomaso, Beltramo, Piomelli 1996; James 1996). The finding that the opioid antagonist naloxone markedly reduces the consumption of sweet foods such as chocolate provides further support for an opioid mechanism (Cleary, Weldon, O'Hare et al. 1996).

Substances in cocoa and chocolate may mimic or potentiate the binding of anandamide to cannabinoid receptors. This might be useful for those taking marijuana for medicinal purposes; administration of medicinal marijuana with chocolate might reduce cost and any side effects although it might impact the patient's waistline (di Tomaso, Beltramo, Piomelli 1996; James 1996).

Clinical Application in Veterinary Behavior Medicine

The use of chocolate as a veterinary psychoactive is, of course, precluded by the fact that it is fatally toxic to cats and dogs. Toxicity is due to the theobromine content of chocolate, which causes cardiac and neurologic stimulation (Frazer 1991). Some veterinary clients may not be aware of this, however, and could be tempted to administer chocolate to their pets. Veterinarians should make a point of clarifying the danger of chocolate to pet owners who may indulge in this favorite food treat and want to share their enjoyment with their pets. Some pet treats are chocolate flavored and contain negligible amounts of theobromine. It would be prudent to discourage pets from developing an affinity for chocolate-flavored foods.

References

Azam S, Hadi N, Khan NU et al. antioxidant and prooxidant properties of caffeine, theobromine and xanthine. Med Sci Monit. 2003;2:BR325–330.

Bastia E, Schwarzschild MA. DARPP chocolate: a caffeinated morsel of striatal signaling. Sci STKE. 2003:2003:PE2.

Benton D, Donohoe RT. The effects of nutrients on mood. Public Health Nutr. 1999;2:403–409.

Bruinsma K, Taren DL. Chocolate: food or drug? J AM Diet Assoc. 1999;99:1249–1256.

Cleary J, Weldon DT, O'Hare E et al. Naloxone effects on sucrose-motivated behavior. Psychopharmacology (Berl). 1996;126:110–114.

Dallard I, Cathebras P, Sauron C et al. Is cocoa a psychotropic drug? Psychopatholigic study of a population of subjects self-identified as chocolate addicts (French). Encephale 2001;27:181–186.

Dillinger TL, Barriga P, Escarcega S et al. Food of the Gods: cure for humanity? A cultural history of the medicinal and ritual use of chocolate. J Nutr. 2000;130:2057S–2072S.

di Tomaso E, Beltramo M, Piomelli D. Brain cannabinoids in chocolate. Nature. 1996;382:677–678.

Dum J, Herz A. Endorphinergic modulation of neural reward systems indicated by behavioral changes. Pharmacol Biochem Behav. 1984;21:259–266.

Fraser CM (ed). Chocolate poisoning. The Merck Veterinary Manual. Merck & Co. Inc., Rahway, NJ. 1991;1643–1644.

Graziano MM. Food of the Gods as mortals' medicine: the uses of chocolate and cacao products. Pharm Hist. 1998;40:132–146.

Hill AJ, Heaton-Brown L. The experience of food craving: a prospective investigation in healthy women. J Psychosom Res. 1994;38:801–814.

Hurst WJ, Tarka SM, Powis TG et al. Cacao usage by the earliest Maya civilization. Nature. 2002;418: 289–290.

James JS. Marijuana and chocolate. AIDS Treat News. 1996;257:3–4.

Macdiarmid JI, Hetherington MM. Mood modulation by food: an exploration of affect and cravings in 'chocolate addicts'. Br J Clin Psychol. 1005;34:129–138.

Moller SE. Serotonin, carbohydrates, and atypical depression. Pharmacol Toxicol. 1992;71(Suppl 1): 61–71.

New Crop Resource Online Program, Purdue University Center for New Crops and Plant Products; Purdue University, W. Lafayette, Indiana; 2003. http://www.hort.purdue.edu/newcrop/

PDR for Herbal Medicines. (2nd ed) Medical Economics Company Inc., Montvale, NJ. 2000;199–201.

Pearson DA, Paglieroni TG, Rein D et al. The effects of flavanol-rich cocoa and aspirin on ex vivo platelet function. Thromb Res. 2002;106:191–197.
Rein D, Lotito S, Holt RR et al. Epicatechin in human plasma: in vivo determination and effect of chocolate consumption on plasma oxidation status. J Nutr. 2000;130(Suppl 8S):2109S–2114S.
Rogers PJ, Smit HJ. Food craving and food "addiction": a critical review of the evidence from a biopsychosocial perspective. Pharmacol Biochem Behav. 2000;66:3–14.
Schramm DD, Karim M, Schrader HR et al. Food effects on the absorption and pharmacokinetics of cocoa flavanols. Life Sci. 2003;73:857–869.
Steinberg FM, Bearden MM, Keen CL. Cocoa and chocolate flavonoids: implications for cardiovascular health. J Am Diet Assoc. 2003;103:215–223.
Wan Y, Vinson JA, Etherton TD et al. Effects of cocoa powder and dark chocolate on LDL oxidative susceptibility and prostaglandin concentrations in humans. Am J Clin Nutr. 2001;74:596–602.
Willner P, Benton D, Brown E et al. "Depression" increases "craving" for sweet rewards in animal and human models of depression and craving. Psychopharmacology (Berl). 1998;136:272–283.
Zhu QY, Holt RR, Lazarus SA et al. Inhibitory effects of cocoa flavanols and procyanidin oligomers on free radical–induced erythrocyte hemolysis. Exp Biol Med (Maywood). 2002;227:321–329.

CHAPTER

6

Suggested Clinical Application of Psychoactive Herbs

"Let us give Nature a chance; she knows her business better than we do."
—*Michel Eyquem de Montaigne* (1533–1592)

This chapter presents tables that summarize the most promising psychoactive herbs in veterinary behavior medicine based upon current information contained in this book. The first table (Table 6-1) is a general summary of the key psychoactive herbs discussed. Additional tables conveniently organize these herbs by specific category of diagnostic application, such as problems of aggressive or compulsive behavior in dogs and cats.

As research around the world delves further into the therapeutic benefits and risks of plant-derived remedies, the application and inclusion of these tabulated herbs will likely require modification. Future editions of this book will update content as necessary. Meanwhile, readers who are not experienced clinicians or herbalists should seek the guidance of an expert before treating themselves or their pets and patients with any medicine. The reader is also reminded that psychoactive medication or compounds are best combined with behavior modification and lifestyle changes in a comprehensive plan designed by a board-certified veterinary behaviorist.

Table 6-1. Suggested Clinical Applications for Psychoactive Herbs Used Alone or in Polyherbal Formulas Discussed in This Book[1]

Symptoms/Category of Misbehavior	Western Herb	Native American	Chinese	Ayurvedic
Agitated States (e.g., excessive vocalization, play aggression, overreactivity, hyperactivity)	*Hypericum perforatum; Lavandula angustifolia; Matricaria chamomilla; Passiflora incarnata; Valeriana officinalis*	*Panax quinquefolius; Piper methysticum; Scutellaria lateriflora*	*Corydalis yanhusuo; Ginkgo biloba; Salvia miltiorrhiza; Scutellaria baicalensis; Zingiber officinale*	*Asparagus racemosus; Centella asiatica; Withania somnifera*
Destructiveness (e.g., digging, scratching, chewing)	*Hypericum perforatum; Matricaria chamomilla; Nepeta cataria; Passiflora incarnata; Valeriana officinalis*	*Panax quinquefolius; Piper methysticum Scutellaria lateriflora*	*Corydalis yanhusuo; Ginkgo biloba; Salvia miltiorrhiza; Scutellaria baicalensis; Zingiber officinale*	*Centella asiatica*
Separation Anxiety Syndrome[2]	*Hypericum perforatum; Lavandula angustifolia; Matricaria chamomilla; Passiflora incarnata; Valeriana officinalis; Vitex agnus-castus*	*Panax quinquefolius; Piper methysticum; Scutellaria lateriflora*	*Corydalis yanhusuo; Ginkgo biloba; Panax ginseng; Salvia miltiorrhiza; Scutellaria baicalensis; Zingiber officinale*	*Albizzia lebbeck; Asparagus racemosus; Centella asiatica; Withania somnifera*
Fear-Related	*Hypericum perforatum; Lavandula angustifolia; Matricaria chamomilla; Passiflora incarnata; Valeriana officinalis*	*Panax quinquefolius; Piper methysticum; Scutellaria lateriflora*	*Ginkgo biloba; Panax ginseng; Scutellaria baicalensis; Zingiber officinale*	*Albizzia lebbeck; Asparagus racemosus; Centella asiatica; Withania somnifera*
Phobia	*Hypericum perforatum; Passiflora incarnata*	*Panax quinquefolius; Piper methysticum; Scutellaria lateriflora*	*Ginkgo biloba; Scutellaria baicalensis; Zingiber officinale*	*Albizzia lebbeck; Asparagus racemosus; Centella asiatica; Withania somnifera*
Generalized Anxiety Disorder	*Hypericum perforatum; Matricaria chamomilla; Passiflora incarnata*	*Panax quinquefolius; Piper methysticum; Scutellaria lateriflora*	*Corydalis yanhusuo; Ginkgo biloba; Panax ginseng; Scutellaria baicalensis; Zingiber officinale*	*Albizzia lebbeck; Asparagus racemosus; Centella asiatica; Withania somnifera*
Feline/Canine Cognitive Dysfunction Syndrome; Senile Dementia	*Agaricus blazei; Lavandula angustifolia; Melissa officinalis; Pausinystalia yohimbe*	*Panax quinquefolius; Piper methysticum; Salvia officinalis*	*Astragalus membranaceus; Ginkgo biloba; Huperzia serrata; Panax ginseng; Salvia miltiorrhiza; Schisandra chinensis; Zingiber officinale*	*Bacopa monniera; Centella asiatica*
Canine Hyperkinesis	*Catha edulis*		*Ginkgo biloba*	
Feline Hyperesthesia Syndrome	*Passiflora incarnata*	*Piper methysticum*	*Ginkgo biloba; Salvia miltiorrhiza; Zingiber officinale*	

(continued)

Table 6-1. Suggested Clinical Applications for Psychoactive Herbs Used Alone or in Polyherbal Formulas Discussed in This Book[1] *(continued)*

Symptoms/Category of Misbehavior	Western Herb	Native American	Chinese	Ayurvedic
Dominance Aggression	*Valeriana officinalis*	*Panax quinquefolius*	*Angelica sinensis; Ginkgo biloba*	*Withania somnifera*
Territorial Aggression	*Lavandula angustifolia; Matricaria chamomilla; Nepeta cataria; Valeriana officinalis*	*Panax quinquefolius*	*Angelica sinensis; Ginkgo biloba*	*Withania somnifera*
Introducing New Pets (e.g., Anxiety +/− Defensive/Offensive aggression)	*Hypericum perforatum; Matricaria chamomilla; Nepeta cataria; Passiflora incarnata; Valeriana officinalis*	*Panax quinquefolius; Scutellaria lateriflora*	*Angelica sinensis; Corydalis yanhusuo; Eleutherococcus senticosus; Ginkgo biloba; Panax ginseng; Scutellaria baicalensis; Zingiber officinale*	*Albizzia lebbeck; Asparagus racemosus; Centella asiatica; Withania somnifera*
Irritable Aggression	*Matricaria chamomilla; Valeriana officinalis*	*Panax quinquefolius; Piper methysticum*	*Angelica sinensis; Salvia miltiorrhiza*	*Withania somnifera*
Introverted Compulsive Behavior (Passive forms; e.g., psychogenic grooming)	*Hypericum perforatum; Melissa officinalis; Vitex agnus-castus*	*Piper methysticum; Scutellaria lateriflora*	*Corydalis yanhusuo; Ginkgo biloba; Scutellaria baicalensis; Schisandra chinensis; Zingiber officinale*	*Albizzia lebbeck; Asparagus racemosus; Centella asiatica; Withania somnifera;*
Extroverted Compulsive Behaviors (Agitated forms; e.g., tail chasing, fly catching)	*Hypericum perforatum; Vitex agnus-castus*	*Piper methysticum; Scutellaria lateriflora*	*Corydalis yanhusuo; Ginkgo biloba; Scutellaria baicalensis; Zingiber officinale*	
Narcolepsy	*Pausinystalia yohimbe*			
Territorial Marking, Litter Box Aversion	*Hypericum perforatum; Valeriana officinalis; Vitex agnus-castus*	*Piper methysticum; Scutellaria lateriflora*	*Corydalis yanhusuo; Panax ginseng; Scutellaria baicalensis; Zingiber officinale*	*Asparagus racemosus; Centella asiatica; Vitex negundo; Withania somnifera*
Urinary Incontinence	*Humulus lupulus; Verbena spp.*		*Panax ginseng; Zingiber officinale*	
Masturbation, Persistent Sexual Behavior	*Vitex agnus-castus*		*Eleutherococcus senticosus*	*Vitex negundo; Withania somnifera*
Aphrodisiac (Promote Breeding)	*Pausinystalia yohimbe; Turnera diffusa*		*Ginkgo biloba; Panax ginseng; Zingiber officinale*	*Albizzia lebbeck; Bacopa monniera; Celastrus paniculatus; Withania somnifera*

[1] Herbal or synthetic psychoactive medicines are not complete treatments for behavior problems; psychoactive substances should be used in conjunction with an appropriate treatment plan for behavior modification that aims to restore balance to the patient's life. Please refer to the text for details of the individual herbs and their suggested clinical applications.

[2] Separation Anxiety Syndrome in dogs and cats can include signs of house soiling, excessive vocalization, destructiveness, self-mutilation, and aggression; these categories of presentation can appear alone or in combination and in varying degrees of intensity and may vary over time.

Table 6-2. Psychoactive Herbs of Potential Use in Aggressive Problems in the Cat and Dog[1]

Symptoms/Category of Misbehavior	Western Herb	Native American	Chinese	Ayurvedic
Agitated States[2] (e.g., excessive vocalization, play aggression, overreactivity, hyperactivity)	*Hypericum perforatum; Lavandula angustifolia; Matricaria chamomilla; Passiflora incarnata; Valeriana officinalis*	*Panax quinquefolius; Piper methysticum; Scutellaria lateriflora*	*Corydalis yanhusuo; Ginkgo biloba; Salvia miltiorrhiza; Scutellaria baicalensis; Zingiber officinale*	*Asparagus racemosus; Centella asiatica; Withania somnifera*
Dominance Aggression	*Valeriana officinalis*	*Panax quinquefolius*	*Angelica sinensis; Ginkgo biloba*	*Withania somnifera*
Fear[3]	*Hypericum perforatum; Lavandula angustifolia ; Matricaria chamomilla; Passiflora incarnata; Valeriana officinalis*	*Panax quinquefolius; Piper methysticum; Scutellaria lateriflora*	*Ginkgo biloba; Panax ginseng; Scutellaria baicalensis; Zingiber officinale*	*Albizzia lebbeck; Asparagus racemosus; Centella asiatica; Withania somnifera*
Introducing New Pets	*Hypericum perforatum; Matricaria chamomilla; Nepeta cataria; Passiflora incarnata; Valeriana officinalis*	*Panax quinquefolius; Scutellaria lateriflora*	*Angelica sinensis; Corydalis yanhusuo; Eleutherococcus senticosus; Ginkgo biloba; Panax ginseng; Scutellaria baicalensis; Zingiber officinale*	*Albizzia lebbeck; Asparagus racemosus; Centella asiatica; Withania somnifera*
Irritable Aggression	*Matricaria chamomilla; Valeriana officinalis*	*Panax quinquefolius; Piper methysticum*	*Angelica sinensis; Salvia miltiorrhiza*	*Withania somnifera*
Masturbation, Persistent Sexual Behavior[4]	*Vitex agnus-castus*		*Eleutherococcus senticosus*	*Vitex negundo; Withania somnifera*
Separation Anxiety Syndrome[5]	*Hypericum perforatum; Lavandula angustifolia ; Matricaria chamomilla; Passiflora incarnata; Valeriana officinalis; Vitex agnus-castus*	*Panax quinquefolius; Piper methysticum; Scutellaria lateriflora*	*Corydalis yanhusuo; Ginkgo biloba; Panax ginseng; Salvia miltiorrhiza; Scutellaria baicalensis; Zingiber officinale*	*Albizzia lebbeck; Asparagus racemosus; Centella asiatica; Withania somnifera*

(continued)

Table 6-2. Psychoactive Herbs of Potential Use in Aggressive Problems in the Cat and Dog[1] (*continued*)

Symptoms/Category of Misbehavior	Western Herb	Native American	Chinese	Ayurvedic
Territorial Aggression	*Lavandula angustifolia; Matricaria chamomilla; Nepeta cataria; Valeriana officinalis*	*Panax quinquefolius*	*Angelica sinensis; Ginkgo biloba*	*Withania somnifera*

[1] Herbal or synthetic psychoactive medicines are not complete treatments for behavior problems; psychoactive substances should be used in conjunction with an appropriate treatment plan for behavior modification that aims to restore balance to the patient's life.

[2] May benefit mild to moderate forms of aggressive behavior characterized by agitation and hyper-reactivity (e.g., jumping, barking); defining the diagnosis and necessary lifestyle changes with training techniques are essential.

[3] May benefit mild to moderate cases of fear aggression because anxiety is a primary component; behavior modification must accompany herbal or synthetic drug therapy.

[4] Persistant sexual behavior in neutered males may be accompanied by aggression toward the sexual surrogate (owner or another house pet); testosterone/LH levels should be verified; behavior modification will ensure a successful outcome to treatment.

[5] Separation anxiety syndrome can occasionally be manifested by aggression directed toward the owners as they prepare to leave; a comprehensive treatment must include appropriate behavior modification and lifestyle changes.

Table 6-3. Psychoactive Herbs of Potential Use in Behavior Problems Associated with House Soiling in the Cat and Dog[1]

Symptoms/Category of Misbehavior	Western Herb	Native American	Chinese	Ayurvedic
Separation Anxiety Syndrome	*Hypericum perforatum; Lavandula angustifolia; Matricaria chamomilla; Passiflora incarnata; Valeriana officinalis; Vitex agnus-castus*	*Panax quinquefolius; Piper methysticum; Scutellaria lateriflora*	*Corydalis yanhusuo; Ginkgo biloba; Panax ginseng; Salvia miltiorrhiza; Scutellaria baicalensis; Zingiber officinale*	*Albizzia lebbeck; Asparagus racemosus; Centella asiatica; Withania somnifera*
Fears (e.g., submissive urination)	*Hypericum perforatum; Lavandula angustifolia; Matricaria chamomilla; Passiflora incarnata; Valeriana officinalis*	*Panax quinquefolius; Piper methysticum; Scutellaria lateriflora*	*Ginkgo biloba; Panax ginseng; Scutellaria baicalensis; Zingiber officinale*	*Albizzia lebbeck; Asparagus racemosus; Centella asiatica; Withania somnifera*
Feline/Canine Cognitive Dysfunction Syndrome; Senile Dementia	*Agaricus blazei; Lavandula angustifolia; Melissa officinalis; Pausinystalia yohimbe*	*Panax quinquefolius; Piper methysticum; Salvia officinalis*	*Astragalus membranaceus; Ginkgo biloba; Huperzia serrata; Panax ginseng; Salvia miltiorrhiza; Schisandra chinensis; Zingiber officinale*	*Bacopa monniera; Centella asiatica*
Territorial Aggression	*Lavandula angustifolia; Matricaria chamomilla; Nepeta cataria; Valeriana officinalis*	*Panax quinquefolius*	*Angelica sinensis; Ginkgo biloba*	*Withania somnifera*
Territorial Marking, Litter Box Aversion	*Hypericum perforatum; Valeriana officinalis; Vitex agnus-castus*	*Piper methysticum; Scutellaria lateriflora*	*Corydalis yanhusuo; Panax ginseng; Scutellaria baicalensis; Zingiber officinale*	*Asparagus racemosus; Centella asiatica; Vitex negundo; Withania somnifera*
Urinary Incontinence	*Humulus lupulus; Verbena spp.*		*Panax ginseng; Zingiber officinale*	
Masturbation, Persistent Sexual Behavior	*Vitex agnus-castus*		*Eleutherococcus senticosus*	*Vitex negundo; Withania somnifera*

[1] Herbal or synthetic psychoactive medicines are not complete treatments for behavior problems; psychoactive substances should be used in conjunction with an appropriate treatment plan for behavior modification that aims to restore balance to the patient's life.

Table 6-4. Psychoactive Herbs of Potential Use in Problems of Compulsive Behavior in the Cat and Dog[1]

Symptoms/Category of Misbehavior	Western Herb	Native American	Chinese	Ayurvedic
Agitated States (e.g., excessive vocalization, overreactivity, hyperactivity)	*Hypericum perforatum; Lavandula angustifolia; Matricaria chamomilla; Passiflora incarnata; Valeriana officinalis*	*Panax quinquefolius; Piper methysticum; Scutellaria lateriflora*	*Corydalis yanhusuo; Ginkgo biloba; Salvia miltiorrhiza; Scutellaria baicalensis; Zingiber officinale*	*Asparagus racemosus; Centella asiatica; Withania somnifera*
Destructiveness (e.g., digging, scratching, chewing)	*Hypericum perforatum; Matricaria chamomilla; Nepeta cataria; Passiflora incarnata; Valeriana officinalis*	*Panax quinquefolius; Piper methysticum Scutellaria lateriflora*	*Corydalis yanhusuo; Ginkgo biloba; Salvia miltiorrhiza; Scutellaria baicalensis; Zingiber officinale*	*Centella asiatica*
Separation Anxiety Syndrome	*Hypericum perforatum; Lavandula angustifolia; Matricaria chamomilla; Passiflora incarnata; Valeriana officinalis; Vitex agnus-castus*	*Panax quinquefolius; Piper methysticum; Scutellaria lateriflora*	*Corydalis yanhusuo; Ginkgo biloba; Panax ginseng; Salvia miltiorrhiza; Scutellaria baicalensis; Zingiber officinale*	*Albizzia lebbeck; Asparagus racemosus; Centella asiatica; Withania somnifera*
Fear-Related	*Hypericum perforatum; Lavandula angustifolia; Matricaria chamomilla; Passiflora incarnata; Valeriana officinalis*	*Panax quinquefolius; Piper methysticum; Scutellaria lateriflora*	*Ginkgo biloba; Panax ginseng; Scutellaria baicalensis; Zingiber officinale*	*Albizzia lebbeck; Asparagus racemosus; Centella asiatica; Withania somnifera*
Generalized Anxiety Disorder	*Hypericum perforatum; Matricaria chamomilla; Passiflora incarnata*	*Panax quinquefolius; Piper methysticum; Scutellaria lateriflora*	*Corydalis yanhusuo; Ginkgo biloba; Panax ginseng; Scutellaria baicalensis; Zingiber officinale*	*Albizzia lebbeck; Asparagus racemosus; Centella asiatica; Withania somnifera*
Introverted Compulsive Behavior (Passive forms; e.g., psychogenic grooming)	*Hypericum perforatum; Melissa officinalis; Vitex agnus-castus*	*Piper methysticum; Scutellaria lateriflora*	*Corydalis yanhusuo; Ginkgo biloba; Scutellaria baicalensis; Schisandra chinensis; Zingiber officinale*	*Albizzia lebbeck; Asparagus racemosus; Centella asiatica; Withania somnifera*
Extroverted Compulsive Behaviors (Agitated forms; e.g., tail chasing, fly catching)	*Hypericum perforatum; Vitex agnus-castus*	*Piper methysticum; Scutellaria lateriflora*	*Corydalis yanhusuo; Ginkgo biloba; Scutellaria baicalensis; Zingiber officinale*	

(*continued*)

Table 6-4. Psychoactive Herbs of Potential Use in Problems of Compulsive Behavior in the Cat and Dog[1] (*continued*)

Symptoms/Category of Misbehavior	Western Herb	Native American	Chinese	Ayurvedic
Territorial Marking, Litter Box Aversion	*Hypericum perforatum; Valeriana officinalis; Vitex agnus-castus*	*Piper methysticum; Scutellaria lateriflora*	*Corydalis yanhusuo; Panax ginseng; Scutellaria baicalensis; Zingiber officinale*	*Asparagus racemosus; Centella asiatica; Vitex negundo; Withania somnifera*
Masturbation, Persistent Sexual Behavior	*Vitex agnus-castus*		*Eleutherococcus senticosus*	*Vitex negundo; Withania somnifera*

[1] Herbal or synthetic psychoactive medicines are not complete treatments for behavior problems; psychoactive substances should be used in conjunction with an appropriate treatment plan for behavior modification that aims to restore balance to the patient's life.

Table 6-5. Psychoactive Herbs of Potential Use in Sexual Problems in the Cat and Dog[1]

Symptoms/Category of Misbehavior	Western Herb	Native American	Chinese	Ayurvedic
Territorial Marking, Litter Box Aversion	*Hypericum perforatum; Valeriana officinalis; Vitex agnus-castus*	*Piper methysticum; Scutellaria lateriflora*	*Corydalis yanhusuo; Panax ginseng; Scutellaria baicalensis; Zingiber officinale*	*Asparagus racemosus; Centella asiatica; Vitex negundo; Withania somnifera*
Masturbation, Persistent Sexual Behavior	*Vitex agnus-castus*		*Eleutherococcus senticosus*	*Vitex negundo; Withania somnifera*
Aphrodisiac (Promote Breeding)	*Pausinystalia yohimbe; Turnera diffusa*		*Ginkgo biloba; Panax ginseng; Zingiber officinale*	*Albizzia lebbeck; Bacopa monniera; Celastrus paniculatus; Withania somnifera*
Dominance Aggression	*Valeriana officinalis*	*Panax quinquefolius*	*Angelica sinensis; Ginkgo biloba*	*Withania somnifera*
Territorial Aggression	*Lavandula angustifolia; Matricaria chamomilla; Nepeta cataria; Valeriana officinalis*	*Panax quinquefolius*	*Angelica sinensis; Ginkgo biloba*	*Withania somnifera*

[1] Herbal or synthetic psychoactive medicines are not complete treatments for behavior problems; psychoactive substances should be used in conjunction with an appropriate treatment plan for behavior modification that aims to restore balance to the patient's life.

Table 6-6. Psychoactive Herbs of Potential Use in Behavior Problems Associated with Canine and Feline Cognitive Dysfunction Syndromes in Geriatric Pets[1]

Symptoms/Category of Misbehavior	Western Herb	Native American	Chinese	Ayurvedic
Feline/Canine Cognitive Dysfunction Syndrome; Senile Dementia	*Agaricus blazei; Lavandula angustifolia; Melissa officinalis; Pausinystalia yohimbe*	*Panax quinquefolius; Piper methysticum; Salvia officinalis*	*Astragalus membranaceus; Ginkgo biloba; Huperzia serrata; Panax ginseng; Salvia miltiorrhiza; Schisandra chinensis; Zingiber officinale*	*Bacopa monniera; Centella asiatica*
Agitated States (e.g., excessive vocalization, overreactivity, hyperactivity)	*Hypericum perforatum; Lavandula angustifolia; Matricaria chamomilla; Passiflora incarnata; Valeriana officinalis*	*Panax quinquefolius; Piper methysticum; Scutellaria lateriflora*	*Corydalis yanhusuo; Ginkgo biloba; Salvia miltiorrhiza; Scutellaria baicalensis; Zingiber officinale*	*Asparagus racemosus; Centella asiatica; Withania somnifera*
Separation Anxiety Syndrome	*Hypericum perforatum; Lavandula angustifolia; Matricaria chamomilla; Passiflora incarnata; Valeriana officinalis; Vitex agnus-castus*	*Panax quinquefolius; Piper methysticum; Scutellaria lateriflora*	*Corydalis yanhusuo; Ginkgo biloba; Panax ginseng; Salvia miltiorrhiza; Scutellaria baicalensis; Zingiber officinale*	*Albizzia lebbeck; Asparagus racemosus; Centella asiatica; Withania somnifera*
Generalized Anxiety Disorder	*Hypericum perforatum; Matricaria chamomilla; Passiflora incarnata*	*Panax quinquefolius; Piper methysticum; Scutellaria lateriflora*	*Corydalis yanhusuo; Ginkgo biloba; Panax ginseng; Scutellaria baicalensis; Zingiber officinale*	*Albizzia lebbeck; Asparagus racemosus; Centella asiatica; Withania somnifera*
Urinary Incontinence	*Humulus lupulus; Verbena spp.*		*Panax ginseng; Zingiber officinale*	

[1] Herbal or synthetic psychoactive medicines are not complete treatments for behavior problems; psychoactive substances should be used in conjunction with an appropriate treatment plan for behavior modification that aims to restore balance to the patient's life.

Table 6-7. Psychoactive Herbs of Potential Use in Anxiety-Related Problems in the Cat and Dog[1]

Symptoms/Category of Misbehavior	Western Herb	Native American	Chinese	Ayurvedic
Agitated States (e.g., excessive vocalization, overreactivity, hyperactivity)	*Hypericum perforatum; Lavandula angustifolia; Matricaria chamomilla; Passiflora incarnata; Valeriana officinalis*	*Panax quinquefolius; Piper methysticum; Scutellaria lateriflora*	*Corydalis yanhusuo; Ginkgo biloba; Salvia miltiorrhiza; Scutellaria baicalensis; Zingiber officinale*	*Asparagus racemosus; Centella asiatica; Withania somnifera*
Destructiveness (e.g., digging, scratching, chewing)	*Hypericum perforatum; Matricaria chamomilla; Nepeta cataria; Passiflora incarnata; Valeriana officinalis*	*Panax quinquefolius; Piper methysticum Scutellaria lateriflora*	*Corydalis yanhusuo; Ginkgo biloba; Salvia miltiorrhiza; Scutellaria baicalensis; Zingiber officinale*	*Centella asiatica*
Separation Anxiety Syndrome	*Hypericum perforatum; Lavandula angustifolia; Matricaria chamomilla; Passiflora incarnata; Valeriana officinalis; Vitex agnus-castus*	*Panax quinquefolius; Piper methysticum; Scutellaria lateriflora*	*Corydalis yanhusuo; Ginkgo biloba; Panax ginseng; Salvia miltiorrhiza; Scutellaria baicalensis; Zingiber officinale*	*Albizzia lebbeck; Asparagus racemosus; Centella asiatica; Withania somnifera*
Fear-Related	*Hypericum perforatum; Lavandula angustifolia; Matricaria chamomilla; Passiflora incarnata; Valeriana officinalis*	*Panax quinquefolius; Piper methysticum; Scutellaria lateriflora*	*Ginkgo biloba; Panax ginseng; Scutellaria baicalensis; Zingiber officinale*	*Albizzia lebbeck; Asparagus racemosus; Centella asiatica; Withania somnifera*
Phobia	*Hypericum perforatum; Passiflora incarnata*	*Panax quinquefolius; Piper methysticum; Scutellaria lateriflora*	*Ginkgo biloba; Scutellaria baicalensis; Zingiber officinale*	*Albizzia lebbeck; Asparagus racemosus; Centella asiatica; Withania somnifera*
Generalized Anxiety Disorder	*Hypericum perforatum; Matricaria chamomilla; Passiflora incarnata*	*Panax quinquefolius; Piper methysticum; Scutellaria lateriflora*	*Corydalis yanhusuo; Ginkgo biloba; Panax ginseng; Scutellaria baicalensis; Zingiber officinale*	*Albizzia lebbeck; Asparagus racemosus; Centella asiatica; Withania somnifera*
Territorial Marking, Litter Box Aversion	*Hypericum perforatum; Valeriana officinalis; Vitex agnus-castus*	*Piper methysticum; Scutellaria lateriflora*	*Corydalis yanhusuo; Panax ginseng; Scutellaria baicalensis; Zingiber officinale*	*Asparagus racemosus; Centella asiatica; Vitex negundo; Withania somnifera*
Urinary Incontinence	*Humulus lupulus; Verbena spp.*		*Panax ginseng; Zingiber officinale*	
Introverted Compulsive Behavior (Passive forms; e.g. psychogenic grooming)	*Hypericum perforatum; Melissa officinalis; Vitex agnus-castus*	*Piper methysticum; Scutellaria lateriflora*	*Corydalis yanhusuo; Ginkgo biloba; Scutellaria baicalensis; Schisandra chinensis; Zingiber officinale*	*Albizzia lebbeck; Asparagus racemosus; Centella asiatica; Withania somnifera*

(*continued*)

Table 6-7. Psychoactive Herbs of Potential Use in Anxiety-Related Problems in the Cat and Dog[1] *(continued)*

Symptoms/Category of Misbehavior	Western Herb	Native American	Chinese	Ayurvedic
Extroverted Compulsive Behaviors (Agitated forms; e.g., tail chasing, fly catching)	*Hypericum perforatum; Vitex agnus-castus*	*Piper methysticum; Scutellaria lateriflora*	*Corydalis yanhusuo; Ginkgo biloba; Scutellaria baicalensis; Zingiber officinale*	
Territorial Aggression	*Lavandula angustifolia; Matricaria chamomilla; Nepeta cataria; Valeriana officinalis*	*Panax quinquefolius*	*Angelica sinensis; Ginkgo biloba*	*Withania somnifera*
Introducing New Pets (e.g., anxiety +/− defensive/ offensive aggression)	*Hypericum perforatum; Matricaria chamomilla; Nepeta cataria; Passiflora incarnata; Valeriana officinalis*	*Panax quinquefolius; Scutellaria lateriflora*	*Angelica sinensis; Corydalis yanhusuo; Eleutherococcus senticosus; Ginkgo biloba; Panax ginseng; Scutellaria baicalensis; Zingiber officinale*	*Albizzia lebbeck; Asparagus racemosus; Centella asiatica; Withania somnifera*
Feline/Canine Cognitive Dysfunction Syndrome; Senile Dementia	*Agaricus blazei; Lavandula angustifolia; Melissa officinalis; Pausinystalia yohimbe*	*Panax quinquefolius; Piper methysticum; Salvia officinalis*	*Astragalus membranaceus; Ginkgo biloba; Huperzia serrata; Panax ginseng; Salvia miltiorrhiza; Schisandra chinensis; Zingiber officinale*	*Bacopa monniera; Centella asiatica*

[1] Herbal or synthetic psychoactive medicines are not complete treatments for behavior problems; psychoactive substances should be used in conjunction with an appropriate treatment plan for behavior modification that aims to restore balance to the patient's life.

Table 6-8. Psychoactive Herbs of Potential Use in Problems of Hyperactivity in the Cat and Dog[1]

Symptoms/Category of Misbehavior	Western Herb	Native American	Chinese	Ayurvedic
Canine Hyperkinesis	*Catha edulis*		*Ginkgo biloba*	
Feline Hyperesthesia Syndrome	*Passiflora incarnata*	*Piper methysticum*	*Ginkgo biloba; Salvia miltiorrhiza; Zingiber officinale*	
Extroverted Compulsive Behaviors (Agitated forms; e.g., tail chasing, fly catching)	*Hypericum perforatum; Vitex agnus-castus*	*Piper methysticum; Scutellaria lateriflora*	*Corydalis yanhusuo; Ginkgo biloba; Scutellaria baicalensis; Zingiber officinale*	
Agitated States (e.g., excessive vocalization, play aggression, overreactivity, hyperactivity)	*Hypericum perforatum; Lavandula angustifolia; Matricaria chamomilla; Passiflora incarnata; Valeriana officinalis*	*Panax quinquefolius; Piper methysticum; Scutellaria lateriflora*	*Corydalis yanhusuo; Ginkgo biloba; Salvia miltiorrhiza; Scutellaria baicalensis; Zingiber officinale*	*Asparagus racemosus; Centella asiatica; Withania somnifera*
Destructiveness (e.g., digging, scratching, chewing)	*Hypericum perforatum; Matricaria chamomilla; Nepeta cataria; Passiflora incarnata; Valeriana officinalis*	*Panax quinquefolius; Piper methysticum; Scutellaria lateriflora*	*Corydalis yanhusuo; Ginkgo biloba; Salvia miltiorrhiza; Scutellaria baicalensis; Zingiber officinale*	*Centella asiatica*
Separation Anxiety Syndrome	*Hypericum perforatum; Lavandula angustifolia; Matricaria chamomilla; Passiflora incarnata; Valeriana officinalis; Vitex agnus-castus*	*Panax quinquefolius; Piper methysticum; Scutellaria lateriflora*	*Corydalis yanhusuo; Ginkgo biloba; Panax ginseng; Salvia miltiorrhiza; Scutellaria baicalensis; Zingiber officinale*	*Albizzia lebbeck; Asparagus racemosus; Centella asiatica; Withania somnifera*
Fears	*Hypericum perforatum; Lavandula angustifolia; Matricaria chamomilla; Passiflora incarnata; Valeriana officinalis*	*Panax quinquefolius; Piper methysticum; Scutellaria lateriflora*	*Ginkgo biloba; Panax ginseng; Scutellaria baicalensis; Zingiber officinale*	*Albizzia lebbeck; Asparagus racemosus; Centella asiatica; Withania somnifera*
Phobia	*Hypericum perforatum; Passiflora incarnata*	*Panax quinquefolius; Piper methysticum; Scutellaria lateriflora*	*Ginkgo biloba; Scutellaria baicalensis; Zingiber officinale*	*Albizzia lebbeck; Asparagus racemosus; Centella asiatica; Withania somnifera*
Generalized Anxiety Disorder	*Hypericum perforatum; Matricaria chamomilla; Passiflora incarnata*	*Panax quinquefolius; Piper methysticum; Scutellaria lateriflora*	*Corydalis yanhusuo; Ginkgo biloba; Panax ginseng; Scutellaria baicalensis; Zingiber officinale*	*Albizzia lebbeck; Asparagus racemosus; Centella asiatica; Withania somnifera*

(*continued*)

Table 6-8. Psychoactive Herbs of Potential Use in Problems of Hyperactivity in the Cat and Dog[1] (*continued*)

Symptoms/Category of Misbehavior	Western Herb	Native American	Chinese	Ayurvedic
Feline/Canine Cognitive Dysfunction Syndrome; Senile Dementia	*Agaricus blazei; Lavandula angustifolia; Melissa officinalis; Pausinystalia yohimbe*	*Panax quinquefolius; Piper methysticum; Salvia officinalis*	*Astragalus membranaceus; Ginkgo biloba; Huperzia serrata; Panax ginseng; Salvia miltiorrhiza; Schisandra chinensis; Zingiber officinale*	*Bacopa monniera; Centella asiatica*
Masturbation, Persistent Sexual Behavior	*Vitex agnus-castus*		*Eleutherococcus senticosus*	*Vitex negundo; Withania somnifera*

[1] Herbal or synthetic psychoactive medicines are not complete treatments for behavior problems; psychoactive substances should be used in conjunction with an appropriate treatment plan for behavior modification that aims to restore balance to the patient's life.

CHAPTER

7

Basic Approaches to Common Behavior Problems in Pet Cats and Dogs

"Come forth into the light of things
Let Nature be your teacher."
—*William Wordsworth* (1770–1850)

This chapter is offered to simplify the clinical approach to some of the principal presenting complaints in small animal veterinary behavior practice that have been noted in this book. The flowcharts that follow are meant to assist in treating the average case of the misbehavior in question. These are outlines only and do not include the many techniques available to veterinary behavior specialists. Furthermore, each clinical case presents its own unique challenges and nuances. Herbal or conventional medications are meant to complement the basic approaches to the common behavior problems that follow. Please refer to a board-certified veterinary behaviorist for expert diagnosis and management of pet behavior problems.

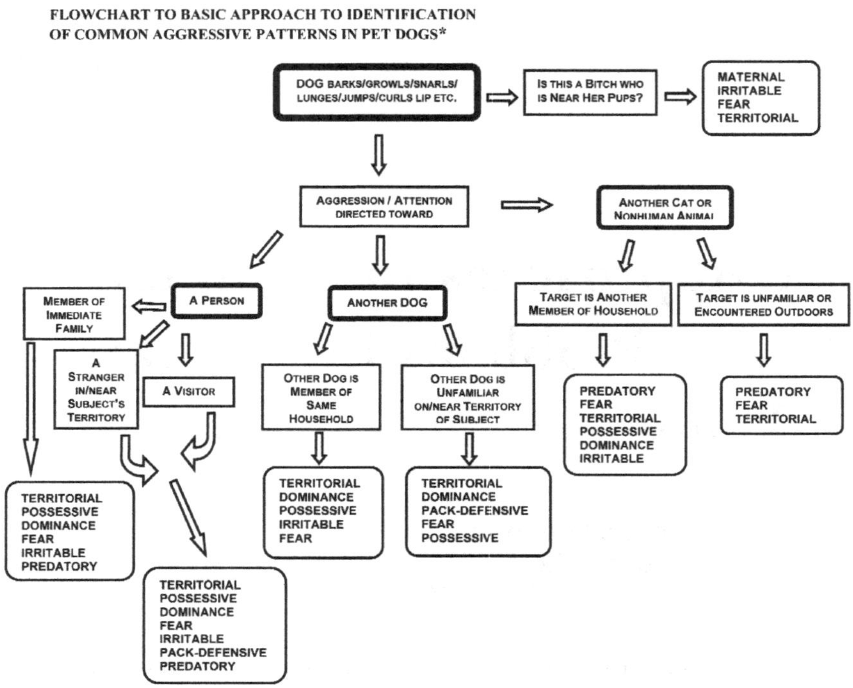

FIGURE 7-1. Flowchart to basic approach to identification of common aggressive patterns in pet dogs.

*This is not an exhaustive list of classifications of aggression; it is meant as a basic clinical guide only. The differential diagnoses are not listed in any order. Please refer to textbooks of veterinary behavior and animal behavior, or discuss your case with a veterinary behaviorist. The basic approaches to specific aggressive problems are available in "Instructions for Veterinary Authors: Canine and Feline Behavior Problems" by Dr. Stefanie Schwartz (Mosby 1997) or at www.dr-cookie.com/quickfxhandouts.htm.

Behavior Modification for Canine Aggression usually includes daily obedience practice; specific application of obedience commands, e.g., sit/stay or down/stay for everything the dog wants/needs at all times and with everyone anywhere; increased exercise (60 min. twice/day for dogs < 10 yrs old, depending on dog's health and the weather extremes); short leash (4 ft. or less); choke collar, Martingale (greyhound) collar, or head collar; dog on leash indoors as necessary; keep dog away from high-risk locations (e.g., owner's bed, under coffee table, in kitchen during preparation of meals); not leaving dog unattended in yard or anywhere; positive reinforcement of desirable behavior! Psychoactive medication must be preceded with hemogram, serum biochemistry, and ancillary tests as suggested by history, signs, and response to treatment.

Basic Considerations for Classifying and Diagnosing Common Types of Aggression:

- WHO are the players? WHO is the aggressor and WHO is the victim?
- WHAT triggers can be identified?
- WHEN did it start and have the patterns changed since then?
- WHERE does it occur? Inside/outside? On/near territory (neighborhood, car, boat, other familiar ground)?
- WHY did the aggression start? This may not be traceable but it usually can be deduced from the evolution and other basic information.

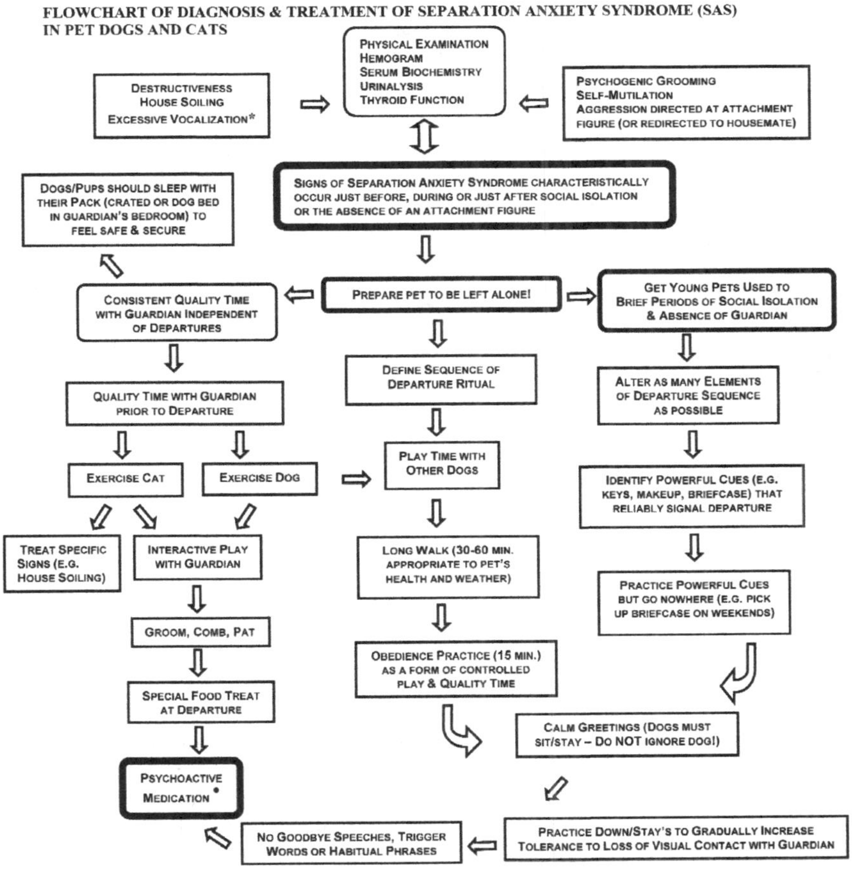

FIGURE 7-2. Flowchart of diagnosis and treatment of separation anxiety syndrome (SAS) in pet dogs and cats.

Most common clinical presentations of SAS; please refer to textbooks of veterinary behavior and animal behavior, or discuss your case with a veterinary behaviorist. The basic approaches to SAS and related problems are available in "Instructions for Veterinary Authors: Canine and Feline Behavior Problems" by Dr. Stefanie Schwartz (Mosby 1997) or at www.dr-cookie.com/quickfxhandouts.htm.

• Drug therapy is considered an adjunct to behavior modification. Please refer to Table A-1 in Appendix for dosages of conventional drug choices (e.g., alprazolam, amitriptyline, clomipramine, clorazepate, diazepam, fluoxetine, gabapentin, paroxetine, sertraline, triazolam) and to Tables 6-1 through 6-8 in Chapter 6 on suggested clinical applications of herbal treatments discussed in detail throughout this book.

FLOWCHART OF BASIC APPROACH TO IDENTIFICATION OF COMMON AGGRESSIVE PATTERNS IN PET CATS*

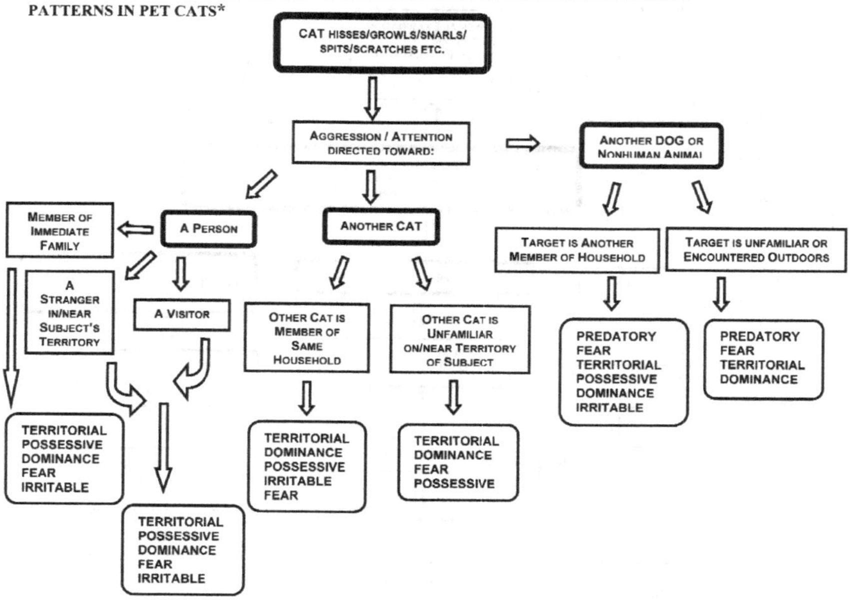

FIGURE 7-3. Flowchart of basic approach to identification of common aggressive patterns in pet cats.

*This is not an exhaustive list of classifications of aggression; it is meant as a basic clinical guide only. The differential diagnoses are not listed in any order. Please refer to textbooks of veterinary behavior and animal behavior, or discuss your case with a veterinary behaviorist. The basic approaches to specific aggressive problems are available in "Instructions for Veterinary Authors: Canine and Feline Behavior Problems" by Dr. Stefanie Schwartz (Mosby 1997) or at www.dr-cookie.com/quickfxhandouts.htm.

Like canine aggression, behavior modification for feline aggression begins with identification of the type of aggression. Any recognized triggers should be controlled as much as possible. If aggression occurs between a cat and another house pet, for example, they should be separated for at least two weeks before gradual reintroduction is attempted. or removal from the problem context. It is always important to rule out the possiblity of underlying illness. A decision to add psychoactive medication to a treatment plan must be preceded with hemogram, serum biochemistry and ancillary tests as suggested by history, signs and response to treatment.

Basic Considerations for Classifying and Diagnosing Common Types of Aggression:

- WHO are the players? WHO is the aggressor and WHO is the victim?
- WHAT triggers can be identified?
- WHEN did it start and have the patterns changed since then?
- WHERE does it occur? Inside/outside? On/near favorite resource (litter box, favorite perch, owner's bed, feeding area)?
- WHY did the aggression start? This may not be traceable but it can be deduced from the evolution and other basic information.

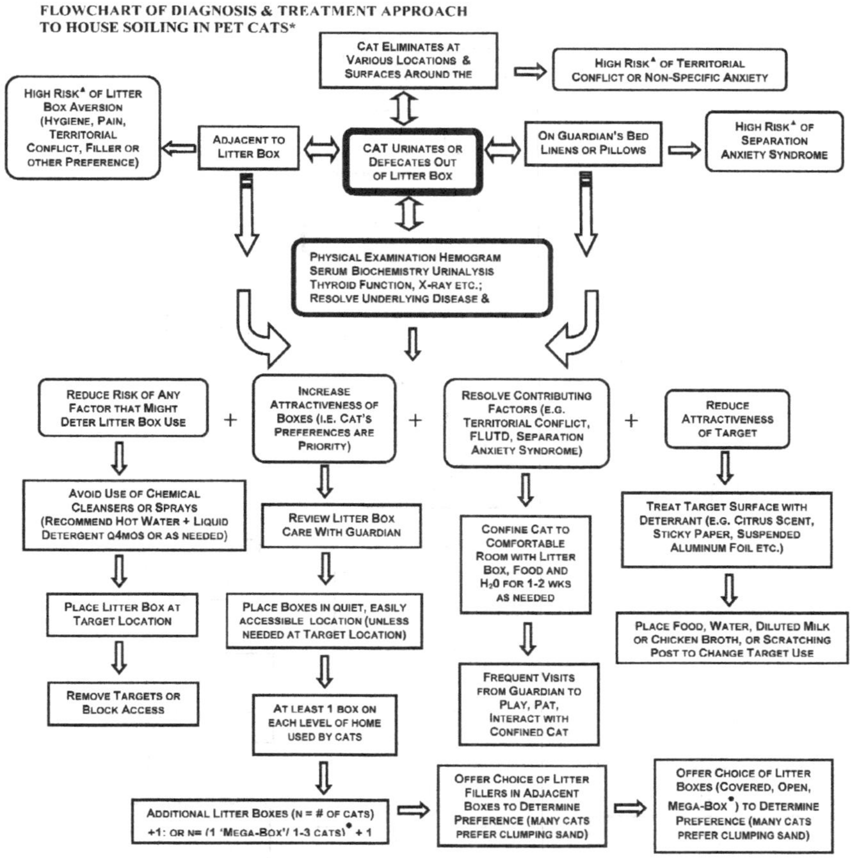

FIGURE 7-4. Flowchart of diagnosis and treatment approach to house soiling in pet cats.

*The basic approaches to feline house-soiling problems are discussed in other books by Dr. Stefanie Schwartz: "Instructions for Veterinary Authors: Canine and Feline Behavior Problems" (Mosby 1997), "Dr. Cookie's Guide to Living Happily Ever After with Your Cat" (St. Martin's Press 2002), or at www.dr-cookie.com/quickfxhandouts.htm. Identification and treatment of underlying physical disease and discomfort must always be considered.

▲ "High Risk" indicates higher probability of initial reason but does not preclude other underlying causes or triggers.

• "Mega-Box" refers to a very large container such as an under-the-bed storage bin that often is particularly attractive to cats; the walls of the container should not be so high as to discourage use.

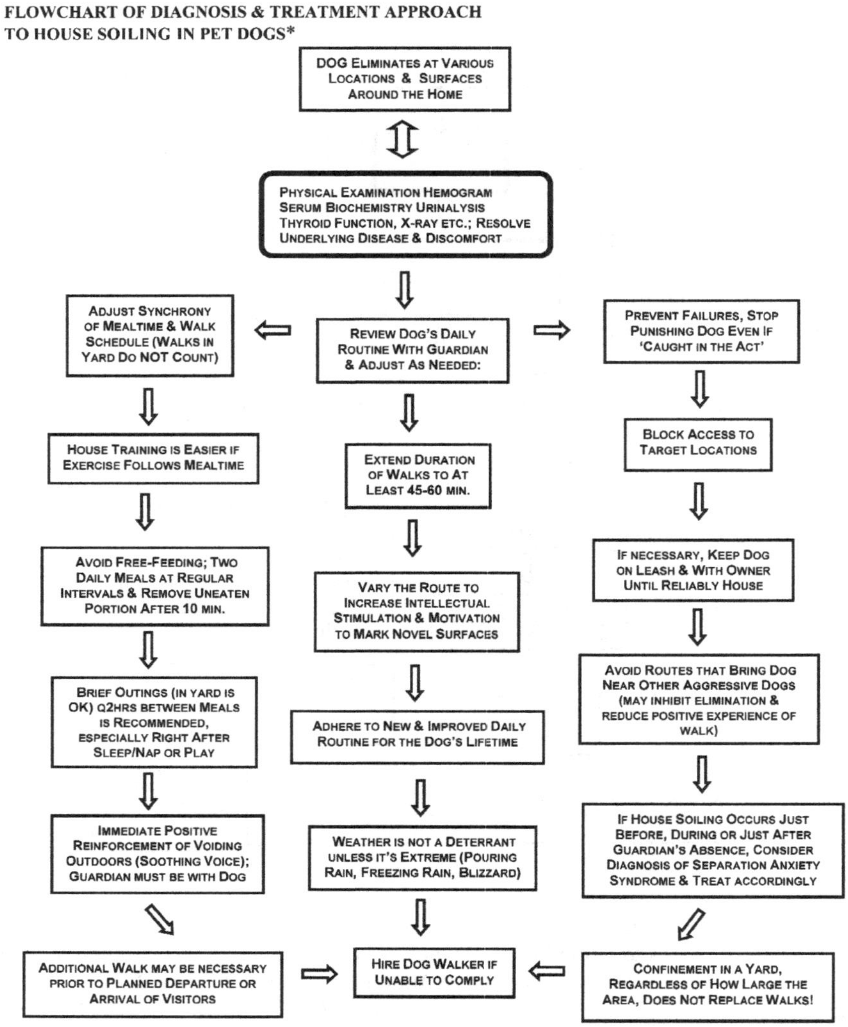

FIGURE 7-5. Flowchart of diagnosis and treatment approach to house soiling in pet dogs.

*Please refer to textbooks of veterinary behavior and animal behavior, or discuss your case with a veterinary behaviorist. The basic approaches to canine house-soiling problems are available in "Instructions for Veterinary Authors: Canine and Feline Behavior Problems" by Dr. Stefanie Schwartz (Mosby 1997) or at www.dr-cookie.com/quickfxhandouts.htm

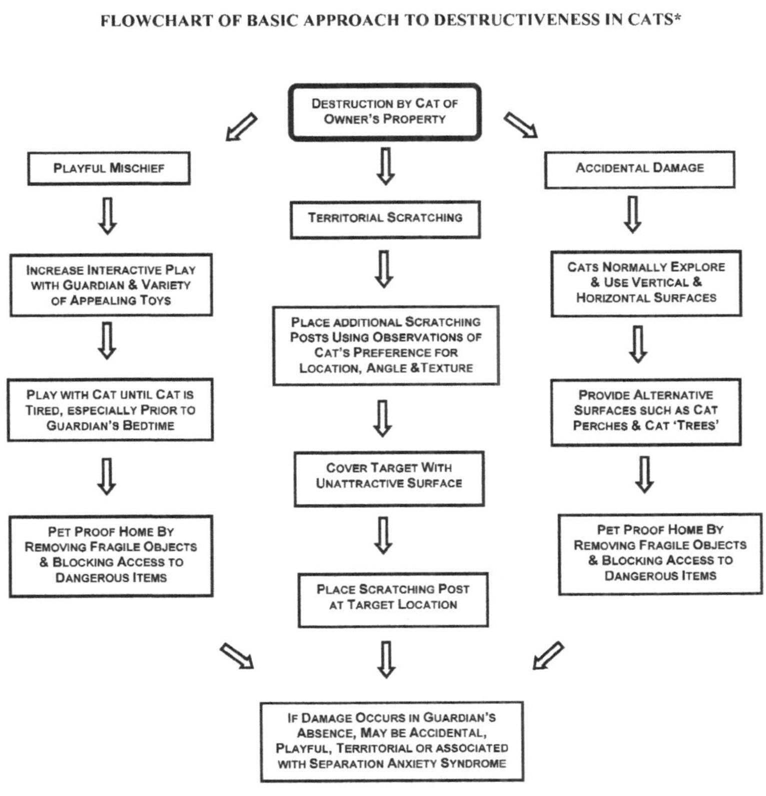

FIGURE 7-6. Flowchart of basic approach to destructiveness in cats.

*The basic approaches to destructive problems in cats and kittens are discussed in other books by Dr. Stefanie Schwartz: "Instructions for Veterinary Authors: Canine and Feline Behavior Problems" (Mosby 1997), "Dr. Cookie's Guide to Living Happily Ever After with Your Cat" (St. Martin's Press 2002), or at www.dr-cookie.com/quickfxhandouts.htm. Identification and treatment of underlying physical disease and discomfort must always be considered.

FLOWCHART OF BASIC APPROACH TO DESTRUCTIVENESS IN DOGS*

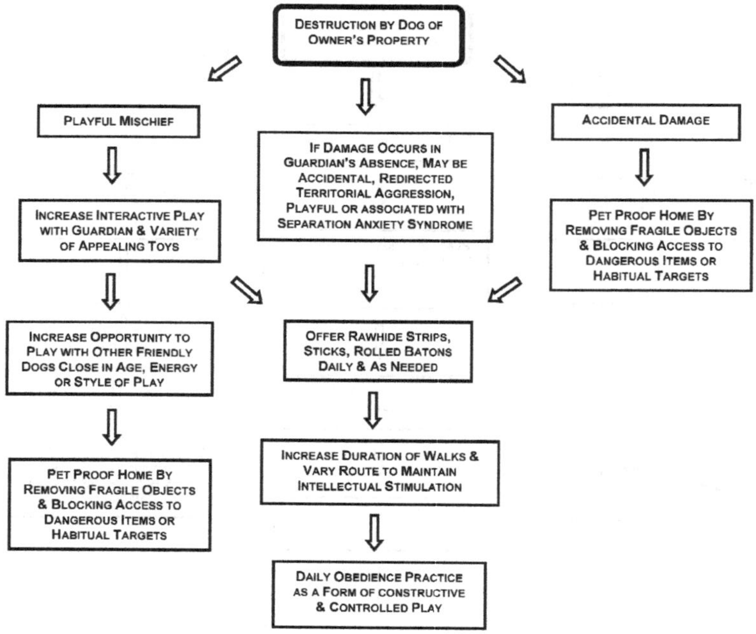

FIGURE 7-7. Flowchart of basic approach to destructiveness in dogs.

*Please refer to textbooks of veterinary behavior and animal behavior, or discuss your case with a veterinary behaviorist. The basic approaches to destructive problems are available in "Instructions for Veterinary Authors: Canine and Feline Behavior Problems" by Dr. Stefanie Schwartz (Mosby 1997) or at www.dr-cookie.com/quickfxhandouts.htm.

APPENDIX

A

Psychoactive Pharmaceutical Drugs in Veterinary Behavior Practice

Herbal remedies are still widely considered to be 'alternative' or 'complementary' from the perspective of Western medicine. This book has attempted to synthesize an enormous range of scattered and under-recognized scientific information in order to highlight the potential of many of these herbal medicines. The mainstream pharmacopoeia of conventional pharmaceuticals dominates the therapeutic choices of most veterinary practitioners and veterinary behavior specialists alike. To be complete, and for the convenience and reference of the reader, this section presents a table of the most commonly prescribed synthetic psychoactive compounds.

As research continues to define and refine the benefits of both conventional drugs and herbal preparations, it seems inevitable that the distinction between the two categories will become increasingly blurred as medical perspectives integrate more fully toward a holistic approach. Ultimately, what is imperative is to prolong and enhance the lives of pets by using whatever legal treatment modality is most effective and most safe regardless of its source.

Accurate diagnosis and treatment aimed at improving the pet's quality of life and resolving the source or cause of misbehavior remain fundamental to the responsible practice of veterinary behavior. In the vast majority of cases, conventional or 'alternative' medication applied as the sole treatment of a problem behavior is inadequate and inappropriate. Please consider referring pets with behavior problems to a board-certified veterinary behaviorist for expert evaluation and care.

Table A-1. Dosages of Commonly Prescribed Psychoactive Pharmaceutical Drugs in Veterinary Behavior Practice

Drug	Application	Oral Dosage	Schedule	Availability *(Brand/Generic)*
Acetylpromazine[1,2] *(Acepromazine®)*	Agitated states associated with anxiety	***Cat*** 1–3 mg/kg ***Dog*** 1–3 mg/kg	SID-BID SID-BID	10, 25 mg tabs
Alprazolam *(Xanax®)*	Anxiety, Generalized Anxiety Disorder, Separation Anxiety Syndrome, phobias, anxiety-related disorders (e.g., housesoiling, submissive urination)	***Cat*** 0.125–0.25 mg/kg ***Dog*** 0.1 mg/kg	BID-TID; PRN BID; PRN	0.5, 1, 2 mg tabs (scored)
Amitriptyline *(Elavil®)*	Housesoiling, Separation Anxiety Syndrome, agitated states associated with anxiety	***Cat*** 5–10 mg/cat ***Dog*** 2–4 mg/kg	SID-BID SID-TID	10, 25, 50, 75, 100, 150 mg tabs
Buspirone *(Buspar®)*	Housesoiling, Anxiety	***Cat*** 2.5–5 mg/cat ***Dog*** 2–4 mg/kg	BID BID	5, 10, 15, 30 mg tabs
Carbamazepine *(Tegretol®)*	Aggression	***Cat*** 25 mg/cat ***Dog*** 400–1600 mg/dog	BID BID	100, 200 mg tabs
Chlorpheniramine *(Chlortrimeton®, Novahistine®)*	Compulsive behavior (e.g., grooming disorders, tail chasing)	***Cat*** 2 mg/cat ***Dog*** 2–12 mg/dog	BID TID	4 mg tab
Clomipramine *(Clomicalm®)*	Anxiety-related disorders (e.g., Separation Anxiety Syndrome, destructiveness, phobias, agitation), aggression, compulsive behavior	***Cat*** 0.5–2 mk/kg ***Dog*** 1–3 mg/kg	SID-TID BID	25, 50, 75 mg tabs (generic); 20, 40, 80 mg tabs (brand)
Clorazepate *(Tranxene®)*	Anxiety, Generalized Anxiety Disorder, Separation Anxiety Syndrome, phobias, anxiety-related disorders (e.g., housesoiling, submissive urination)	***Cat*** 0.5–1 mg/kg ***Dog*** 0.5–2 mg/kg	SID-BID, PRN SID-BID, PRN	3.75, 7.5, 15 tabs (scored)
Cyproheptadine *(Periactin®)*	Housesoiling, inappetance	***Cat*** 1–2 mg	SID-BID	4 mg tab
Diazepam *(Valium®)*	Anxiety, Generalized Anxiety Disorder, Separation Anxiety Syndrome, phobias, anxiety-related disorders (e.g., housesoiling, submissive urination)	***Cat*** 0.2–.4 mg/kg ***Dog*** 0.5–2 mg/kg	SID-BID, PRN BID-TID, PRN	2, 5, 10 mg tabs
Fluoxetine *(Prozac®)*	Anxiety-related disorders (e.g., Separation Anxiety Syndrome, destructiveness, phobia, agitation), aggression, compulsive behavior	***Cat*** 0.1–1.0 mg/kg ***Dog*** 1 mg/kg	SID SID	10, 20, 40 mg tabs/caps
Gabapentin [2,3] *(Neurontin®)*	Neuralgia (relevant to compulsive grooming, tail chasing), social phobia, Generalized Anxiety Disorder, anticonvulsant (psychomotor seizures)	***Cat*** 2–10 mg/kg[4] ***Dog*** 25–50 mg/kg	BID TID	100, 300, 400 mg caps; 600, 800 mg tabs
Hydrocodone *(Hycodan®)*	Compulsive licking	***Dog*** 0.22 mg/kg	BID-TID	5 mg tab

Table A-1. Dosages of Commonly Prescribed Psychoactive Pharmaceutical Drugs in Veterinary Behavior Practice (*continued*)

Drug	Application	Oral Dosage	Schedule	Availability (*Brand/Generic*)
Megestrol acetate[1] *(Ovaban®)*	Territorial marking, psychogenic grooming	***Cat*** 2.5–5 mg/cat ***Dog*** 1–2 mg/kg	SID, EOD, PRN SID, PRN (1–2 wks)	5 mg tab
Methylphenidate *(Ritalin®)*	Narcolepsy; hyperkinesis	***Dog*** (Narcolepsy) 5–10 mg/dog ***Dog*** (Hyperkinesis) 2–4 mg/kg	BID-TID PRN	5, 10, 20 mg tabs
Naltrexone *(Trexan®)*	Compulsive tail chasing	***Dog*** 2-4 mg/kg	SID	50 mg tabs
Oxazepam *(Serax®)*	Anxiety-related anorexia, inappetance	***Cat*** 0.2–0.5 mg/kg	SID-BID	10, 15, 30 mg caps
Paroxetine *(Paxil®)*	Anxiety-related disorders (e.g., Separation Anxiety Syndrome, destructiveness, phobias, agitation), aggression, compulsive behavior	***Cat < 10 lbs*** 2.5 mg/cat ***Cat > 10 lbs*** 5 mg/cat	EOD; 1/2 dose SID	10, 20, 30, 40 mg tabs
Selegiline *(Anipryl®)*	Feline Cognitive Dysfunction Syndrome; Canine Cognitive Dysfunction Syndrome	***Cat*** 0.5 mg/kg ***Dog*** 0.5–1 mg/kg	SID AM only SID AM only	2, 5, 10, 15, 30 mg tabs/caps
Sertraline *(Zoloft®)*	Anxiety-related disorders (e.g., Separation Anxiety Syndrome, destructiveness, phobias, agitation), Aggression, Compulsive behavior	***Dog*** 1–3 mg/kg	SID	25, 50, 100 mg (scored)
Triazolam *(Halcion®)*	Anxiety-related disorders (e.g., Separation Anxiety Syndrome, destructiveness, agitation), aggression	***Cat*** 0.03 mg/cat	SID-TID	0.125 mg tab (scored)

[1] These medications with greater risk of adverse effects have been largely replaced with newer, more specific drugs but may be used as a last resort.

[2] Avoid use in animals or breeds prone to agitation or aggressiveness.

[3] Begin at 1/3 dose and increase gradually over 4 wks; max. 1200 mg/dose.

[4] Dr. Ilana Reisner, University of Pennsylvania, personal communication 2004.

References

Hall LW, Clarke KW. Veterinary Anaesthesia. (9th ed) Bailliere Tindall, Philadelphia, PA. 1991;52–54.

Matar JM, Nicholls PH, Tekle A et al. Effect of vigabatrin and gabapentin on phenytoin pharmacokinetics in the dog. Eur J Drug Met Pharmacokin. 2000;25:189–193.

Overall KL. Pharmacologic treatments for behavior problems. In: Houpt KA (ed). Progress in Companion Animal Behavior. WB Saunders, Philadelphia, PA. Vet Clin of N Amer: Sm Anim Pract. 1997;27:637–664.

PDR for Herbal Medicines. (2nd ed) Medical Economics Company Inc., Montvale, NJ. 2000.

Podell M. Antiepileptic Drug Therapy. Clin Tech Sm Anim Pract. 1998;13:185–192.

Simpson BS, Papich MG. Pharmacologic management in veterinary behavioral medicine. In: Houpt KA, Virga V (ed). Update on Clinical Veterinary Behavior. WB Saunders, Philadelphia, PA. Vet Clin of N Amer: Sm Anim Pract. 2003;33:365–404.

Schwartz S. Use of cyproheptadine to control urine spraying in a castrated male domestic cat. JAVMA. 1999;215:501–502.

Schwartz S. Use of cyproheptadine in the control of urine spraying and masturbation in a domestic cat. JAVMA. 1999;214:369–371.

Schwartz S. Carbamazepine in the control of aggressive behavior in cats. J Am Anim Hosp Assoc. 1994; 30:515–519.

Vollmer, von Hodenberg A, Kolle EU. Pharmacokinetics and metabolism of gabapentin in rat, dog and man. Arzneim-Forsch. 1986;36:830–839.

APPENDIX B

Traditional Jewish Medicine: Parallels to Ayurveda and Traditional Chinese Medicine

"So its waters will grow from the Sanctuary,
so its fruit will be for food
and its leaves for healing"

—Book of Ezekiel 47:12

The basic concepts of traditional Jewish medicine and mystical healing have been alluded to at various places in this book and are outlined in this addendum for the reader's interest. It is important to include a discussion of Jewish spirituality in this book because of important parallels with Ayurvedic and Traditional Chinese Medicine (TCM). In the discussion that follows, the reader will note that "ch" is pronounced with the guttural "h" in the English presentation of Hebrew words. In preparing this addendum, which is meant only as a brief overview of the subject, the author is grateful for the guidance of two special mentors. Simcha Gottlieb, MS, L.Ac., Diplomate in Acupuncture and Chinese Herbal Medicine, NCCAOM and faculty at the prestigious Pacific College of Oriental Medicine in New York City, is a Chabad Chassid based in Rockland County, New York. Thanks also to Yehuda Frischman, MS Acupuncture and Oriental Medicine, certified in craniosacral therapy and graduate of Yeshiva University; he is a Biala Chassid, teacher, and therapist practicing in Los Angeles, California.

Healing and Health in the Torah and Scriptures

Although there is no formal system of Jewish medicine, Jewish scriptures and traditions are steeped with a profound reverence for all forms of life and the importance of balance in living a healthy and meaningful life. These include foods to avoid, laws of hygiene, and many others.

The Torah (Five Books of Moses, "instruction"), the sacred scriptures of the Jews, was taught by God to Moses on Mount Sinai some 5,000 years ago and presented to 3,000,000 Jews who had made a desperate escape after centuries of slavery to the pharaohs of Egypt. The oral teachings of Torah, embodied in what we know today as the 38 volumes of the Talmud, were subsequently transcribed about 1,500 to 2,000 years ago to preserve their integrity. It is said that Moses received additional instruction from God at a desert oasis called Mara ("bitter"), where the water was undrinkable until Moses purified it with a piece of bitter wood. It was here that Moses also learned lessons about the medicinal properties and spiritual impact of plants and herbs. Unfortunately, most methods of Jewish healing handed down in oral form have been lost in time.

The Torah makes specific mention of the role and responsibility of the healer. The messages may be summarized by three fundamental concepts: (1) All healing is divine in origin; (2) the physician (or veterinarian, may we add) is God's agent and is obliged to pursue every possible treatment and research all options possible to heal the patient and is forbidden to harm the patient; and (3) each individual is responsible to honor and preserve his or her own physical and spiritual health. In Judaism, illness is perceived as a signal from God that we must pause to review our lives and make necessary adjustments.

The Talmud is the rabbinical commentary of the word of Torah, interpreting and applying the messages of the Hebrew Bible for application to living the life prescribed by Judaism. The Talmud tells the story of King Chizkiyahu, who lived in Israel about 2,500 years ago. It is said that an extraordinary text (The Book of Remedies) was in use for some 300 years until the time of King Chizkiyahu, who took it upon himself to hide the book away. It is unknown who wrote this book, and it is controversial as to why King Chizkiyahu felt obliged to conceal it. One interpretation is that the book's medical answers were so complete that people forgot their humility and the divine source of all healing. This wise king understood that both the body and soul must be cured at the same time for true healing to occur. Another possible explanation is that the book was based in the occult and therefore forbidden.

The Talmud is rich with practical medical advice as it pertains to Jewish law. Although it is not a medical text, it contains discussions and laws pertaining to hygiene, diet, exercise, elimination, and sex. Direct reference can also be found to specific remedies for toothache, stomach pain, fever, and heart ailments. The scriptures address the organs and body systems. The Talmud describes bloodletting, for instance, and recommends it for conditions similar to those described in TCM.

The first Hebrew medical text is attributed to the seventh-century physician Asaph Harofeh; he was followed by the writings of the great Jewish physicians of Arabia in the ninth, tenth, and eleventh centuries. The most famous of twelfth-century Jewish physicians was Moses Maimonides, who was chief physician to the Sultan of Egypt. His text *Pirkei Moshe* taught of anatomy, physiology, pathology, gynecology, etiology of disease, diagnosis and therapeutics, surgery, hygiene, exercise, bathing, diet, drugs, and more. He wrote more books on hemorrhoids, seizures, cohabitation, asthma, and poisons and their antidotes. He is the author of a materia medica that details the flavors and temperatures of the herbs, and an authoritative yet brief treatise on diet and lifestyle (*Hanhagat Habriut*). He described four tastes (sweet, sharp, salty, and bitter) and discussed their specific qualities in healing herbs and foods. Although not as complex, this is distinctly similar to the systems of TCM. Maimonides was so revered as a physician and healer that his legend persists in the Arab world to this day. Dr. Maimonides was also a revered Jewish scholar and leader of the Jewish community far beyond Egypt. Referred to as the Rambam (a contracted form of Rabbi Moses ben Maimon), he produced extensive commentary about Jewish law and ethics that continue to influence modern Jews. The Jewish medical tradition has thrived wherever Jewish culture has flourished, and Jewish doctors remain prominent today.

Other important parallels can be drawn between traditional Jewish medicine and Oriental medicine. In TCM, the use of pulse detection and qualification to diagnose disease is based on three paired pulse points on each wrist and 18 diagnostic positions used to define 28 different pulse patterns. In the mystical Jewish tradition of the Kabbalah, there are 10 main pulse patterns that are used to detect physiological as well as spiritual imbalance; each pulse pattern indicates a specific vital energy flowing into the body via the soul. Ayurveda also describes in detail the use of pulse patterns to diagnose disease. All three traditions emphasize function over structure, and harmony in the flow of spiritual energy. They also share a belief that happiness, and even pleasure, are essential to a happy Heart and Soul, and a clear Mind. Mental, Spiritual, and Physical health are one.

Additional similarities between TCM and Judaism can be found in Jewish scriptures. In the Gemara section of the Jewish Talmud (Brachot:61a), for example, the rabbis address the different functions of the organs from a metaphysical perspective. They teach that the two kidneys influence a person's thought processes by challenging them to rethink what might otherwise be uninhibited thinking and reacting. They are the seat of the individual's deepest inclinations and attitudes. One kidney gives good advice and is thought to represent the *yetzer tov* (the good side) of the individual; the other kidney gives bad advice and represents the *yetzer hara* (the dark side). In addition to the intellectual influence of the kidneys, they also noted that the heart understands; it is the source of conscious emotions such as fear and love. The lungs draw up different liquids, the trachea produces sound, the mouth and lips express what the tongue articulates, the esophagus takes and expels food, the liver gets angry, the spleen causes laughter, the gall bladder secretes bile to soothe the liver's anger, the stomach causes sleep, and the nose wakes up. If the roles of stomach and nose reverse, disease will follow; if both assume the same function, death will follow. The rabbis even mention the maw or rumen, which they recognized as grinding food in animals.

Historical Perspective of the Kabbalah

Kabbalah ("received") is the study of Jewish mysticism. It is thought to have originated with Adam, who was inspired when he named the animals. The first volume of the Kabbalah (*Sefer Hayitzerah*) is attributed to Abraham. On Mount Sinai, the sacred discourse between Moses and God included the mystical interpretation of the words, letters, and wording of the Torah including the Gematria (sacred numerology). The *Zohar* is a lyrical commentary attributed to the second-century mystic Rabbi Shimon bar Yochai and includes teachings of the great rabbis of fourteenth-century Spain such as Rabbi Moses de Leon. In sixteenth-century Israel, Rabbi Moses Cordovero wrote his treatise (*Pardes Rimonim*) that first organized the ten sefirot. His successor Rabbi Yitchak Luria continued the conceptualization of the ten *sefirot* described below and refined kabbalistic thought to an unprecedented level. In seventeenth-century Ukraine, Rabbi Israel ben Eliezer (*Baal Shem Tov*) emerged to make the Kabbalah more accessible to the average person and not just the scholarly elite; he emphasized the enactment of loving-kindness and joy of life over exclusive intellectual focus. Rabbi Schneur Zalman of Liadi, a student of a Baal Shem Tov disciple, later recorded the great text known as the *Tanya,* which systematically elaborated on the teachings of the Kabbalah to make them even more understandable.

Basic Concepts of the Kaballah

In the kaballah, God is referred to as *Ein Sof* (without end, meaning boundless or infinite). There is a slight similarity here with the Ayurvedic concept of Ether, which is viewed as an ever-expanding primal energy. God has qualities that are partially represented by the ten *sefirot,* the Divine Attributes by which we identify God's presence in the world (Table B-1). The ten sefirot are often portrayed in diagrams or illustrations as branches of the Tree of Life (*Etz Chaim*). The powerful symbolism of the Tree of Life also hints at the reverence for herbal sources of healing from the perspective of Traditional Jewish medicine, and a profound respect for Nature in Judaism.

The ten sefirot have been divided into groups according to their function: *Chochmah* (wisdom), *Binah,* (intelligence, understanding), and *Da'at* (knowledge, connection, connectedness) are all associated with intellect and pure thought; *Chessed* (kindness), *Gevura* (strength), and *Tiferet* (beauty) provide substance to the action; the practical implication of the deed: *Netzach* (victory or lasting endurance) and *Hod* (awe) contribute to the practical implication of the action; *Yesod* (foundation) is the planning of the act itself; and *Malchut* (kingship) is the enacted deed. The Tree of Life organization of the sefirot corresponds metaphorically to parts of the body as well. There are many similarities between the kundalini chakra system of Ayurveda and the body parts correlated with the sefirot (Table B-1).

Table B-1. The Ten Divine Attributes (Sefirot) of the Kaballah's Tree of Life and Their Corresponding Body Parts

The Ten Sefirot[1]	Translation	Significance	Physical Correlation
Chochmah	Wisdom	The spark of an idea; intuition, insight	Right cerebral hemisphere
Binah	Understanding	Conceptual analysis, idea development, deductive reasoning, comprehension; discernment of truth vs. falsehood	Left cerebral hemisphere; Ears
Da'at	Knowledge	The bridge between concept and reality; the conscious reflection of *ketef;* directly influences and energizes the emotions of the heart with the life force	Memory, concentration, sensitivity
Chessed	Kindness	An initial act of loving-kindness that is performed without expectation, as with the first act of Creation; *chessed* embraces the perfect love and harmony in all of Creation	Right arm
Gevura	Strength	Will power; self-discipline; self-determination; balances selflessness and unlimited giving (and receiving) of *Chessed* with accountability, judgment, and truth; the power to implement the innate desire to perform acts of loving-kindness	Left arm
Tiferet	Beauty, glory	Beauty is expressed through acts of focused compassion (*Chessed* + *Gevura*); it also results from the integration of talents and traits to make a whole being who has depth and character	Upper torso, heart
Netzach	Persistence, victory, eternity	Conquest derived from *Gevura;* the ability to overcome obstacles that stand in the way of *Chessed*	Right leg
Hod	Awe, devotion	Retribution against evil forces; determination to reach one's goals; acknowledgement of a supreme purpose to life lived according to Torah	Left leg
Yesod	Foundation	Spiritual connection; the bridge that connects humankind to God	Male genitalia; Female genitalia
Malchut	Monarchy, kingship	God acts through us; when we absorb the first nine sefirot, we are transformed; self-fulfillment verifies one's commitments and ideals; acting and communicating with divine inspiration	Mouth; vaginal labia; corona of the penis

[1] The Tree of Life is sometimes presented in the following order: *Keter*—crown (divine aura or superconscience); *Chochmah*—wisdom; *Binah*—understanding; *Chessed*—kindness; *Gevura*—strength; *Tiferet*—beauty; *Netzach*—victory; *Hod*—awe; *Yesod*—foundation; *Malchut*—monarchy, kingship.

"The body is the tree,
the medicine is the fertilizer,
the physician is the tiller of
the soil"

—*Midrash Sh'muel,* Chapter 4

Jewish mysticism also includes discussions of masculine and feminine principles that are not unlike the fundamental Chinese principle of yin-yang. For example, Chochmah, Chessed, and Netzach possess a primarily masculine quality, whereas Binah, Gevura, and Hod have a more predominantly feminine or receptive nature (Table B-2). These abstract concepts are the source of more tangible polarities that we see in the physical world, such as heat and cold, that are also inherent to TCM.

Each of the ten sefirot are further subdivided and analyzed in great detail in the great collections of Jewish kabbalistic thought. The sefirot may also be grouped into triads that consist of right and left polarities and a central harmonizing entity: the "intellectual sefirot" (Keter/Da'at, Chochmah, Binah); the "emotional sefirot" (Gevura, Tiferet, Chessed); and the "functional sefirot" (Netzach, Hod, Yesod). The "functional sefirot" triad (Malchut is sometimes also included in this group) includes reproductive and communicational functions.

In the metaphorical anthropomorphic representation of the sefirot, each sefira (singular of sefirot) has other physical associations. For example, the sefirot of Netzach, Hod, and Yesod correlate with the human reproductive system, including the kidneys (which are understood functionally in TCM as reproductive organs) as well as the gonads and genitals. Netzach and Hod are placed below Chessed (love/attraction/kindness) and Gevura (respect/awe/separation). This association links sexual or reproductive motivations to a person's emotions. It also implies that persistence and devotion are based in love and respect.

Da'at is the harmonizing entity between the polarities of Chochmah (abstract thought, intuition) and Binah (analytical, rational mind). It is divided into several levels of functioning. Its lowest aspect is its role in integrating intellect with emo-

Table B-2. The Three Classic Groupings of the Ten Sefirot of Kaballah and Their Corresponding Emotional or Spiritual States (in Parentheses)

Sefirot of the Heart	*Sefirot of the Mind*	*Sefirot of Behavior*
	KETER Divine Inspiration	
BINAH Joy *(Ta'anug)*	DA'AT Unification *(Yichud)*	CHOCHMAH Selflessness *(Bitul)*
GEVURA Fear *(Yirah)*	TIFERET Mercy *(Rachamim)*	CHESSED *Love (Ahavah)*
HOD Sincerity *(Temimut)*	YESOD Truth *(Emet)*	NETZACH Confidence *(Bitachon)*
	MALCHUT Humility *(Shiflut)*	

tion; however, its highest aspect is to integrate the two intellectual sefirot of Chochmah and Bina with the divine illumination that emanates from Keter. Da'at is the pivotal core of the sefirot; it receives energy and information from beyond the conscious mind and connects, focuses, and integrates all aspects of human experience.

Kabbalistic philosophy classifies 248 positive commandments (the "do's" of Jewish law) that correspond to the 248 viscera and limbs. These give substance to a person and enable him or her to perform the do's. There are also 365 negative commandments (the "don'ts") that correspond to the 365 sinews, tendons, ligaments, and major nerves. These give foundation and structure to a person's actions and life.

Jewish mysticism teaches that all things on earth were infused with Divine or Holy Sparks. Food, for example, is merely packaging for divine sparks that nourish us. The metaphor of "man cannot live by bread alone" suggests that we need spiritual nourishment, but it also implies that there is divine energy in the food. This resembles the concept of qi in TCM, which teaches that consumption of foods such as meat enhance yang or male energy whereas eating food such as fish or chicken boosts yin or female energy. In Ayurveda, specific foods contain characteristic energy that must be taken in balance to properly nourish the body and maintain health. From the Jewish perspective, everything that we use during life releases a divine spark that is returned to the source. We are responsible for eating healthy food ourselves to remain healthy, but also to feed ourselves with spiritual practices and acts of loving-kindness. In the Kabbalah, there are three levels of Divine or Life Force (*koach, chayut, ohr*), which are reminiscent of the concepts of qi and prana.

Kabbalah and Psychiatry

The kabbalistic perspective on mental health, the equivalent to veterinary behavior medicine, is that of imbalance. If an individual focuses too heavily on his or her own thoughts, needs, and experiences, there is an imbalance between egocentricity and theocentricity. The cure lies in refocusing oneself in divine pursuits according to Jewish laws and customs. In this way, the troubled mind is reoriented toward healthier and more fulfilling paths. On the other hand, to unburden one's self and to prevent overwhelming psychological stress, regular intimate discussions with a mentor or special confidante are encouraged.

Three biblical texts are considered to be therapeutic in nature. The Book of Proverbs is a textbook of ethics written by King Solomon and is filled with analogies of good and evil, light and darkness, joy and sorrow. It hints at treatments for anxiety in Proverb 12:25; for example, it suggests three methods of dealing with anxiety: talk about it (the subconscious mind is the source of darkness and primal urges, and the conscious mind is the source of light and clarity), ignore it (this suggest healthful distractions and replacing worry with positive thoughts or actions), or transform it into joy through prayer and selflessness. The basic premise is that the mind will fill itself with all kinds of negative contents such as evil, dark, depressive, obsessive, anxious thoughts if it is not intentionally filled with holy thoughts as well as the planning and enactment of holy deeds. The Book of Psalms, written by King David, is traditionally recited in times of sorrow when inspiration is sorely needed. The Book of Job is one of the greatest stories ever told and describes the deepest soul-searching of a man submerged in an existential crisis who has lost everything, including his belief in the beauty of Creation and the healing power of God. Job, too, returned to Nature for inspiration and healing, much as we do today.

> "But ask now the beasts, and they shall teach thee; and the fowls of the air, and they shall tell thee: Or speak to the earth, and it shall teach thee; and the fishes of the sea shall declare unto thee . . . With the ancient is wisdom; and in length of days understanding."
> —*Book of Job 12:7–8,12*

References

Aish ("Fire" in Hebrew) Jewish Spirituality. http://www.aish.com/spirituality/kabbala101/

Baal Shem Tov Foundation. http://www.baalshemtov.com/

Exploration in Jewish healing: A self-paced guided learning program. http://www.healingjewish.org

Glazerson M. Torah, Light and Healing. Mystical Insights into Healing based on the Hebrew Language. Jason Aronson Inc., Northvale, NJ. 1996.

Judaism 101. http://www.jewfaq.org/kabbalah.htm.

Kabbalah and Jewish medicine: The healing of body and soul. http://www.inner.org/healing.htm

Olitzky KM. Jewish Paths toward Healing and Wholeness. Jewish Lights Publishing, Woodstock, VT. 2000.

Scholem G. Kabbalah. The New American Library, New York, NY 1974.

Scholem G. Major Trends in Jewish Mysticism. Schocken Books, New York, NY. 1961.

The Inner Dimension: A Gateway to the Wisdom of Kabbalah and Chassidut. http://www.inner.org/

APPENDIX

C

Online Resources

There is an infinite range of Web sites devoted to herbal medicine, alternative systems of healing, and veterinary medicine. The list that follows is meant to provide a basis for the reader's preliminary ventures in search of information contained or alluded to in this book. Reference lists of texts and journal articles are provided at the end of each section or chapter and are important sources of knowledge.

Native American Ethnobotany

Native American Ethnobotany Database	http://herb.umd.umich.edu
Native American Herbs and Plants of the Southwest	http://www.angelfire.com/art/nativeherb/index.html
Indigenous Knowledge Pages	http://www.nuffic.nl/ik-pages/
Native American Herbal, Plant Knowledge	http://www.kstrom.net/isk/food/plants.html

Ayurveda—Traditional Indian Medicine

National Institute of Ayurvedic Medicine	http://www.niam.com
History of Traditional Indian Medicine	http://www.mic.ki.se/India.html
Ayurveda Infocenter	http://www.holistic-online.com/ayurveda/ayv_home.htm
Everyday Ayurveda	http://www.everydayayurveda.com
Life Positive	http://www.lifepositive.com/ayurveda.html
All Ayurveda	http://www.allayurveda.com
The Ayurvedic Institute	http://www.ayurveda.com

Western Herbal Medicine

American Botanical Council & Journal	http://www.herbalgram.org
European Society of Ethnopharmacology	http://www.ethnopharma.free.fr
Traditional Chinese & Western Herbal Medicine in Humans & Animals	http://homepage.tinet.ie/~progers/herblink.htm
Michael Moore – South Western School of Botanical Medicine	http://www.all-natural.com/herbindx.html
Botanical.com	http://www.botanical.com/botanical/mgmh/comindx.html
Herb Research Foundation	http://www.herbs.org
Botanical Pathways Online	http://www.botanicalpathways.com
Evidence-based Complementary and Alternative Medicine (Oxford University Press)	http://www3.oup.co.uk/jnls/list/ecam/
HerbMed	http://www.herbmed.org
Herb Data Free Library	http://www.herbdatanz.com

Henriette's Herbal	http://www.ibiblio.org/herbmed/index.html
Index of Herbal Resources	http://www.herbalists.on.ca/resources/freeman
Plants for Our Future Database	http://www.scs.leeds.ac.uk/pfaf/database/latinA.htm
International Centre for Phytotherapy	http://www.phytotherapy.info
Killer Plants Online Botanical Knowledge	http://www.killerplants.com

Traditional Oriental Medicine

Traditional Chinese Veterinary Medicine	http://www.tcvm.com
Traditional Chinese Medicine (TCM) & Acupuncture	http://www.tcm.health-info.org/Herbology.Materia.Medica/HerbsWebPage.htm
Chinese Medicine and Acupuncture	http://tcm.health-info.org
Committee on Chinese Medicine and Pharmacy	http://www.ccmp.gov.tw/index-e/1.htm
New Century Nutrition Chinese Herbal Libraries	http://newcentury.vegsource.com
Herbasin Database	http://www.herbasin.com/herbs.htm
The Pulse of Oriental Medicine	http://www.pulsemed.org
TCM Student Resource for Acupuncture & Chinese Medicine	http://www.tcmstudent.com
International College of Traditional Chinese Medicine of Vancouver	http://www.tcmcollege.com
The Register of Chinese Herbal Medicine	http://www.rchm.co.uk
Pacific College of Oriental Medicine	http://www.pacificcollege.edu
RMHI Chinese Medicine School	http://www.rmhiherbal.org/index.html
Acta Pharmacologica Sinica	http://www.lifescience.org.cn/qikanbj/aps
Honso USA Inc. – Japanese Kampo	http://www.honsousa.com/Products/H01.htm
Kampo Today – News of Japanese Herbal Medicine	http://www.tsumura.co.jp/english/kampo/today/
Department of Oriental Medicine, Keio University, Japan	http://web.sc.itc.keio.ac.jp/kampo/english/what_en.html

Miscellaneous Sites of Interest

Dr. Stefanie Schwartz (Dr. Cookie®) Veterinary Behaviorist	http://www.dr-cookie.com
American Veterinary Medical Association	http://avma.org
American College of Veterinary Behaviorists	http://veterinarybehaviorists.org
Veterinary Botanical Medical Association	http://www.vbma.org
Alternative Medicine On-Line Journals	http://dir.yahoo.com/Health/Alternative_Medicine/Magazines/
Phytotherapies—Herbal Database and Monographs	http://www.phytotherapies.org
US Department of Agriculture, Natural Resources Conservation Service Plant Database	http://plants.usda.gov/cgi_bin/
Botanical Pathways—Information & Research	http://www.botanicalpathways.com
Iknowledgenow On-line Library of Veterinary Medicine	http://www.iknowledgenow.com
International Veterinary Information Service	http://www.ivis.org/home.asp
International Academy of Medical Acupuncture	http://www.iama.edu
Dr. Phil Rogers' Reference Lists of TCM, Acupuncture, Holistic & Conventional Life Sciences	http://homepage.eircom.net/~progers/searchap.htm
National Animal Supplement Council	http://www.nasc.cc/index.htm
Environmental News Network	http://www.enn.com
Neot-Kedumim—The Biblical Landscape Reserve in Israel	http://www.n-k.org.il/public/index.htm
Rain-tree Nutrition Database of the Rain Forest	http://www.rain-tree.com/plants.htm
Herb Pictures	http://www.herbselect.com/herbpictures.htm

Fine Digital Herb Photography	http://www.alternative-herbalmedicine.net/herb_photographyAB.htm
Free Herb Pictures	http://www.freeherbpictures.com
TraditionalJewishMedicine and TCM	http://health.groups.yahoo.com/group/TraditionalJewishMedicineandTCM/
Aish Jewish Spirituality	http://www.aish.com/spirituality/kabbala101/
Basics in Kabbalah & Chassidut	http://www.inner.org/sefirot/sefchesd.htm
The Upledger Institute	http://www.upledger.com/home.htm
Dr. Ihor Basko, Holistic Veterinarian, Hawaii	http://drbasko.com

Commercial Herbal Sites

Ayurveda Herbal Remedy	http://www.ayurveda-herbs.com
Ayurveda Retreat	http://www.ayurveda.org
Ayurvedic Herbs	http://www.iherb.com/ayurvedic.html
Richters Herbs Specialist	http://www.richters.com
Horizon Herbs	http://www.horizonherbs.com
Blue Poppy Enterprises	http://www.bluepoppy.com
1st Chinese Herbs	http://www.1stchineseherbs.com
Acuxo Acupuncture Reference Software	http://www.acuxo.com
MediHerb (Practitioners only)	http://www.mediherb.com
Botanicum—Chinese Herbal Medicine, Extract Granules, Herb Concentrates	http://www.botanicum.com
Ancient Way Acupuncture & Herbs	http://www.ancientway.com
Tsumura Kampo Herbs	http://www.tsumura.co.jp/english/products/index.htm
Herbasin	http://www.herbasin.com/herbs.htm
Herbal medicines	http://www.biopsychiatry.com/herbalmedicines.htm
Greater China Herbs	http://www.herbsnsenses.com/eng/index.html
DaMo Chinese Medicine World	http://www.herb.damo-qigong.net
Chinese Natural Herbs	http://www.chinesenaturalherbs.com
Chinese Herb Shop	http://www.herbalshop.com/tcm/ChineseHerb_Channels.html
China Herbs	http://www.china-herbs.com
Chinese Natural Therapy Centre	http://www.medicineconference.com
Chinese Herbal Medicine, Country Life Vitamins, and Massage Supplies	http://www.morningstarhealth.com
Crane Herb Company Chinese Herbs and Acupuncture Supplies	http://www.craneherb.com
Cathay Herbal Laboratories	http://www.cathayherbal.com/index.cfm
Chinese Herbs	http://eng.herb.com.tw/main
Sacred Seed—Seed List	http://www.sacredseed.com
Earth Lodge Herbals Nutritional Supplements for Horses	http://www.earthlodgeherbals.com
Godshaer	http://www.godshaer.co.uk
MotherNature	http://www.mothernature.com

Index of Psychoactive Herbs

General Index

Printed in the USA/Agawam, MA
September 17, 2026

910661.036